The Jewish Tradition and Choices at the End of Life

A New Judaic Approach to Illness and Dying

Lewis D. Solomon

University Press of America,® Inc.
Lanham · New York · Oxford

4720 Boston Way
Lanham, Maryland 20706

12 Hid's Copse Rd.
Cumnor Hill, Oxford OX2 9JJ

Printed in the United States of America
British Library Cataloging in Publication Information Available

Library of Congress Cataloging-in-Publication Data

Solomon, Lewis D.
The Jewish tradition and choices at the end of life : a new
Judaic approach to illness and dying / Lewis D. Solomon.
p. cm
Includes bibliographical references and index.
1. Death—Religious aspects—Judaism. 2. Death—Moral and
ethical aspects. 3. Terminal care—Religious aspects—Judaism.
I. Title.
BM635.4 .S64 2001 296.3'3—dc21 2001027001 CIP

ISBN 0-7618-1959-2 (cloth : alk. paper)
ISBN 0-7618-1960-6 (pbk. : alk. paper)

™The paper used in this publication meets the minimum
requirements of American National Standard for Information
Sciences—Permanence of Paper for Printed Library Materials,
ANSI Z39.48—1984

In memory of my father

Contents

Acknowledgments

I want to single out two individuals for their help. Beatrice Bruteau, Ph.D. read a complete draft of this book and gave me extensive comments that guided me in my revisions. Nell B. Taylor typed the manuscript, provided editorial suggestions, and helped index the book. Claire Feinson and Robert E. Shepard also aided in editing the manuscript.

John P. Miller and Todd G.E. Melnick, Reference Librarians at the Jacob Burns Law Library of The George Washington University Law School, assisted in locating hard-to-find materials. Rabbi Jan Caryl Kaufman of The Rabbinical Assembly provided useful research materials as did Maria Candy Sarinas Caballero.

Chapter 1

Introduction

Have you ever seen the face of a dying person - a relative or friend - who is suffering and observed his or her fragility and vulnerability? One day, you or a loved one may wear this agonizing face, you or a beloved's body or mind may become a source of suffering or even horror.

More than two million, three hundred thousand Americans die each year.[1] The process of dying is often messy, filled with anguish and sorrow.

You're probably familiar with at least one miserable death. You've seen or heard about the deaths of people who were choking, struggling, thrashing about in their final days and hours. Perhaps you've heard someone groan with each out-breath, repeatedly pleading, "Please let me go." Most of us know someone whose dying went awry, whether through inadequate pain care or overzealous treatment. You may have also witnessed the prolonged discomfort resulting from the slow physical or mental disintegration. The dependence, the loss of control and dignity, the complete helplessness accompanying the wasting away of one's body or mind.

This is a very personal book. It deals with intimate concerns - life, death, dying. Some of you may now be diagnosed with a terminal illness or a chronic, degenerative condition; others are loved ones of sufferers. All of us wonder about what our process of dying will be like - when, how, where we will die, will our final illness be long and painful, will we be able to deal with our pain and suffering, will our pain and suffering be controlled, will we be a burden on others?

Some will encounter inoperable cancer and experience constant, excruciating pain. Others face a chronic, nonterminal, debilitating condition but have years to live, or some form of dementia -- slow, insidious mental deterioration.

Medical care at the end of one's life often involves wrenching decisions. I've written this book for three reasons. First, it will help you and your loved ones make better, more informed choices as you face: the onset of a terminal illness or an incurable, chronic, debilitating condition; a lengthy period of debility and frailty, with ever greater and more demeaning physical and mental weakness and dependency; or a hopeless medical condition marking the final agony of a fatal illness. To put it bluntly: do you want to engage in a preemptive, self-chosen death at any point along the trajectory of your illness or condition?

For nearly all of us, it's not, nor should it be, a straight line decision -- fight on to the bitter end or let's get it over with now. Arriving at a rational choice, actually, a series of choices along the way, represents a slow, often tangled, process. You'll repeatedly ask yourself: Is my decision to control and to time the manner of my death an acceptable act of stewardship over my life? In this book I hope to explore the meaning of life-and-death with you -- your life-and-death -- and to inquire into what gives value to human life. More specifically, what do you personally value in life and in death and is your end of life decision consistent with your values?

You and your loved ones will go through periods of doubt and be filled with numerous questions. You want to attain the goal of dying in character, integrating your values into the process.

Each of us differs in our approach to death and dying. A few find comfort when faced with death; most are filled with terror. Some may fear the process of dying because of the prospect of experiencing unimaginable pain and suffering; others welcome death because of the expectation of relief from their pain and suffering.

This is not a book with simple, pat answers to the complex choices we face at the end of life. It's not neatly etched in black or white. Would that it could be so, but it's not. As we'll see, it's a spiritual, emotional and psychological matter of considerable ambiguity. Through this book, I hope to provide the tools you and your loved ones need to make sound, rational, intelligent choices, rather than decisions shaped by a large measure of hysteria, guilt, or despair.

Second, I want you to face the process of dying and death in the twenty-first century informed, but not straightjacketed, by the Jewish tradition. In helping you make informed end of life choices, enlightened, responsible Jewish-oriented decisions, and deal with your angst and ambivalence and that of your loved ones, this book presents a wide spectrum of viewpoints from the various strands of contemporary Judaism -- traditional (Orthodox) and more modern and flexible (Conservative and Reform). In providing the guidance offered by the Jewish tradition, I draw upon modern Jewish commentators from the last quarter of the twentieth century, who while looking to ancient sources, witnessed the contemporary transformation of death and dying. They're aware of the realities of the current process of dying and the complexities of life-and-death in the context of modern, high tech medicine.

As we'll see in Chapter 5, these modern Jewish commentators generally accept some or nearly all forms of passive euthanasia -- the withholding or withdrawing of medical treatment -- popularly put, "pulling the plug." Yet, as considered in Chapter 6, with near unanimity, they oppose any form of physician aid-in-dying.

The hard and fast opposition of the contemporary Jewish commentators to assisted dying, forces persons who wish to cut short their suffering from life threatening illnesses and their loved ones to stand outside their religion. Often they follow their own hearts and act, regardless of the Jewish tradition. Furthermore, the pressure for a self-determined demise will continue to grow, given the aging of the American population and the ever mounting number of deaths from degenerative diseases. The growing magnitude of the problem in the twenty-first century will open an ever wider gulf, a form of spiritual separation, for many from Judaism unless the Jewish tradition adjusts in some creative way.

Whether, as a compass for decision-making at the end of life, the current position of the Jewish tradition comes up short, I leave to you. As you read this book, ponder the conclusion of one observer, a practicing psychologist: "Traditionalist medical ethics, like traditionalist Judaism, is seen by most [American Jews] as something old to revere and respect. It is like a fine fossil or an elegant piece of cracked statuary; it is venerable, but it is not relevant today. It comes from a culture that no longer exists. It was produced by ancient or at least ancient-thinking people who knew nothing about science. . . . [Traditional] Jewish medical ethics is also perceived as an approach to medical moral questions that, like traditional Judaism, is regarded as harsh, ponderous, and unpleasant."[2] Increasingly, we may challenge or disregard entirely the unbending, traditional approaches to end of life decision-making, further weakening the essence of Judaism for many of us.

The life-and-death issues raised by modern medicine, for me, also point to the necessity of rethinking the Jewish tradition and its reliance on the commanding authority of biblical and rabbinic sources. In place of legalistic guidelines taking the form of a prescribed set of rules, I offer the perspective of Spiritual Judaism, a nonlegalistic approach to living and dying. Spiritual Judaism rests on: our faith in God, our Creator and Sustainer; our immortal soul; and on our autonomy, grounded in our Godlike nature and our ongoing relationship with the Eternal in improving the world.

Third, in coming decades, recognizing the possibility for responsible, rational choices in end of life matters, progressive Jewish institutions and organizations should take the lead in offering nondirective, nonpaternalist counseling for sufferers and their loved ones. Counseling would help patients explore what their real wishes are, focusing on their values. From the perspective of Spiritual Judaism, this type of counseling would encourage the search for meaning and purpose in life and achieving of closure through a sufferer's expression of unconditional love and forgiveness during the dying process.

The Transformation of Death and Dying

Death has always been with us. We all share in common this fate.

Until the development and availability of modern pharmacology and high tech medicine, beginning roughly about 1940, physicians provided what comfort and support was possible, but they let diseases take their natural course to recovery or death. Treatments were often ineffective.

The advances of medical science have transformed the causes of death and where we die, both of which contribute to why we dread the modern way of dying.

At the beginning of the twentieth century, most adults died rather quickly, without warning, in a matter of days, from infections, such as pneumonia or influenza, or accidents.[3] Our ancestors despaired of lives snuffed out too early. An extended period of dying was an exception, not the rule. People died at all ages of things that killed swiftly. For women, it meant death in childbirth, or from warfare, infections or accidents. For men, death resulted from warfare, infections or accidents. Most people died of their first major illness. People who got cancer, for example, usually knew it only when it was widespread and untreatable. Except for tuberculosis, dying represented a very brief episode immediately preceding one's demise.

Over the last sixty years, life sustaining and life prolonging technologies and drugs have led to a vast expansion of life expectancy and have given us a sense that death can be defeated, or, more realistically, postponed. The discovery and use of antibiotics marked medicine's first successful effort to treat formerly common, but lethal, conditions followed by a variety of biotechnological innovations. People now no longer succumb to pneumonia or strep throat. As a result of heart bypasses, organ transplants, cancer treatments, kidney dialysis and joint replacement, how we die has changed.

Modern medicine works wonders in extending life spans. Physicians now successfully treat diseases that previously extinguished lives, swiftly and relentlessly. Medical intervention not only holds death at bay but also elongates -- and to a considerable extent deforms -- the process of dying. Modern medicine can keep people alive for weeks, months, even years.

We face an epidemic of chronic diseases and conditions in the twenty-first century. As our aging population continues to increase, with longevity aided by healthier lifestyles and medical advances, more and more deaths will result from physical or mental infirmities. Most of us will succumb at the end of a long life to lingering, progressively debilitating diseases -- heart attack, cancer, stroke or Alzheimer's.

Chronic health problems, such as those that affect the heart, which until recently would have claimed patients' lives relatively early in the course of the disease, are now subject to aggressive treatment measures. Technology and pharmacology routinely prolong the lives of patients who then face severe, and often multiple, chronic conditions. An ever larger number of elderly, ill people will experience the prospect of a lengthy dying process, marked by a long downhill decline. More and more of us will gradually die by inches.

Modern medical breakthroughs have proven a mixed blessing. Physicians prolong life, bringing patients back from the brink of death, but often making the last chapter of life a protracted struggle. Those living longer encounter diseases and conditions, physical or mental, diminishing the quality of their lives. In particular, we face a tidal wave of dementia among the elderly, with the prospect of their mental slide into oblivion. As more elderly, ill people, who experience prolonged periods of frailty and disability, are kept alive, they become are part of the daily world of many families -- perhaps your everyday existence -- posing ever mounting strains on their loved ones.

Many of us have had "bad" experiences watching our beloved die. We fear protracted deaths including years of incapacitation, marked by a lengthy period of disability and discomfort, even anguish, depriving us of our dignity. Modern medicine extends life but often makes it a living hell.

Many dread the indignities of becoming an elderly patient: increasingly dependent, feeling hopeless and helpless, facing a loss of self-esteem and control, becoming a burden of others, despondent from one's bodily deterioration and the loss of mental clarity. Facing a lengthy and humiliating dying process, many of us wonder: is life in such a condition worse than death?

Where we die has also undergone a remarkable transformation. Up to the middle of the twentieth century, without any possibilities of prolonging life or affecting a cure, most Americans died at home, in a familiar environment, under their loved ones' care. They died surrounded by family members and friends.

Now fewer than 20% of deaths occur at home. Nearly 80% percent of us die in a hospital or a nursing home.[4] There's a simple explanation for the new venue: technology. The equipment and personnel to provide modern, high tech care are located in hospitals. We spend our final days in a hospital often attached to sophisticated, life-support systems extending the most fragile of existence and enabling physicians to forestall death for a period of time.

Hospitalized patients are often connected by dozens of tubes to machines doing most of their living for them. In an intensive care unit, you see more machinery than patients, more flashing lights than healthcare professionals. Patients are explored by a legion of physicians -- medical specialists -- none of whom the sufferer knows in any meaningful way.

Many of us have visited an intensive care unit. We've seen a loved one, with a withered body, tethered to a web of wires and tubes pumping oxygen, medicine and nutrients into her, draining out various fluids and used air, in the midst of the beeping monitors and the hissing respirators, life-support systems noisily and continuously functioning. We realize we're merely delaying the inevitable.

Extrapolating from our personal experiences with our beloved, here is a scenario many of us personally dread: Dying in a hospital desperately ill, subject to overly aggressive treatment, a high tech, medicalized death.

By our side a respirator, helping us breathe. Tubes run into our nose and stomach, providing nutrition and hydration to keep us alive. In such a situation, we're dependent, helpless, and passive.

In our quiet moments of reflection, we fear that we'll be forced to accept more medication and technology than we want. We question the desirability of living an unrelieved, pointless, humiliating suffering, extended through the efforts of modern medicine. We fear that our physicians will over treat us with the life prolonging techniques at their disposal. Because doctors possess the means to forestall death, the technological imperative, marked by invasive procedures and extensive treatments, often runs wild. Therapeutic belligerence typically serves as the order of the day for critical care medicine.

Physicians often fight the tides of time with the machines and drugs at their command. Many seem unable to give up and admit death. Yet, at some point, death, the enemy, wins.

We dread medical interventions setting us up for a lingering death, accompanied by an absence of any meaningful control over our destiny, long after any return to reasonable functioning is possible. In addition to a dying process needlessly protracted by technology and pharmacology, many of us have difficulty with the medical bureaucracy isolating the dying in intensive care units among strangers, where they are left, abandoned to healthcare professionals who barely know them. The hospital, especially, the intensive care unit, has become a place of isolation and solitary death. We fear dying alone.

Our healthcare system often fails to provide humane care at the end of life. Dying in our modern technological age comes with previously unknown horrors, particularly a callous, dehumanized, institutionalized end of life. As Norman Cousins writes, "Death is not the ultimate tragedy of life. The ultimate tragedy is depersonalization - dying in an alien and sterile area, separated from the spiritual nourishment that comes being able to reach out to a loving hand, separated from a desire to experience the things that make life worth living, separated from hope."[5]

Many of us have witnessed the massive, daily failures of medicine to provide humane care at the end of life. We've seen impersonal medical interventions directed at postponing others' deaths and extending the dying process beyond the point that living has any meaning for sufferers and their loved ones. In short, hospitals have too often become torture chambers for patients and their dear ones.

It's important to realize that physicians are increasingly considering the comfort of those whose death can't be averted. Comprehensive comfort care, more technically known as palliative care, is fast becoming standard for many patients suffering from progressive, advanced diseases, who have a limited prognosis.

Yet even the best available palliative care may prove ineffective to remedy patients' profound emotional and spiritual suffering. Although medicine can neither avert all pain or ensure a tranquil course illness (nor will it in the foreseeable future), generally adequate pain control is not the problem. Encountering the process of dying, whether prolonged at home or at the end in a hospital, each of us undergoes a unique form of torment and doubt. Many will face a cruel irony. Technology and pharmacology have provided us with the capacity to prolong life before we have determined how to value our existence.

We see what others have gone through. We feel our death will not come gently. More often than not, despite the highest quality medical care, patients face personal dilemmas: living as long as possible or living as meaningfully as possible. Many feel that the sacredness traditionally marking the end of life seems missing.

Until medicine, and more generally, society, bring back the human and spiritual dimension into the dying process, many of us will seek alternatives. Although physicians promise a gentle death, some of our experiences with family members and friends suggest the contrary. Thus, when the time comes, you or a loved one may consider choosing to accelerate the time of death rather than merely surviving in an unacceptable life situation -- a deformed process of dying. You or a beloved may want to determine the time and place of your death. For those who want to take control of their destiny by actively speeding up their demise, the mainstream of the modern Jewish tradition offers no alternative to a resounding "No, don't do it, suffer!"

A Personal Note: Putting My Cards on the Table

As I noted earlier, this is a very personal book. It focuses on sound decision-making for you and your loved ones at the end of life. It's basically not about public policy, judicial decisions, legislative changes, new administrative or medical ethics rules, although these are briefly summarized where appropriate by way of background. At the outset, let me express my own preferences with respect to the role physicians should be able to play in the dying process.

A degree of realism is in order. Despite various legal restrictions throughout the United States on physician-assisted suicide (except in Oregon) and voluntary active euthanasia, patients commit countless quiet suicides, aided to some degree, as we'll see in Chapter 6, aided by physicians. Aid-in-dying, through passive euthanasia, also takes place daily. The sale of more than one half million copies of Derek Humphry's *Final Exit*,[6] a recipe book for fatal drug doses, provides perhaps the most telling incidence of the prevalence of suicide, assisted suicide and various forms of voluntary euthanasia in the United States.

We need to ask: should assisted suicide or voluntary active euthanasia remain covert procedures or be open and properly documented, with legal safeguards against abuse? Today, patients and their dear ones daily struggle to make end of life decisions while courts, legislators, activists of all stripes, and the public at large wrestle with a difficult question: should the government should make it easier for physicians to help sufferers?

My preferred public policy approach is quite simple. The American legal system and medical ethical guidelines should let physicians help their patients to die, subject to two basic limitations: first, carefully protect a sufferer's real wishes to ensure he or she is making an informed, rational and unpressured decision; and second, avoid an unwitting choice for death by patients when there is a real chance for recovery and an acceptable quality of life. For me, on the policy level, the answers to end of life issues represent matters of individual choice, not social control, subject to these limitations.

Fears of uninformed, nonconsensual deaths -- involuntary active euthanasia -- are vastly overblown. We must study and debate the form the law should take so that we can assure ourselves that physician-aided death, will be voluntarily undertaken and in accordance with each patient's wishes.

Selecting an appropriate course between prolonging life as long as possible and maintaining a personally desired quality of life should happen one patient and one physician at a time. It's a very personal decision, involving a patient, his or her loved ones and physicians, who struggle with the uncertainties surrounding the dying process under a specific set of circumstances at a particular point in time.

For me, whether on a policy or a personal level, autonomy represents the most important value. Self-determination, exercised responsibly, lets each of us make a life-or-death decision. Autonomy enables you to make important decisions about your life according to your values and what you conceive as a good life. In exercising self-determination, people are encouraged to take a considerable degree of responsibility over their lives.

Thus, generally I want to strengthen personal autonomy in decision-making. Neither government nor religion should dictate how people are to see meaning in their lives or in their deaths. You should be able to make the profound decisions about how to live and how to die for yourself. Choices regarding life-and-death should not be imposed on you by a judge, a legislator, a bureaucrat, a rabbi, a physician, or a hospital ethics committee.

My emphasis on personal autonomy in end of life decision-making, exercised in a rational, responsible manner, may repel some. It certainly does not comport with the mainstream of the Jewish tradition. However, I urge the exercise of self-determination from the perspective of Spiritual Judaism,[7] its view of the immortal soul, the virtues of love, compassion, forgiveness, and the quest for meaning and purpose in one's life. In other words, autonomy should rest on a large measure of responsibility grounded in our relationship to God, certain interpersonal virtues, and the search for a meaningful life. We need to face these issues, not deny or avoid them. We need to hear one another at length and in depth as we explore the meaning of life-and-death and our possible choices at the end of life.

With some basic safeguards, as developed in Chapter 6, legalizing physician-assisted dying, would offer patients a safety valve. It would reassure individuals wanting physician aid-in-dying, so as to avoid a protracted dying process, that they could, but need not, obtain it. The availability of a legal escape is important to some patients, allowing them to focus on other things, such as the search for meaning and purpose in life. Legalization would reassure sufferers that they need not endure what they regard as an unnecessarily prolonged ending to their lives. For people who are dying, the possibility of assistance, having a measure of control such as that afforded by a physician's prescription for a lethal drug, would provide sufficient assurance and offer more peace of mind. As Lonny Shavelson, an emergency room physician, writes, "They will rest assured of comfort as they progress to their natural deaths, perhaps never needing the fatal dose that is ready."[8]

An Overview of This Book

In the context of medical advances and our fears about death and dying, Chapter 2 explores two Jewish approaches to life-and-death: one, a text-oriented methodology and a second, focusing on our autonomy, grounded in our Godlike nature and our partnership with the Eternal in perfecting the world. Traditionally, Judaism has accorded considerable, if not total, weight in end of life decision-making to the intrinsic worth of each and every human life. An abstract principle, the sanctity of biological life, reigns supreme, no matter what the quality of one's life. We are told that it is never right to intentionally take an innocent human life. An absolute prohibition is said to exist; however, as we'll see, exceptions exist.

Although I respect and revere the sanctity of our earthly life and find enduring and transcendent meaning to our existence through our immortal souls, I reject the notion of biological idolatry, underpinning most of the Jewish tradition's teachings in which the only, or at least the primary, concern of healthcare focuses on keeping the physical body alive, regardless of its condition. I also reject the position that whatever may be done by means of drugs and technology ought to be done, often resulting in malignant over treatment.

As you read not only Chapter 2 but also the rest of this book, I want you to ask yourself: Is physical life as a well-tended vegetable, often unable to think, what God has in mind for us?

In Chapter 2, I also develop the need to exercise our autonomy subject to restraints, but not those embodied in the sanctity of life concept. Rather, following the principles of Spiritual Judaism, certain interpersonal virtues, namely, love, compassion and forgiveness as well as our quest for meaning and purpose in our life, should guide our decision-making as we face the end of life.

In Chapter 3, I present a Jewish perspective on suffering. We need to inquire into why a good and loving God requires so much misery on our part. For some, suffering may lead to a fatalistic acceptance of what befalls them in life. Others look to the afterlife, the World to Come, where God will reward and punish. Even in our present earthly existence, however, we can learn and grow spiritually from our anguish. The process of dying, for all its attendant suffering, can be a time of spiritual awareness and growth as well as renewal, personal connection, and transcendence. We can come to express lovingkindness, forgive others, and find meaning and purpose in our lives. As we explore these issues, we need to remain open to the possibility of meeting the challenge, learning and growing from hardship, but acknowledge the possibility of intolerable, unrelenting suffering prior to death and an absence of meaningfulness.

Chapter 4 affords insights into how the Jewish tradition views the dying process, as part of the spiritual and physical ebbing of life, and the concept of death in the context of our immortal souls. The chapter focuses on the transformation of the definition of death in both the American legal system and the contemporary Jewish tradition, marked by the general acceptance (with the notable exception of some Jewish traditionalists) of what is known as the whole brain definition of death. Looking to the future, the chapter explores the likely impact, as well as the advantages and disadvantages, of another definition, namely, the higher brain concept of death.

Chapter 5 deals with the problem of patients in a hopeless condition. Most of us don't wish to be subjected to futile attempts to maintain our life. We're concerned about the excessive, even the inhumane, high tech medicine and other interventions.

Most hospital deaths in the United States now are anticipated and controlled. Healthcare professionals engage in passive euthanasia. They withdraw or withhold medical treatment; they sedate patients to unconsciousness. In addition to discussing the impact of judicial decisions and the transformation of medical ethical standards, this chapter considers how the Jewish tradition tries to answer the question: when shouldn't we do all that we can do? After presenting an overview of the general approaches to this question, three situations are examined in detail: first, the withholding or withdrawing of machines, medication, and other medical treatments; second, the withholding or withdrawing of artificially administered food and water; and third, the use of pain medication.

There's no need for heroic measures to prolong the life of a terminally ill patient. We can gently and mercifully stop it. Increasingly, most modern Jewish commentators permit the withholding or withdrawal of life-support treatments at the end of life, when it is pointless to continue and these interventions only prolong the dying process. Most contemporary Jewish observers regard the cessation of treatment and allowing death to occur as compatible with the overarching sanctity of biological life principle. Once a decision is made to let nature take its course, new dilemmas present themselves, however, around the removal of artificial food and water as well as the use of terminal sedation. If at all possible, I recommend a conscious, spiritually-oriented dying.

Chapter 6 considers how we face a terminal illness or a chronic condition. A terminal diagnosis often brings with it fear of a future dominated by severe pain and other physical symptoms. We dread the debilitation brought about by a chronic condition. We face suffering in all of its dimensions, together with the specter of dependence, humiliation, and disintegration of self. Some of us think we know what lies ahead prior to death; we do not want to prolong our existence. Because technological and pharmacological developments enable physicians to maintain biological life functions, but not cure underlying disorders, we may view the process of dying as worse than death itself.

In the context of a terminal illness or an incurable, debilitating chronic condition, this chapter explores what the Jewish tradition says about suicide, physician-assisted suicide, and voluntary active euthanasia as modes of controlling the time and manner of our demise. As more of us face death from protracted, degenerative diseases, our choices throughout the process of dying will become major issues in the twenty-first century. Compassion may lead to a shortening of life. Because souls come into biological life and again depart from it, remaining in themselves immortal, death need not equate with harm if life holds only unrelenting misery. The cessation of biological functions does not constitute the end of life, but a transition to another phase of one's existence. We can (and should be able to) bring life to a close in keeping with our own values, as inspired by the teachings of Spiritual Judaism.

Departing in style from the legal precedents considered in Chapters 4 through 6, Chapters 7 and 8 provide suggestions for and a series of questions designed to promote better decision-making by patients. Whichever side of the bed we're on, we want a sufferer's choice to be rational, to reflect his or her deeply held feelings and values, and to be made calmly over the weeks and months given to him or her.

Life's final installment, no matter how messy and painful, offers important opportunities, from the perspective of Spiritual Judaism, for a life review, forgiveness, reconciliation, and closure -- provided one's pain and other physical needs are addressed. In their dying, patients may use a newfound approach to life in order to reframe their anguish.

Questions are posed in Chapter 8 designed to elicit answers and to assist sufferers to think about, rationally and responsibly, whether they want to accelerate their deaths. These choices involve a profound, very personal assessment of one's values, encompassing spiritual and religious issues, the physical and mental quality of one's life, and emotional, social and financial concerns. One size -- one abstract principle -- does not fit all.

Chapter 9 looks at a patient's death and dying from the perspective of his or her loved ones. In addition, examining the various strains caregivers face, this chapter offers dear ones suggestions for meeting a dying person's physical, emotional and spiritual needs.

Chapters 7 and 9 also contain prayers, meditations, visualizations, and exercises, as well as practical and spiritual suggestions, designed to help patients and their loved ones. In short, Chapters 7, 8 and 9 strive to help someone who is dying and his or her beloved achieve emotional and spiritual acceptance and completion regarding the conclusion of life.

Chapter 10 deals with the need and techniques for planning ahead by all of us, even the most healthy, using healthcare proxies and living wills (so-called advance care directives) as well as making provision for postmortem organ donations. It may be overly idealistic on my part, but I believe we must stop avoiding these issues and squarely face our mortality. I encourage discussions between and among you, your loved ones, and your physicians regarding medical care choices in various circumstances, if in the future you should lack decision-making capacity. Talk with those closest to you and with your doctor; put your wishes in writing about how you want to be treated. I urge you, whatever your physical and mental health, to make plans now not only regarding your future medical care but also for an array of financial and legal details. In addition to designating a healthcare proxy and detailing your written instructions regarding the medical treatments you wish (or don't want), give your loved ones a written statement of your values and beliefs regarding end of life care. Chapter 10, together with Chapter 8, will help you think out, in advance, how you want your life to end.

Chapter 11 offers a brief conclusion, focusing on our search for a "good" death.

Notes

1. Bureau of the Census, *Statistical Abstract of the United States, 1999*, 119th ed. (Washington, D.C.: Government Printing Office, 1999), 95, table 130; Joyce A. Martin et al, "Births and Deaths: Preliminary Data for 1998," *National Vital Statistics Reports* 47:25 (October 1999): 5, table D.

2. Matthew (Menachem) Maibaum, "A 'Progressive' Jewish Medical Ethics: Notes for an Agenda," *Journal of Reform Judaism* 33:3 (Summer, 1986): 29.

3. *Oxford Textbook of Palliative Medicine*, ed. Derek Doyle, Geoffrey W.C. Hanks, and Neil MacDonald, 2d ed. (New York: Oxford University Press, 1998), 33, table 2; Gregory L. Armstrong, Laura A. Conn, and Robert W. Pinner, "Trends in Infectious Disease Mortality in the United States During the 20th Century," *Journal of the American Medical Association* 281:1 (January 1999): 61-66.

4. National Center for Health Statistics, *Vital Statistics of the United States 1992*, vol. 2, part A (Washington, D.C.: Government Printing Office, 1996), 374, table 1-30.

5. Norman Cousins, *Anatomy of an Illness as Perceived by the Patient: Reflections on Healing and Regeneration* (New York: Norton, 1979), 133.

6. Derek Humphry, *Final Exit: The Practicalities of Self-Deliverance and Assisted Suicide for the Dying* (Eugene, Oreg.: The Hemlock Society, 1991).

7. The principles of Spiritual Judaism are developed in Lewis D. Solomon, *Jewish Spirituality: Revitalizing Judaism for the Twenty-First Century* (Northvale, N.J.: Jason Aronson, 2000).

8. Lonny Shavelson, *A Chosen Death: The Dying Confront Assisted Suicide* (Berkeley: University of California, 1998), 66.

Chapter 2

Looking to Jewish Law and Beyond in Matters of Life-and-Death

From a Jewish perspective, there are two basic approaches to medical care decision-making at the end of life.[1] First, the traditional text oriented approach builds on the sanctity of biological life: God as the Author of Life reigns supreme in all matters. This approach accords paramount authority to the Jewish tradition, particularly Jewish law as interpreted and applied by rabbis over the ages. The strictures of Jewish legal rules and principles set limits on self-determination.

Second, the alternative approach focuses on our autonomy grounded in our Godlike nature and our partnership with the Eternal in perfecting the world. A considerable degree of decisional autonomy is implicit in the notion of being created in God's image. Looking to autonomy, not authority, rests on one's ability to make important decisions shaping his or her life -- life-and-death decisions -- for oneself. Autonomy recognizes the ability of each of us to express our own distinctive character - our own values, interests, and commitments; it allows us to shape our lives according to our personality. It permits us to lead our own lives, not subject to or being led along by a textual tradition, no matter how ancient, or rabbinical authority.

As we will see, in addition to using divergent modes of reasoning and often yielding different conclusions, these two approaches differ in who makes a life-or-death medical decision. It is a rabbi under the first approach. It is a patient or his or her loved ones under the second approach.

In this chapter and throughout this book, I develop the nonlegalistic notions of Spiritual Judaism, an approach rooted in our autonomy.

Spiritual Judaism focuses on: the One Divine Presence; the adherence to ethical standards in our conduct with others; and the pursuit of personal virtues. The prophet Micah expressed it so well more than two thousand five hundred years ago: ". . .[D]o justice, and . . . love goodness, and walk humbly with your God" (Micah 6:8). In striving to formulate an approach to a Jewishly "successful" life-and-death, Spiritual Judaism guides and helps us exercise our autonomy. In making end of life medical care decisions, it is important to act on personal values, rooted in the interpersonal virtues of love, compassion, and forgiveness underpinning Spiritual Judaism as well as the individual search for meaning and purpose in life.

The Traditional Text-Centered Approach

The traditional approach of Jewish bioethics, and more generally, Jewish ethics, identifies precedents from biblical and rabbinic sources to arrive at Jewish principles and prescriptions applicable to a specific situation. Thus, a qualified rabbi, as the ultimate decision-maker, first turns and looks to primary authorities, biblical and rabbinic.

Biblical texts include the Five Books of Moses, namely, Genesis, Exodus, Leviticus, Numbers, and Deuteronomy, known as the Pentateuch (or the Torah), as well as the Prophets and various writings including the Psalms and the Proverbs. These biblical texts were mainly written from the tenth to the fifth century B.C.E. The Torah is often referred to as the written law in contrast to the oral law representing unwritten traditions interpreting and applying the Five Books of Moses.

Rabbinic Judaism was born out of the destruction of the Second Jewish Temple in Jerusalem some one thousand nine hundred years ago. For the next 500 to 900 years of the Common Era, up until the medieval period in Europe, a vast body of literature developed reflecting the creative ferment of the rabbis. The rabbinic literature consists of two parts. First, the Talmud, mainly a legalistic discourse on all aspects of Jewish life, representing a reduction to writing of the oral law consisting of the opinions and teachings of numerous rabbis who analyzed and commented on the Torah as well as various nonlegal materials. Second, the Midrash, written interpretations of Biblical passages using allegories, parables, analogies, and stories to illustrate the meaning of a Torah verse.

Rabbinic sources from the medieval period include various

commentaries and legal codes. These medieval rabbinic sources function today as statutory materials. The major medieval commentary on the Hebrew Bible and the Talmud is that of Rabbi Shlomo ben Isaac, who lived from 1040 to 1105, known to us today as Rashi. Rashi's commentaries had an enormous influence on the development of modern *Halakhah*. The most illustrious Jew of the Middle Ages was Maimonides, a rabbi, philosopher, physician and ethicist, who lived from 1135 to 1204. His most famous work, the classic and authoritative multivolume *Mishneh Torah*, represents a monumental compilation and systematization of biblical, Talmudic, and post-Talmudic law. The *Shulchan Aruch (The Code of Jewish Law)*, a unified code compiled by Rabbi Joseph Karo, who lived from 1488 to 1575, serves as the standard work of Jewish law. It has become Judaism's most authoritative legal code.

The major rabbinic literature of the last four centuries consists of responsa -- case law, if you will -- which are formal replies to legal questions about individual cases addressed to rabbinic scholars. Numerous rabbis authored volumes and volumes of responsa over the centuries.

Previous responsa, in which rabbis applied concepts derived from the primary biblical and rabbinic authorities to specific problems, as well as various Jewish codes, such as constructed by Maimonides or Karo, serve as the precedents for traditionally-oriented modern day rabbis. Although these responsa constitute precedents and describe the specific situation necessitating a decision, no two cases are exactly identical. The specifics of each case, of course, play a large role. The writings of more contemporary rabbis are also analyzed thereby clarifying the purpose and meaning of earlier Jewish materials.

In grappling with a current situation, rabbis reason by analogy. They consider not only prior holdings on a comparable issue and their reasoning but they also apply principles derived from somewhat similar fact patterns deemed appropriate to the situation at hand.

Divergences in opinion arise from how one reads, stringently or leniently, prior precedents. Opinions also differ as to which sources are analogous to the instant situation. For some, precedents may be excluded from consideration as irrelevant; while for others the same precedents may be viewed as extremely relevant, if not controlling.

As we will see in Chapter 4 when we examine the evolution of the definition of death, a text may be read literally or in accordance with the principle of purposive interpretation (that is, a text's "true" intent) looking, in this case, to medical evidence and scientific advances to inform Jewish legal interpretation. Thus, giving rabbis the discretion to use principle of purposive interpretation or other extra-legal factors, such as the Holocaust, often leads to a broader, more flexible construction of ancient texts. However, some traditionalists maintain that the sources must be read narrowly and quite literally leading to harsh, unpleasant, need I say almost inhumane conclusions in the context of end of life decision-making that may be psychologically or physically painful for a patient and his or her loved ones.

In short, traditionalists sift through Jewish sources, both primary authorities and precedents, in deciding into what category a specific situation falls. They then apply, by analogy, these primary authorities and precedents. Thus, even when authorities use the same methodology and read the same sources, they may read the same texts differently and reach quite different conclusions. The predilections and values of different rabbis, as well as their theological assumptions, their implicit views about what it means to be human, moral considerations, the social-historical situation in which they find themselves, and their accompanying psychological state, play a role, often a key role, in the interpretative process.

Application of the Traditional Text-Center Approach to Matters of Life-and-Death

In the medical context, when facing an ethical dilemma, the sanctity of biological life principle, based on the notion that God created and owns our physical bodies, takes precedence. According to the author of the Book of Deuteronomy (10:14), "To God belong even the highest heavens, the earth and everything on it." Also God declares in Deuteronomy (32:39), "I kill and I give life." In Job 33:4, Job expressed this same belief when he proclaimed in the midst of his suffering, "God's spirit made me and the Divine breath sustains me." The Eternal, according to the Hebrew prophet Ezekiel, declares, "All lives are Mine." (Ezekiel 18:4)

Although each of us has stewardship over our bodies on the earthly plane, according to the traditionalists, we do not have ownership of them. Our bodies remain the property of the Holy One; thus, the decision of when to end anyone's life rests in Divine hands alone.

For text-centered traditionalists, earthly life is a gift from God to be held in trust. Only the Eternal gives life; only the Supreme Sovereign can take it away. In response to the question: "Whose life is it?", the traditionalist answers, "God's, not yours." Thus, we should leave life-and-death to God; death represents the Holy One's decision, not ours.

For traditionalists, this conclusion rests on the affirmation of all human life. Every life is precious in God's eyes. Each biological life is "infinite in value." As Lord Immanuel Jakobovits, the late Orthodox Chief Rabbi of the United Kingdom, put it, ". . . every fraction of life is worth as much as the totality of life."[2] Seconds, minutes, hours, days, and months have equal value because of the indivisibility of infinity. Also, all human life is equally valuable and absolutely inviolable regardless of its quality. Every moment of earthly life is of inestimable value, even if one is terminally ill or permanently unconscious. Because the preservation of biological life takes precedence over everything, according to rigorous traditionalists (there are, of course, more flexible interpretations), we should preserve every last wisp of life at all costs (subject to one very limited exception of virtually no practical significance, as discussed in Chapter 5), even if it is of no benefit to a patient. (There are other exceptions for self-defense, war, and capital punishment.) Why? Because biological life, as a gift from God, has value to the Eternal. The Holy One remains the final arbiter over matters of life-and-death.

For text-centered traditionalists following the sanctity of biological life approach, a rabbi (a *posek* in Hebrew), who has studied and mastered Jewish sources and is committed to "tradition," serves as the medical decision-maker. Rabbinical authority rests on Deuteronomy 17:8-13, where we read that each generation's questions about Jewish "law" must be addressed to that generation's judges, in modern terms, rabbis. Thus, a qualified rabbi, acting as a legal arbiter, makes the life-and-death medical decision, taking the form of a Halakhic directive, for a patient seeking to apply Jewish legal rules and principles, on an individualized, case-by-case basis. In other words, it is really not up to patients or their loved ones, at least for those who submit to the continuing authority of Jewish law.

A More Liberal Text-Centered Approach

More liberal (Conservative and Reform) rabbis and commentators apply a similar text-centered methodology in approaching bioethical issues. The Conservative Movement has appointed the Committee on Jewish Law and Standards to provide interpretations of Jewish law. The Committee validates acceptable options on issues that individual rabbis raise. It also adopts standards binding on Conservative rabbis and synagogues. The Reform Movement's Central Conference of American Rabbis has created a Committee on Halakhic Inquiry and has published several books of Reform responsa, now available on-line at ccarnet.org, which function in an advisory capacity for Reform Jews.

Continuing to use a text-focused approach, for these more liberal authorities, a decision flows whenever possible from an interpretation of legal precedents derived from Jewish texts and sources, aided and enlightened, however, by an assessment of historical and cross-cultural materials. Thus, these less literal commentators take into consideration the variety of meanings texts have as well as their historical and literary context and the new settings arising from significant changes in medical practice in the area under consideration.

For these liberal authorities, accommodation can occur within the Jewish legal system. Jewish law can undergo appropriate changes thereby preserving and enhancing the *Halakhah*. One of the most thoughtful of the modern interpreters of the Jewish tradition, Conservative Rabbi Elliot N. Dorff, Rector and Professor of Philosophy at the University of Judaism in Los Angeles, strives to find a dynamic methodology able to "accommodate the revolutionary changes occurring in the world of medicine on an almost daily basis and yet remain unmistakably Jewish." Dorff wants to "root a contemporary Jewish medical ethic in the Jewish conceptual and legal structures of the past but recognizing that to do so honestly and wisely, we will have to make difficult judgments as to when and how to apply that material to substantially new settings."[3]

However, despite these efforts to move away from literal textual interpretations, any text-centered approach, particularly with respect to the questions of suicide, physician-assisted suicide or voluntary active euthanasia, as we'll see in Chapter 6, leads back to one key principle: the sanctity of biological life. Any form of suicide is forbidden; voluntary active euthanasia is prohibited. Why? Even for these more liberal authorities, human life has infinite and inestimable value. Each moment of earthly life, regardless of its quality or usefulness, is sacred. Thus, judgments cannot (and should not) be made as to the quality of any given life. We must not consider whether a person is valuable or worthless to society.

Some commentators, as we will see, allow certain departures from this seemingly inviolable rule, the supreme value of biological life, particularly with respect to passive euthanasia, the withholding or withdrawing of medical treatment. These more flexible interpretations of the Jewish tradition permit the withdrawal of machines and other artificial life-support systems, when these measures serve only to prolong a patient's dying process. As Dorff concludes, Jewish law embodies a "strong push for life as a consistent policy. . . , but not an unbreakable rule."[4] In reaching this conclusion, Dorff reasons that we are not commanded to save earthly life at all costs and in every situation.

Dorff sees a legalistic approach as carrying traditional Jewish concerns into and responding to contemporary medical situations. He maintains, "We should retain a legal method with its inherent discipline, authority, continuity, coherence and educational utility in making our moral decisions and in teaching moral sensitivity, recognizing after all that the law must be continually tempered by its traditional and necessary interaction with morality."[5]

A text-centered approach, whether in the hands of traditional or liberal commentators, suffers from one fundamental weakness: the Jewish texts on which they rely were not Divinely revealed. They are human documents reflecting our spiritual creativity.

Jewish Texts Were Not Divinely Revealed

In going back to and using Jewish sources to guide us in making medical care decisions in the twenty-first century, it's important to realize that the Torah and subsequent rabbinic interpretations were not Divinely revealed. Jewish traditionalists, particularly Jewish fundamentalists, never want to discuss or face the virtually unanimous conclusion of scholars that the written law (the Torah) and oral law (the Talmud and later rabbinic interpretations) were not revealed by God to Moses on Mount Sinai. Rather, the Torah achieved its familiar shape and dimensions by various human hands as the result of an evolutionary process. The books of the Hebrew Bible were recorded at different times by various writers. Thus, the Torah, the Talmud, and the Jewish law (*Halakhah*) are the products of human beings striving to understand God and the Eternal's ways.

For the past four hundred years, critical biblical analysis has found the following: numerous duplications and repetitions in the Pentateuch typical of writings recording oral traditions; variations in the name of the Divine; and a broad diversity of language and style and contrasting viewpoints in the text of the Torah.

The discovery of duplication extending across a considerable body of the Five Books of Moses, starting with two stories of creation in the Book of Genesis (Genesis 1:1-2:3 and Genesis 2:4-24), led to the claim, going back to the seventeenth century, that the Torah had its own history of composition. Specifically, it had been compiled from a number of documents.

Variations in God's Hebrew names, Elohim and Yahweh, used in the Pentateuch provide further evidence of different sources.

Three parallel sources (E, J, and P) and the addition of a fourth source, D, gave rise to what has become known as the four-source documentary hypothesis.[6] Although scholars vigorously dispute the dates and the exact nature of the four sources, the view that four sources underpin the Torah, as we know it today, holds the field.

Thus, modern, critical biblical scholarship has undermined the traditional understanding of the Torah as Divinely revealed by God to Moses. Biblical scholarship called and continues to call into question two bedrock doctrines: first, a literal revelation and second, the covenant between God and the Jews, as the Eternal's chosen people, on which much of traditional Jewish law is based.

The authors of the Five Books of Moses wove together various source material: a collection of traditions, semi-historical stories, and sheer fantasies, originating at different times in ancient Israel and neighboring cultures. The Pentateuch, as a human work, was authored by many humans and was subject to editing and re-editing over long periods of time.

Although the Torah has special significance for the Jewish people, these writings are not absolutely or ultimately true or a superior form of Divine revelation. Therefore, I suggest that we view the Torah as a record of the spiritual life of the Jewish people and as evidence of their quest to know God and the Eternal's ways.

Viewing the Pentateuch as a product of humans, an unverifiable mix of myth and historical fantasy, not the commanding voice of God, we in the twenty-first century need not accept as binding, definitive authority for our lives either the Torah or the two thousand years of rabbinic interpretations. We need not live in accordance with all of the supposed 613 Divine commands designed to take Jews through all aspects of living and dying.

We are thus led to a most difficult and challenging inquiry. If not rabbinic authority and the *Halakhah*, what is to guide Jews in the twenty-first century? Specifically, in the context of end of life decision-making, can we formulate a new approach to surmount the new form of idolatry, namely, biological idolatry, centered on keeping the physical body "alive" regardless of its condition?

An Alternative Approach Focusing on Personal Autonomy

Perceiving the inadequacies of a text-centered methodology for developing a Jewish viewpoint to contemporary bioethical quandaries, some commentators have formulated a new approach, focusing on personal autonomy, based on three factors. First, in light of dazzling advances in medical technology in recent years and the differences between medical conditions of fifty years ago (let alone one thousand five hundred years ago) and now, particularly, the ability of physicians to help people live and thereby to prolong the dying process, the Jewish tradition cannot retain as an absolute, unmodified principle, the sanctity of biological life as determined by the Holy One. Modern medicine's remarkable ability to extend life and let us time one's demise by giving or withdrawing treatment refutes the notion that biological life is a gift of God, to be given and taken at the time of the Eternal's choosing, and that our bodies belong to the Supreme Sovereign. When we use medical technology and knowledge to keep patients alive, the humans behind the machines "play" God through their interventions.

A person, who is permanently and irreversibly unconscious, who exists as a mindless body, does not seem to me to further the wonders of human life. God's purposes are not served by the plastic tubes and chemicals keeping that person alive. In such a situation, as well as others discussed later in this book, death may respect and sanctify the value of human life. A quick, earlier, more peaceful death, in contrast to a prolonged demise, may in fact show greater respect for biological life. Thus, we need to ask: will sustaining life benefit or harm a patient? Implicitly, as we'll see in Chapters 5 and 6, quality of life questions surface and enter into the end of life decision-making process.

Second, we need to focus on: What does it mean to be alive? What is our essential nature as human beings? We need to think deeply about this question, as we will do in Chapter 4. For me, it is our immortal soul.

Third, we are led to ask: What is humanity's relationship to God? The formulation of an alternative approach to the sanctity of biological life doctrine moves from the basic premise of the Messianic Era, namely, that humanity serves as God's partner in shaping, improving, and perfecting the world. The Messianic Era will usher in not only a time of peace and justice but also human self-realization. All humans will be treated like the Divine and will become Godlike.

The notion that in perfecting the world the Eternal requires human help, in turn, rests on two fundamental Jewish values: first, humans are created by the Eternal and in God's image and second, humans are autonomous. We read in the Book of Genesis: "God created humans in the Eternal's image. . . ." (1:26-27; 5:1). At least three meanings flow from this concept. First, each human being created in the Divine image has unlimited value. As the Talmud (Babylonian Sanhedrin 37a) says, if you save one life, it is like saving the entire world. Second, all humans, as children of God, are equal. Third, each one of us, created in the Divine image, however, is unique.[7]

Humanity's role in perfecting the world rests on personal autonomy, namely, our free will and our freedom to live the life we choose. We are morally free and we have the ability to distinguish right from wrong and to act accordingly. The author of the Book of Deuteronomy tells us (30:15): "I [God] place before you a choice between good and evil, between life-and-death." Each of us possesses the rather perilous privilege of freedom of choice, perhaps God's greatest gift to us, and with it we must assume full responsibility for our decisions.

In the Jewish tradition, a soul's earthly incarnation involves a mixture of God's control, Divine providence and mercy, and human free will. Charting the soul's future course, the Jewish mystics suggest, God tells each soul in the womb, particularly less developed souls, what its mission will be and how to fulfill it.[8] The soul obtains its instructions and the specific lessons it needs to learn to achieve a higher degree of perfection. A soul may be assigned a spirit guide. More advanced souls may receive only a general outline. Each soul is reborn with the task of mending itself and also helping improve the world.

At the same time, the Jewish tradition insists on free will. The Holy One's power is restricted so that we may exercise our freedom of choice.

We are not puppets. We are free to respond to the circumstances in which we find ourselves, how we perceive and experience them, how we interpret what happens to us, and the choices we make in life. Using our creative imagination and our constructive will, each of us is responsible for who we are and what we make of our life.

Through our mind and our way of thinking, we create the world we see. How each of us interprets what happens to us determines our inner peace (or lack of it). Thus, our future is not made in the womb or at birth, rather it is within our will to create it, subject, of course, to certain boundaries.

Because humans are created in the image of God, we are morally free. We partake, on a small and often on a rather imperfect scale, of the Eternal's attributes. Our reason and our consciousness give us freedom and make us Godlike. We have a considerable degree of power over our decisions. However, responsibility serves as a corollary of freedom, a rather strange thought in our modern era of irresponsibility. Each of us has responsibility for our choices -- to make the most thoughtful decisions that improve humanity.

Because of our Godlike nature as well as our freedom and our capacity for thoughtfulness, we are called to participate in the ongoing process of improving the world and completing the work of creation. Each generation does what it can; then the task is taken up by the next generation and so on, until perfection will be realized. Each of us has a part to play in the human chain designed to shape the world and remove imperfections.

Humans become more and more Godlike as a result of their ongoing partnership with the Holy One. As Reform Rabbi Peter Knobel writes, "In such a . . . relationship human freedom is not overwhelmed by divine will. Such a relationship is characterized by mutuality and respect for the integrity of each partner."[9]

This approach to decision-making impacts on who serves as the ultimate decision-maker regarding end of life choices. A rabbi, if desired by the patient and his or her loved ones, may provide input into the decision-making process. Acting as a consultant and an advisor, a rabbi may provide the patient, family members, friends, and healthcare professionals with information drawn from the Jewish tradition. The patient, possessing the mental capacity (or if incompetent, his or her surrogate) will, however, ultimately make medical decisions and determine the course of his or her treatment, not a rabbi or a physician. Thus, because of humanity's relationship with God, this alternative approach accords a key role to each patient's autonomy.

In exercising our self-determination, what should we look to and follow if not the authority of the Torah, the Talmud and the Jewish law which have provided a sense of security and order, a feeling of tradition and community? How can we create a sense of Jewish identity?

Refashioning Our Approach to Matters of Life-and-Death in Light of Spiritual Judaism

I write this book within the context of Judaism -- what I call Spiritual Judaism, an ethical, virtue-oriented, monotheistic system -- beyond the minutiae of the traditional legalistic rules and rituals designed govern everyday living.[10]

Striving to fill our spiritual hunger, to offer meaning to our existence and a connection with the Transcendent, Spiritual Judaism represents a nondogmatic, nonlegalistic path, not relying on Jewish legal rules and principles. It is a way of thought, feeling, and belief, not centered on rules, about God and the spiritual depths of our being. It welcomes all people who seek to attune Divine Presence in their lives. It offers the vision of a personal, intimate experience of the Eternal as the source of health, joy, love, abundance, and wholeness. It is designed to help us meet the crises we all face in living and dying.

Spiritual Judaism focuses on practical spirituality, spiritual living that's liberating, promoting and unfolding our inner human possibilities, helping each of us realize his or her highest self and that of others around us, and aiding each of us to find his or her meaning and purpose in life. What then does Spiritual Judaism mean for decision-making at the end of life?

Because humans are created in God's image, they share power with the Eternal. The perspective of human beings must be taken into consideration in reaching conclusions with respect to bioethical matters. Implicit in the notion of being created in God's image is a considerable measure of free will. Human autonomy reflects the dignity of both God and the Eternal's worldly creation. The ability of humans to make and act on their decisions about their lives, including what happens to our physical bodies, rests on the freedom of choice the Holy One gives each of us. By empowering humans, we become more Godlike.

Humans can assert a large and ever growing measure of control over their lives. The greater a patient's say in matters impacting his or her life, the more Godlike is the patient. As the Modern Orthodox Rabbi Irving Greenberg reminds us, "The patient is in the image of God; then the greater the role in the patient's own therapy, the greater the patient's own dignity. The greater the patient's say in those matters which affect the patient's life, the more Godlike is the patient."[11]

This line of reasoning leads to each patient determining the nature and extent of his or her medical care, the type and duration of medical treatment, and what actions healthcare professionals may perform on his or her body. Each of us is free to make medical choices throughout life, particularly at the end of life, in accordance with our own values, recognizing the uniqueness of each of us. One size -- one rule -- does not fit all.

Self-determination represents, for most of us, the most basic characteristic of being human. Most people want to decide for themselves: what goals and values they bring to a situation; how they feel and should act when facing a difficult, if not a tragic, situation.

From my experience, most of us want to minimize our physical and psychological agony and lessen our suffering. We don't want some sort of gruesome or callous medical process or result so as to satisfy God Who, text-oriented commentators tell us, "owns" our bodies; nor do we want an abstract rule, not Divinely ordained, but merely promulgated by humans. We're concerned with the problem of over treatment of a terminal illness, stemming from the mind set of "whatever can be done medically should be done" and leading to inhumane healthcare decisions. Except for the strictest of traditionalists, as we face a chronic, debilitating condition, marked by a slow physical or mental decline, nearly all of us want an approach from the heart, not merely from the intellect. Biological life, an important value, should not override everything else. Keeping physical life going may be an assault on human dignity.

Rather, I propose that a Jewish approach to matters of life-and-death should focus on our relationship with God and the values implicit in such a relationship. We need to reexamine our values. We can (and should) bring our values to the fore and expand the range of values beyond reaffirming one simple, though admittedly fundamental, concept -- the sanctity of biological life -- which nevertheless may only reflect submerged anxieties and the inability of many commentators to come to terms with death, in general, and their own finiteness, in particular.

In making life-and-death decisions within the general framework of autonomy, what sort of action should one pursue as a Jew? What is the relation of our actions to our values? The timeless interpersonal virtues underpinning Spiritual Judaism, namely, love, compassion, and forgiveness, as well as our search for meaning and purpose in our life, even if one is terminally ill, provide a framework for the exercise of our autonomy preventing our descent in anarchy and narcissism.

Love, Compassion, and Forgiveness: Keys to Spiritual Judaism

It is important for Judaism to emphasize our ethical responsibilities as a corollary of and as a guide for our autonomy and the exercise of our free will. We need to conduct ourselves ethically even in the most complex and difficult moments of our lives, for instance, choices at the end of life.

The ethics of Judaism, which have become part of our Western heritage, are as necessary and as relevant in the twenty-first century as when first delivered. Judaism should mold our daily conduct, influence our relations with our neighbors, and make us more honest with the world, zealous for justice and righteousness.

In addition to being just and truthful in all of our relationships and interactions, we should strive to do the "good and beautiful" by living in a loving, compassionate, and forgiving manner. We need to act with love and compassion and to speak kind words. We need to forgive others and to deal with our unresolved emotional issues and botched relationships before we die.

Love and Compassion. Spiritual Judaism rests on bringing us into an ideal relationship with others. We are here to express love which draws people together. We are here to be the presence of love.

Each day we need to be more and more loving and compassionate.[12] We need to realize that anyone we meet represents a holy encounter. We need to recognize that we love best when we have as much regard for others as we have for ourselves.

This is part of our Godlike nature. We are endowed with the power of love by God. Love is inherent in all of us. It is intertwined with the roots of our being. God's Presence within us causes us to love. Our love flows from the Holy One's love; the Eternal is love, unconditional and all-embracing.

Love implies warm-heartedness and kindness. The Torah tells us, "Love your neighbor as yourself. . . ." (Leviticus 19:18). This admonition represents one of the oldest expressions of the "Golden Rule."

At the beginning of the Common Era, when Hillel, one of the greatest of the early sages, was asked to sum up the Torah in a single sentence, he replied, "What is hateful to you, do not do to your fellow." (Babylonian Talmud Shabbat 31a).

Loving your neighbor means feeling a deep connection with and compassion for others. Feel toward others as you would have them feel toward you. As a famous Hasidic rabbi, Shmuel Shmelke of Nikolsburg, who lived from 1726 to 1778, expressed it, "What is hateful to you in your neighbor, don't do yourself."[13]

We can all learn how to love truly, as did Rabbi Moshe Leib of Sassov, the Sassover Rebbe, who lived from 1745 to 1807, the most prominent disciple of Rabbi Shmelke of Nikolsburg, when he went to an inn and overheard the following conversation between two peasants:

First Peasant: "Tell me, do you love me?"

Second Peasant: "Certainly, I love you. I love you like a brother."

First Peasant: (shaking his head): "You don't love me. You don't know what I lack. You don't know what I need."

As the Sassover Rebbe so well understood: "To know the need of others and to bear the burden of their sorrow, that is true love."[14]

Each of us must strive to be compassionate and sympathetic. Compassion is a matter of feeling with and for others. It rests on the notion that your heart will break and that you cannot bear what another is going through. By acknowledging and opening your heart to others' pain and suffering, you feel your unity with others.

Being compassionate, according to the Jewish tradition, enables us to be Godlike. According to the rabbis: "Resemble the Holy One, please! Just as God is merciful and gracious, you too must be merciful and gracious." (Mekhilta de Rabbi Ishmael on Exodus 15:2). As Rabbi Joshua interpreted in Rabbi Levi's name: "God imparts the Divine attribute of mercy to humans so that they may be merciful like the Holy One." (Midrash Rabbah Genesis 33:3). As God is merciful and compassionate, so too you should be merciful and compassionate.

Forgiveness. Love and forgiveness are interrelated.[15] You experience love by extending forgiveness to others. By forgiving others, you open your heart and rediscover the capacity to love that is within. Forgiveness represents the capacity to love when your mind resists love.

Every situation offers you the chance to reunite with the love within you that is your true nature and the true source of your joy and fulfillment. Every human has the same need and longing for love, the essence of our being. See the pure spiritual soul which is inherently good, the holiness, the spark of the Divine in others who are calling out for love from you. We are all united with and connected to God. We all want to experience happiness, avoid pain and suffering, and make a worthwhile contribution to life.

In the Talmud, Jewish sages discussed forgiveness. For instance, Mar Zutra daily said: "If anyone has hurt or wronged me, they are forgiven" (Babylonian Megilah 28a). Just as God forgives, so we, as Godlike beings, should be forgiving. We read in the Talmud: "Only if you forgive others will God forgive you." (Babylonian Rosh Hashanah 17a).

Whatever is not an expression of love on the part of another -- selfishness, anger, or cruelty -- represents a cry for help, a cry for love. You experience love by extending forgiveness to others -- by accepting them and letting go of the past.

In forgiving others, we cannot pretend that we are not affected by someone's acts or speech. Forgiveness is not permissiveness, it is not an expression of "anything goes." By forgiving, you do not pronounce as acceptable someone's past cruelty, thoughtlessness, or inhumanity.

Almost all of us sometimes utter words or do things, whether intentionally or negligently, out of ignorance or forgetfulness, perhaps out of fear, that are unkind and unloving. These actions or statements bring suffering not only to the actors or speakers, but also to those to whom the actions or words are addressed. Forgiveness does not mean condoning or justifying such actions or statements. You cannot ignore others' difficult qualities or hurtful acts or words.

Forgiveness means saying "no more" from a calm, quiet place. It means sharing your issues and your concerns with another person, confiding how you have felt hurt.

Through your forgiveness, you accept people who have disappointed you by not being perfect. You show that you are willing to let go of your focus on another's behavior and of the way you have been looking at a situation, an interpersonal problem or a relationship, and not hold on to the past. Do not retain your anger and your hate, for they will continue to poison you.

Strive to see things differently and look beyond another's body, behavior, and personality. Try to go beneath the surface differences that seem to separate us to the more profound reality, to the deep truth of the love each of us shares with our fellow human beings.

See others in the light of love. Perceive another's essence, his or her innocence, wholeness, and fundamental worth, deserving of your compassion, understanding, and lovingkindness.

Try to see others for who they really are. See others as the children of God.

The Search for Meaning and Purpose in Our Lives: Another Key to Spiritual Judaism

All of us, whatever the state of our health, need to start by reflecting on what our life is all about. There's much more than our every day physical world. There's transcendent meaning to our existence beyond our materialistic culture and our physical bodies.

As we search for our deeper needs, increased knowledge and awareness, from the Jewish tradition and other belief systems, provide a means to rethink our values and our goals. As we become more aware of our potential and our essence, we become cognizant of the trade-offs we have made and continue to make in our daily quest for material existence and progress.

Many of us search for a calling, even near the end of life. We want to do something meaningful and significant. We seek to find our bliss -- here and now -- which will enable us, fully using our capabilities, however, physically or mentally limited they may be, to make a genuine contribution, not only to our personal development but also to the well-being of humanity. Striving to be of genuine service to others, we want to make the world a better place than when we found it.

Each of us needs to discover his or her bliss, his or her destiny. Each of us has a unique and special place in God's creation. A place only each of us can fill.

It is up to each of us to decide what role we want Jewish sources and values to play in our end of life decision-making process. I want to encourage each of us to take responsibility for our life and to think for ourselves, making life-and-death decisions for ourselves as enlightened by, but not shackled by, the Jewish tradition and its modern interpreters. We can make these critical decisions about our lives consonant with our values, illuminated by the interpersonal virtues underpinning Spiritual Judaism, namely, love, compassion, and forgiveness as well as the quest to find meaning and purpose in life. An approach founded on our Godlike nature and on our partnership with the Eternal in perfecting the world calls for a balance between the respect for human life flowing from our belief in God and the principle of human autonomy and free will, not servility. In other words, both God and humans play roles in formulating a Jewish approach to resolving our end of life quandaries.

If you see yourself as a partner with God, this arrangement presumably permits an ongoing negotiation (and renegotiation) of its terms and conditions. What you perceive as the poor quality of your life and its meaninglessness then become relevant arguments in the negotiation process. If you revere life, you may not want to exist in a humiliating or degrading form. Each of us should be allowed to make judgments about the value of his or her life based on each one's quality of life as actually lived and experienced.

Throughout this book, we need to think about: What is the meaning and value of human life, in general? What is the meaning and value of any particular human life -- my life? Specifically, what is the meaning and value of a life that is human only in a biological or a physical sense? Beyond reciting texts, we need to think seriously and deeply about what it means for humans to belong to God and whether in making medical decisions in conformity with this notion sanctifies (or deprecates), in some sense, our relationship with the Holy One.

As autonomous beings, we have a primary interest in self-determination in selecting and pursuing our own plan for life-and-death, founded on our Godlike nature and our ongoing relationship with the Eternal in perfecting the world. Each immortal soul should possess the ability to extend or terminate its earthly existence as its proper share of the responsibility of the ongoing creative activity. Within the context of the virtues of love, compassion, and forgiveness, we need to ponder, as we'll do later in this book, whether sufferers, in exercising their self-determination, may choose the time and manner of their death. When and under what conditions is such action appropriate? To anticipate our discussion, let me suggest that accelerating the end of one's life may represent an act of respect for the Holy One when a human's likeness to God becomes markedly distorted because of physical or mental disability. Each immortal soul should possess the ability to extend or terminate its earthly existence as its proper share of the responsibility for the ongoing creative activity. But before focusing on these questions, let's first consider our concept of God, the purpose of suffering in our lives, and how each of us responds to anguish.

Notes

1. I have drawn on David H. Ellenson, "How to Draw Guidance From a Heritage: Jewish Approaches of Mortal Choices," in *A Time to be Born and a Time a Die: The Ethics of Choice*, ed. Barry S. Kogan (New York: Aldine de Gruyter, 1991; reprinted in *Contemporary Jewish Ethics and Morality: A Reader*, ed. Elliot N. Dorff and Louis E. Newman, New York: Oxford, 1995), 129-139; Eugene B. Borowitz, *Choices in Modern Jewish Thought: A Partisan Guide* (New York: Behrman, 1983), 243-289.

2. Sir Immanuel Jakobovits, Ph.D., "Ethical Problems Regarding the Termination of Life," in *Jewish Values in Bioethics*, ed. Rabbi Levi Meier (New York: Human Sciences, 1986), 88.

3. Elliot N. Dorff, *Matters of Life and Death: A Jewish Approach to Modern Medical Ethics* (Philadelphia: Jewish Publication Society, 1998), 415, 417.

4. Ibid., 203; Elliot N. Dorff, "A Jewish Approach to End-Stage Medical Care," *Conservative Judaism* 43:3 (Spring 1991): 15; Daniel B. Sinclair concludes in his book *Tradition and the Biological Revolution: The Application of Jewish Law to the Treatment of the Critically Ill* (Edinburgh: Edinburgh University Press, 1989), 81 ". . . Jewish law does not adopt the notion of sanctity of human life, at least not in its strong form. . . . [In the Jewish tradition], it is generally accepted that life in itself is not endowed with intrinsic holiness; rather, holiness is a state to be achieved by dint of sustained effort."

5. Dorff, *Matters of Life and Death*, 416.

6. The scholarly insights on documentary hypothesis are brilliantly summarized by Richard Elliott Friedman in *Who Wrote the Bible*? (Englewood Cliffs, NJ: Prentice Hall, 1987).

7. Rabbi Irving Greenberg, Ph.D., "Toward a Convenantal Ethic of Medicine," in *Jewish Values in Bioethics*, 125-126.

8. Lewis D. Solomon, *The Jewish Book of Living and Dying* (Northvale, NJ: Jason Aronson, 1999), 236-238.

9. Peter Knobel, "Suicide, Assisted Suicide, Active Euthanasia: A *Halakhic* Inquiry," in *Death and Euthanasia in Jewish Law: Essays and Responsa*, ed. Walter Jacobs and Moshe Zemer (Pittsburgh: Rodef Shalom Press, 1995), 31.

10. See generally, Lewis D. Solomon, *Jewish Spirituality: Revitalizing Judaism for the Twenty-First Century* (Northvale, N.J.: Jason Aronson, 2000).

11. Greenberg, "Convenantal Ethic," 142.

12. The interpersonal virtues of love and compassion are developed more fully in Solomon, *Jewish Spirituality*, 63-78.

13. Adapted from *The Hasidic Anthology: Tales and Teachings of the Hasidim*, trans. Louis I. Newman (Northvale, N.J.: Jason Aronson, 1987), 222.

14. Adapted from Maurice Friedman, Ph.D., *A Dialogue with Hasidic Tales: Hallowing the Everyday* (New York: Insight Books, 1988), 86 and *Hasidic Anthology*, 221.

15. For further details on the virtue of forgiveness see Solomon, *Jewish Spirituality*, 79-91.

Chapter 3

Why Me? Why Now? Why This? Looking at Suffering from the Perspective of the Jewish Tradition

Facing a life threatening illness, you naturally ask: "Why me? Did I do something wrong that made this happen?"

Sometimes one's anguish seems contrary to human understanding. We wonder, why do virtuous, innocent people suffer, in so many different ways? Why do the wicked seem to prosper? We grieve at our loss and envy the good fortune of those who seem so unloving, so unforgiving, so ready to "cut corners" in their dealings with others. We feel very angry at God; it's a normal reaction.

The question of suffering and its meaning represents a central problem for humans. We need to face the harsh realities of earthly existence, particularly the problems our torment poses for our faith and trust in a good and loving God. We ask: Why does a good and loving God allow so much anguish? What's the value of misery for a patient and his or her loved ones?

As we ponder these questions, let's begin to approach our inquiry into suffering from the perspective of modern medicine. Biomedical technology is defined by its triumphs; however, it also produces pain and suffering. The culture of modern biomedicine values diagnosis and the treatment of pathology, not really looking at the core illness experience and the accompanying degradation.

Pain, a physical signal, must be distinguished from suffering, one's response to the signal provided by pain. Pain which is chronic, or dire, yields suffering.

On a physical level, physicians often relieve suffering in the presence of continued pain by making the source of pain known, changing the meaning of pain, controlling pain, or demonstrating that an end of pain is in sight. However, our anguish goes beyond its physical aspects. It reflects the meaning an illness has for one who is sick. Suffering often stems from a variety of major concerns about the future.[1]

Suffering connotes the emotional and spiritual distress threatening one's wholeness -- what one loses in relation to others and the Eternal. It cuts one off from others; it restricts one's ability to do things as well as the range of one's activities. Suffering thus represents a perceived threat to one's physical and psychosocial integrity, involving a profound feeling of helplessness and a sense of loss.

Today, physicians can generally, but not totally, control pain and other physical symptoms, such as nausea and vomiting; however, the remediation of suffering, a subjective experience, remains difficult. Suffering on its various levels -- existential, emotional, spiritual -- is not readily amenable to biomedical or pharmacological intervention.

As we will see at the end of this chapter, suffering may serve not only as a source of positive change -- regeneration -- but also, perhaps even more routinely, negative transformation -- bitterness, pessimism and despair. The downside of anguish, in the context of a terminal illness or a chronic, debilitating condition, may lead patients, as we will consider in Chapter 6, to contemplate suicide, physician-assisted suicide, or voluntary active euthanasia.

Patients seriously ill with cancer, heart difficulties, stroke, kidney or liver diseases often experience major depressive disorders, a pervasive feeling of hopelessness. Studies indicate, for example, that about 25% of patients with advanced cancer are clinically depressed; more than half of these patients (and perhaps upwards of 80%) feel sad, anxious, and irritable.[2] They often come face-to-face with nihilism, the notion that nothing really matters anyway, that continued life is without meaning or purpose. The agony inflicted by a long drawn out struggle, whether with, for instance, cancer or Alzheimer's, presents for many a seemingly meaningless and undeserved torment.

As a hospitalized seventy-eight year old artist with leukemia put it: "I'm ready to die; but they won't let me, it seems. It makes sense in my case: this disease can't be cured. I've had all the treatments. Nothing's worked. Now [it's] time to let me die on my own terms. Oh, I'm not always convinced another try with yet some other treatment won't give me a few more days or weeks. And my family is just as uncertain. But really what's the point. . . . A psychiatrist told me I was depressed. Of course, I am. Isn't that what suffering is supposed to be? I want to bring it all to a close. Do I have to go with a smile on my face? That seems to me ridiculous, and insulting."[3]

This chapter examines the meaning of suffering in the Jewish tradition, particularly, whether it has any redeeming value. On one level, our anguish may lead us to accept life fatalistically. We may come to stop expecting fairness or meaningfulness, at least in this earthly life, looking rather to the World to Come. Or, our anguish may enable us to refocus our attention on concerns of the spirit: to express lovingkindness, forgive and receive forgiveness, and find meaning and purpose in our life. Misfortune may afford us the opportunity to learn and grow spiritually.

Before exploring the meaning of suffering, let's first consider our concept of God from the perspective of Spiritual Judaism. If we see the Eternal as both omnipotent and omnipresent and as good and loving, why is there so much misery in the world? In the Jewish tradition, we move from the dual premises that God is both all powerful and good. But are these notions sound?

Spiritual Judaism and Our Concept of God

In striving to grapple with suffering and its meaning, we cannot bypass the question of God. Although the Eternal transcends human knowledge, we continue to ask: Is God omnipotent? Is the Holy One good? Does the Supreme Sovereign care about us?

Is God Omnipotent and Omnipresent?

God is the Source and the Creator of all reality and the Sustainer of all life. As the Sustainer, God's love and care makes all existence possible.

The Hebrew prophets speak of God's power, the Eternal's omnipotence as manifest in the Divine act of creation. The Holy One, the Essence of all that exists, represents an all-pervading presence in the universe. As the prophet the Second Isaiah tells us (Isaiah 40:22, 25):

> God lives above the circle of the earth, its inhabitants look like grasshoppers.

> . . . "To whom could you liken Me and Who could be my equal?" says the Holy One. Lift your eyes and look. Who made these stars if not the Eternal? Who drills them like an army, calling each by name? So mighty is the Supreme Sovereign's power, so great the Eternal's strength that not one fails to answer.

God, Who gave and continues to give life and existence to every being, guides the cosmos. The Supreme Sovereign is the origin of all things: past, present, and future. The Eternal called all reality into existence. The stream of life, in its many shapes and forms, flows from the Eternal.

God is omnipresent, filling the universe. The Holy One is present throughout the cosmos, charging the atmosphere with vital elements and life sustaining energy. The Divine is present in the heavenly bodies, directing their course, and supplying them with substance. The Eternal is present in every living being. God is a vitalizing force, the Life Principle of all that exists.

For the Psalmist, God dwells everywhere and in everything, permeating all reality. As we read in Psalm 139:7-10: "Where shall I go from Your spirit? Where shall I flee from Your presence? If I ascend into heaven, You are there; if I descend into the netherworld, You are there, too. If I take wing with the morning and come to rest on the western horizon, even there Your hand shall lead me and Your right hand will hold me fast." In Psalm 145:13, the Psalmist also states: "Your sovereignty embraces all the world and Your rule extends over all generations."

The Hebrew prophets were also deeply conscious of God's presence. According to the Second Isaiah (Isaiah 66:1-2), God declares: "Heaven is My throne and the earth is My footstool. Where is the house that you built for Me? Where is the place that may be My resting place? For all these things My hand made and all these things came to be."

Wherever there is life and existence, God is in action. As the Eternal is omnipresent, the Almighty exists everywhere at the same time, penetrating all things and permeating all worlds. The Supreme Sovereign is at the heart of all beings.

Undeserved suffering appears to represent a direct assault on God's omnipotence. How can we understand the Eternal's powerfulness?

Some modern, post-Holocaust commentators seek to limit God's power. Rabbi Harold Kushner, whose son died in his teens of a rare aging disease, authored a best-selling book, *When Bad Things Happen to Good People*.[4] For Kushner, God is sometimes impotent. Expounding a theme of comfort, Kushner sees the Eternal as angered and saddened at suffering but unable to do anything to prevent or stop the misery resulting from natural causes.

In his book, Kushner distinguishes between the evil perpetrated by humans -- social evil -- and the evil of natural catastrophes or diseases -- natural evil. For Kushner, human tragedy does not result from God punishing us, but results partly from individuals harming each other. The Eternal gives humans free will and cannot stop us from hurting each other without taking away our freedom.

In answer to the question about the sickness of innocent people, Kushner sees their misfortune resulting from the laws of nature which apply equally to each of us. The laws of nature, for Kushner, decree that we are subject to accidents, sickness, and disease. We possess a physical body, subject to decay and pain, and ultimately, to death and destruction. God rarely intervenes to countermand the workings of physical laws. Kushner writes: "I don't believe that God causes mental retardation in children, or chooses who should suffer from muscular dystrophy. The God I believe in does not send us the problem; [God] gives us the strength to cope with the problem."[5]

Many have difficulty with Kushner's answers to the perplexing riddle of evil as well as the pervasiveness of pain and suffering in the midst of human existence. We question: the notion of a limited God; an inoffensive deity, removed or in some sense shielded from evil and suffering, isolated from humans and the world; that things happen outside of the Divine will; or, the large role assumed by the laws of nature, bad luck, or randomness. Kushner's view also defies our desire for a sense of universal order and purpose.[6]

Thus, we are left with the question which generations of Jewish sages have pondered. How can there be an imperfect world -- which is obvious to us all -- if a perfect and all-powerful God is everywhere?

Let's go back some four hundred years to the sixteenth century, to Safed, in Northern Palestine as it was then known. There, a mystical Jewish thinker, Rabbi Isaac Luria, sought to resolve the question of how a perfect God created an imperfect world out of nothing. His attempt to resolve this quandary provides the foundation for much of Jewish mystical thought for the past four centuries.

As Luria saw it,[7] God was compelled to make room for the world by abandoning a region within the Eternal, creating a kind of primordial space from which the Divine withdrew in order to return to it in the act of creation. The first act of creation, therefore, was not a traditional view of God expanding but rather the Holy One withdrawing a part of the Divine essence from a portion of space. Thus, prior to creation came a contraction of God.

Luria then spun out a rather elaborate theory of creation in which humans occupy space left open by the Eternal's contraction. God created the world out of a clash between the powers of mercy and judgment. Creation witnessed the breaking of vessels made of light. Evil became embedded in the "dark shells" of the shattered vessels that mask the reality of the Divine endless light.

Luria's concept of creation as a contraction, not an expansion, may help explain the continued presence of evil and suffering in our earthly existence. The remaining earthly "dark shells" lead, according to Luria and his followers, to evil and misery. God restricts the Holy One's power so that we may exercise our free will and enhance our autonomy. If noninterference were removed, then meaningfulness would be diminished almost to vanishing. Yet, as developed in Chapter 2, we possess the ability to serve as co-partners with the Eternal in improving and completing the world.

Is God Good?

If God is omnipotent and omnipresent, is the Eternal responsible for both good and evil? Some Jewish commentators view human misfortune as deriving from God. In other words, the Holy One is responsible for both evil and undeserved suffering.[8] These commentators, look to the prophet, the Second Isaiah, who indicates that God proclaims: "I create both light and darkness; I bring both blessing and disaster. . . ." (Isaiah 45:7, also Lamentations 3:38). In the Book of Deuteronomy (32:39) we read: "I [God] kill and I give life, I wound and I heal. . . ." For most of us, however, the Eternal as force for both good and evil represents a difficult notion to accept.

From the perspective of Spiritual Judaism, God, as the all powerful, all pervasive Divinity, manifests an all-sustaining care for humanity. In the words of the Psalmist, the Eternal is our compassionate, loving parent (Psalm 103:13), Who desires our happiness. God is the loving Helper, Who cares for everyone. The Holy One has a beneficent interest in each of us. God watches over and is concerned with everyone the Eternal has created. Each of us matters to the Supreme Sovereign; each of us is precious to the Holy One.

For spiritually-oriented Judaism, the main attribute of God is unconditional love. The Eternal serves as the source of all love, compassion, and goodness in the world. As the Psalmist (Psalm 116:5) reminds us, ". . . [O]ur God is compassionate."

God's will is for love, joy, and our inner peace. We are an extension of God's love and creative energy.

Through love God called, and continues to call, everyone into existence. The Holy One created humans to lavish goodness and love on them. The Eternal's love sustains the world. The Holy One offers hope and happiness for everyone.

The Hebrew prophets saw God's goodness and mercy. According to Ezekiel (Ezekiel 18:23): "Have I any pleasure at all that the wicked should die?" says God. "It is rather they should repent and live." Hosea (14:5) views the Divine mercy as follows: "I will heal them freely, generously will I take them back in love; for My anger is turned away from them."

When God, the Eternal Goodness, answers the Psalmist's prayers, his difficulties vanish, his despair leaves him. In Psalm 30:12, we read that the Supreme Sovereign is the source of goodness and the fountain of all joy. The Psalmist writes: "You did turn for me my mourning into dancing, You did loose my sackcloth and girded me with gladness...." In Psalm 106:1, the Psalmist declares: "God is good, the Eternal's love and mercy endures forever."

God's beneficence for humanity perhaps best expresses the Eternal's goodness. God the Sustainer is near to us. The Holy One has a benevolent interest in each of us. In the midst of our suffering, God remains the Sustainer to whom we can turn for guidance and for help.

Why Is Suffering Pervasive?

In the Jewish tradition, suffering is accepted as a fact of human existence. It is real. It is not an illusion, a figment of our imagination. It is part of the way the world happens to be. It exists in the world -- in considerable and often overwhelming abundance. It must, therefore, be dealt with as reality.

If God is all powerful and totally in control of the situation, loving and beneficent, why do people suffer and how is it meted out? How could the

Divine abide so much human misery? How could the good, loving, and all powerful Holy One allow all this anguish?[9]

The traditional answer focuses on suffering as a form of punishment for one's wickedness: sin, wrongdoing, or some imperfection. As the prophet Isaiah warns (3:10-11), "Happy is the righteous person, for she will feed on the fruit of her deeds; woe to the wicked, evil is on him, he will be treated as his actions deserve." The author of the Book of Proverbs (10:27) tells us: Obeying God adds length to life, the years of the wicked will be cut short. In other words, the Hebrew Bible points to a cause-and-effect explanation of human distress. The good triumph; the wicked are doomed.

Over the centuries, this simple explanation has run into one formidable objection: it's simply not true, at least from the perspective of this earthly plane and any human being's lifetime. The wicked seemingly don't get cut off; the ruthless often prosper. Why?

The prophet Jeremiah, who lived some two thousand five hundred years ago, asked God: "Why is it that the wicked live so prosperously? Why do the treacherous enjoy peace?" (Jeremiah 12:1). Although Jeremiah remained firmly convinced that somehow the Eternal was in control, he found few answers to his questions.

The author of the Book of Proverbs typifies one answer; namely, although the punishment of the wicked and the sinful is delayed on this earthly plane, it will occur. As Proverbs advises us, "Do not be indignant about the wicked, do not be envious of evil doers, because there is no tomorrow for evil persons, the lamp of the wicked will be extinguished." (Proverbs 24:19-20). In Psalm 37, the Psalmist tells us the virtuous will be rewarded, the wicked punished (37:25 and 28). Despite these promises, the righteous still continue to suffer. Why, we continue to ask, is our anguish a riddle beyond human understanding, never mind our control?

Perhaps the cynical note of the author of the Book of Ecclesiastes provides a degree of realism in our quest:

> And then I saw the wicked brought to burial and people come from the Temple to honor them in the city for having been the people they were. . . . Because the sentence on wrong doing is not carried out at once, peoples' inmost hearts are intent on doing wrong. The sinner who does wrong a hundred times survives even so. I know very well that happiness is reserved for those who obey God, because they obey the Eternal; that there will be no

happiness for the wicked and that they will only eke out their days like a shadow, because they did not obey God. But frustration occurs on earth. The good receive the treatment the wicked deserve; the wicked the treatment the good deserve. (Ecclesiastes 8:10-14).

...

Just as one fate comes to all, to the virtuous as to the wicked, to the pure and the impure, . . . so it is with the good person and the sinner. . . . This is the evil that inheres in all that is done under the sun: that one fate comes to all. . . . The race does not go to the swift, nor the battle to the brave; there is no bread for the wise, wealth for the intelligent, nor favor for the learned; all are subject to time and mischance. People do not know their hour; like fish caught in a net, like birds taken in a trap, so are people overtaken by misfortune suddenly falling on them. (Ecclesiastes 9:2, 11-12).

As we continue to struggle for an explanation of the torment encountered by seemingly virtuous, innocent people, we are left with the biblical Job, a good man, who faced a calamity, the loss of his family, his wealth, his status and his health. The Book of Job, perhaps the most probing of all ancient Jewish sources on the topic of human suffering, presents the dialogue between Job, the prototypical innocent, God-loving, upright, righteous person, who shunned evil, and his three friends, who try to explain to him the reasons for his adversity which seemingly serves no useful purpose. Following the traditional punishment for sin equation, they admonish him to repent.

Yet, even in the worst of his afflictions, for all of his anguish and doubts, his sense of abandonment not only by God but also by his wife, family, friends, and society at large, Job did to deny the Eternal's existence or power. Yet like Job, we, in our suffering, feel enraged, somehow rejected by the Almighty. We can't make sense of our plight. We too want to judge God.

Job, in his despair, becomes depressed. Yearning for death, Job cries out (3:11, 20, 21): "I wish I had died in my mother's womb or the moment I was born. . . . Why does God give light to the sufferer and life to those in grief? They wait for death but it does not come; they prefer a grave to any treasure."

The righteous Job affirms his innocence and castigates his Maker: "If it be a matter of power, the Holy One is the strongest, but if of justice, who will make God go to court? I am blameless, but I no longer care, I am sick of living. It is all one; I say, 'The blameless and the wicked, the Eternal destroys alike.' . . . The land is given over to the hand of the evildoer, who is able to bribe the judges. If not God, who then is guilty?" (Job 9:19, 21-22, 24).

The Prologue to the book suggests that Job's suffering represented a test of his faith (Job 1:6-12). The Epilogue suggests, however, that Job made his anguish redemptive by faithfully accepting it, despite his doubts about God's ways.

Job never received any reply to his charge that God was "cruel" to him. The only answer received was the Holy One's appearance in a whirlwind and the Divine nearness to him. We are told that Job came to "know" God (Job 42:2) and that the Eternal became aware of Job's plight.

Job was shown the magnificence of God's universe extending far beyond human understanding. Job saw that our world is but a tiny part of the cosmos, too vast and magnificent to be grasped by human minds. Realizing his own small place in the glorious universe, Job found his consolidation. Reasons exist for our misfortune we cannot understand. It's part of a Divine design we cannot fathom. Job had to be satisfied with that. His faith reaffirmed, Job arrived at an implicit trust in God's goodness.

Perhaps then, we cannot provide a ready answer to the riddle of suffering. Each of us is too small to discern the overall design. We cannot possibly comprehend God's overarching plans. In comparison to the Eternal, each of us is an ignorant, insignificant being. As the Supreme Sovereign tells Job: "Where were you when I [God] laid the earth's foundations? Tell me, since you are so well-informed! Who decided the dimensions of it, do you know? Or, who stretched the measuring line across it? Do you know all the answers?" (Job 38:4-5).

The Holy One advises Job to accept how the Eternal runs the world even if it does not make sense to him. We are to take it on faith that most things happen for a reason.

In the face of the miracles of creation and of life itself, Job turns to God, declaring: "I know that You are all-powerful; what You conceive, You can perform. . . . I have been holding forth on matters I cannot understand, on marvels beyond me and my knowledge. . . . I retract all I have said, and in dust and ashes I repent." (Job 42:2-3, 6).

The Book of Job enables us to gain valuable insights in our attempt to understand suffering. We cannot understand God and the Eternal's ways. The core mystery persists. The author of the Book of Job portrays the frailty of human commitments and bonds in response to prolonged misfortune. God restored nothing of what Job lost -- things, loved ones, time or trust.

Yet the Book of Job offers us a hopeful, yet realistic, perspective. Persevere in our faith in the Eternal and in the Divine plan for human existence. God's ways are sometimes incomprehensible to us. The Eternal declares, in the prophecy of Isaiah (55:8): "For My plans are not your plans; My ways are not your ways." There's a larger context lending meaning to tragedy which we do not fully understand. As the noted writer Reynolds Price reminds us, "Observe that all of creation is the vehicle upon which you pursue the Creator's will. Attempt any change of pace or direction at your own dire peril. Relish the journey for however long it lasts and wherever it goes. . . . See the splendor of all I [God] have made and savor that, for the time you have."[10]

Surrender to the Almighty, recognizing that we cannot understand the mysterious ways in which the Divine operates. God's reasons, known only to the Eternal, are hidden from us. Much is beyond our scope. The bigger picture may become apparent over time; although there is a core enigma in human tragedy.

If we live life joyfully and if we appreciate that God's ways are not our ways and the Eternal's knowledge is not our knowledge, then perhaps we will find our torment somewhat more bearable. Our lives are in the Holy One's hands, subject to the Eternal's will. We are left with our faith and trust in God's ultimate goodness and mercy that get worked out somehow. Tragedies do not happen in the Eternal's absence. However, faith remains difficult, especially for those facing a life threatening illness or even a chronic, debilitating condition. They ask plaintively: "Why me?"

Beyond this rather passive acceptance of suffering, the Jewish tradition offers other explanations. In the Book of Job there is no suggestion that a solution to the riddle of human despair may exist in life after death, that the seeming inequities and miseries in this life will be righted in the afterlife, in the World to Come, or through the soul's future reincarnation in another earthly human embodiment. For Job, the future beyond the grave offered no compensation. But is the future so bleak? Because the death of our physical body does not bring an end to our immortal soul, the notion that all will work out well in the afterlife may enable us to better face the harsh realities of our present existence.

Our Earthly Suffering and the World to Come

In the afterlife, what Jewish mystics refer to as the World to Come, everything may make sense. People will receive what they deserve. In the Babylonian Talmud we read about Rabbi Joseph, the son of Rabbi Joshua ben Levi, who after falling ill, became temporarily unconscious. When he recovered, his father asked him, "What did you see?" "I saw a topsy-turvy world," he replied. He continued, "I saw in the World to Come those who were above (on earth) below, and those who were below -- above." His father observed, "My son, you saw a clear world." (Pesahim 50a). We are also told in the Talmud by Rabbi Eleazar, the son of Rabbi Zadok, that God brings affliction on the righteous so that they may inherit the World to Come (Kiddushin 40b). In short, justice -- reward and punishment -- may prevail for each of us after our earthly demise.

Although death terminates physical life, the mystical Jewish teachings have long taught that death does not end a soul's existence.[11] Death represents a transition from one state of consciousness to another level of consciousness, a nonmaterial, spiritual realm where each immortal soul undergoes a series of transformational experiences. During this postdeath period, each decedent's soul is tempered and healed, culminating in reincarnation -- the soul's rebirth in another human body.

An Overview of the Jewish Mystical Tradition

Before we take a quick tour through the postdeath World of Souls, let's step back and briefly consider the Jewish mystical tradition. Long ago, the Jewish mystics began to focus on a person's soul, our invisible essence, linking each of us to God. These Jewish mystics recognized that we are more than our earthly body. Death only marks the departure of the soul from the physical body and its entry into the World of the Souls.

This approach takes us back to mystical Jewish teachings (the *Kabbalah* in Hebrew), products of academies of Jewish mysticism in the thirteenth to fifteenth century Spain and France and sixteenth century Palestine. These writings, particularly the *Zohar* (The Book of Splendor), a mystical commentary on the biblical Five Books of Moses, which appeared in the late thirteenth century of the Common Era, provide some of the most sophisticated Jewish views on life-and-death, particularly the afterlife and the survival of the soul.

The mystical literature also encompasses the tales produced by the Hasidim, a populist Jewish movement emphasizing ecstasy and joy in prayer and worship, which emerged in the eighteenth century and continues to our own day. The Hasidic movement brought mysticism to the Jewish masses and spawned the Hasidic tale, telling in story form of the wondrous lives and deeds of various charismatic Hasidic rabbis (rebbes - or *zaddikim* - highly evolved, righteous spiritual leaders) beginning with the Baal Shem Tov (Master of the Good Name), the founder of the Hasidic movement, who lived in Poland from 1698 to 1760. In addition to glorifying the lives and deeds of deceased rebbes, the Hasidic tales provide a rich source of afterlife teachings and beliefs about immortality and the postdeath survival of the soul.

A Quick Tour Through the World to Come

According to the Jewish mystical tradition, the afterlife World to Come involves six stages: first, the soul separates from the physical body; second, the soul undergoes a purification of the emotions in Purgatory; third, one's personality is further refined in Lower Paradise; fourth, the soul receives its rest and reward in Upper Paradise; fifth, the soul returns to the Divine Treasury; and sixth, the soul is reborn on earth in a new physical body; in other words, it is reincarnated.

Stage One. Separation from the Physical Body. Stage One of the World of Souls involves the surrender of the soul's attachment to the physical body and the gradual acceptance of the reality of death. A soul experiences what Jewish sages describe as the "pangs of the grave." For a three to seven-day period after death, a soul remains close to its physical body, struggling to hold onto life, and only slowly releasing its attachment to its body and the material world. Individuals who refuse to relinquish their attachment to their physical body or their material possessions or those who have died suddenly, for instance, as a result of suicide or a physician-assisted death, or violently, may remain in this world of confusion for more than seven days.

For most of us, the soul's withdrawal from the body and gradually giving up the entrapments of the material plane, usually results in an emotional, often tormenting, upheaval. According to Jewish mystics, the soul of one who lived a life too focused on the body's physical aspects or its sensual delights, or who was too attached to the material world or its pleasures, experiences a severely difficult time in overcoming the pangs of the grave. Conversely, the separation from the physical body is much easier for those who have avoided earthly addictions, for those who have cultivated the spiritual, nonmaterial dimensions of life, not overly identifying with the physical body and the material world.

Eventually, however, for each of us, the soul surrenders to the reality of death, separating from its physical body, and entering the World to Come passing through various stages on its postdeath journey, experiencing the torments of Purgatory and the bliss of Paradise.

Stage Two. Emotional Purification in Purgatory. The soul, after surrendering any attachment to its physical body, next undergoes emotional purification in Purgatory for its earthly defilements. Purgatory as a realm for the postdeath punishment, or in modern terms, a healing transformation, for those who did not live a righteous life, a life filled with good deeds and words and ethical actions, represents a central notion for the afterlife teachings in the Jewish mystical tradition. Purgatory heals a soul's various impurities, including destructive thoughts and words as well as negative emotions and harmful actions, such as hate, aggression, anger, fear, hostility, shame, guilt, resentment, and an inability to forgive.

Jewish sages graphically portrayed Purgatory as consisting of seven realms, each offering a punishment of a different tormenting nature. Particular categories of sinners are said to be consigned to one or more of the seven regions of Purgatory to receive specific types of purification based on their respective "sins." These realms are viewed as characterized by a blazing fire of abnormal intensity designed to purify each soul's accumulated contamination as well as snow, seen as freezing out the sins of calculation and the failings of an unloving, unforgiving heart.

The description of Purgatory, and the processes occurring there, serve as metaphors for the purifying, tempering and transforming of the soul. The soul's torment in Purgatory serves as a symbolic representation of the soul's state of consciousness or awareness, not as a physical locale or an actual place.

The Jewish mystics view Purgatory as finite in time, not eternal. The soul completes its period of purification after a maximum of twelve months. One year represents the length of time needed to extract most of the soul's impurities and prepare it for its ongoing journey. Because time does not exist in the World to Come, however, who knows what one year feels like in Purgatory. Eventually, the soul's journey through Purgatory ends. The vast proportion of souls, after the transitory experience in Purgatory, are sufficiently purified and enter the realm of Paradise where they continue their journey of emotional, intellectual and spiritual growth.

Stage Three. The Journey in Lower Paradise: The Completion of an Individual's Personality. In the Jewish mystical tradition, Paradise, consisting of both lower and upper levels, represents a realm where purified souls reside for an unspecified, but not an eternal, time period. Souls who do not immediately merit entry into Upper Paradise are assigned to a subordinate realm, Lower Paradise, according to their merits accumulated in their immediate past earthly lifetime.

Lower Paradise serves as a transit stage between Purgatory and Upper Paradise. The period a soul spends in Lower Paradise represents a time for refining, completing and working out an individual's personality. The last vestiges of one's most recent earthly personality slowly ebb. Souls experience the emotional, intellectual and spiritual bliss in Lower Paradise appropriate to their respective attainments and experiences during life. The more spiritually developed a soul, the higher the realm in Lower Paradise in which it resides.

In Lower Paradise, each soul continues its purification process and prepares for entry into Upper Paradise. Thus, Paradise serves as neither a static experience nor a resting place. On its postdeath journey, each soul progresses through various realms, advancing to ever more transcendent spiritual heights.

Stage Four. Upper Paradise: The Soul's Rest and Reward. Eventually, the soul leaves Lower Paradise and experiences the heavenly bliss of Upper Paradise. After the last vestiges of a deceased's personal life play out in Lower Paradise, the soul basks in the realm of Upper Paradise, a region reserved for the even more righteous, which brings to the fore an even higher level of spiritual fulfillment.

Jewish mystics regard Upper Paradise as a world of transcendental bliss. There the soul experiences the spiritual, emotional, and intellectual rewards it merits. Each soul dwells in a level of Upper Paradise according to the merits of and as a reward for its deeds, words, and thoughts accumulated during its immediate past earthly existence.

In Upper Paradise, the soul experiences the great ecstasy of knowing God. Like-minded souls gather together in a Celestial Academy where each soul attains a joyful understanding of the Eternal. The Holy One is said to appear daily in the Celestial Academy and share the Divine wisdom with the souls dwelling there.

In Upper Paradise, a sense of transpersonal awareness exists. Each soul is said to gain a richer, deeper understanding of life on earth. This realm opens the soul to be more inclusive. The soul perceives the universe as an integrated, unified whole. The world is seen as inherently good and bountiful. Perceptions of awe and wonder abound in the face of a grand, magnificent order. The distinctions between an individual's soul and the infinite God become blurred.

Stage Five. Return to the Source. After the soul's time in Upper Paradise is complete, before being reborn again, it gathers together with other souls in a realm awaiting birth. Each soul returns to the Storehouse of the Souls, the Divine Treasury, a postdeath gathering place for souls in the highest spheres. It is in this region that each soul receives its assignments for its next incarnation before it reenters the earthly life plane in a new physical body.

Stage Six. Preparation For Rebirth and Reincarnation. The sixth stage, reincarnation, marks the rebirth of the soul and its reemergence on earth in a new physical body. Through a physical rebirth, a soul can improve its good deeds, words, and thoughts as well as attain further spiritual perfection, perhaps remedying any wrongdoing committed in a previous life. Also, through reincarnation a righteous person may help others attain a higher degree of spiritual perfection.

With new opportunities for meritorious deeds, words, and thoughts, reincarnation enables each soul more fully to actualize its potential and continue its spiritual evolution. A soul continually reincarnates, ultimately achieving its complete purification and perfection. Through successive rebirths, each soul progresses to its final goal, union with God.

In addition to things getting worked out in the World to Come, Spiritual Judaism also offers the notion that our earthly suffering represents a learning experience, as advocated by some of Job's consolers. The misery we encounter represents an opportunity for emotional and spiritual growth. Although difficult, we can use our anguish in a meaningful way, making it a positive experience, a topic we will return to in Chapter 7.

Learning to Reframe Your Pain and Suffering

Profound reasons exist for our being and what happens to us in our earthly sojourn, although we may be unable to discern them. Each experience contains a lesson; every relationship has its lesson; each task presents a lesson. There are no accidents in God's plan for us. Each situation provides a means for us to become more aware of the Eternal's presence and love. A time of challenge, hardship, and difficulty offers the chance to discover (or rediscover) our own deeper essence and transcendence as well as to enhance our spiritual life. In other words, where does out plight lead us? What can we do now and in the future?

God sends us a vast array of experiences: the people we meet; the relationships we form; the physical, emotional, and spiritual pain and suffering we encounter; the other adversities we face as learning opportunities, often quite difficult and demanding, designed to help us grow spiritually and to purify and perfect ourselves.

How you interpret and respond to your pain, a physical signal, and suffering, your response to the signal provided by pain, may make you stronger, at least from a spiritual perspective. Try to reframe your situation, searching out positive ways of viewing your physical or mental plight.

Rabbi Nachman of Breslov, the grandson of the Baal Shem Tov, lived from 1772 to 1810, attaining exceptional levels of saintliness and wisdom. In one of Rebbe Nachman's tales, "The Seven Beggars,"[12] all of the seven heroes are beggars, they're on the lowest of most scales of success. Each of them is terribly disabled. One is blind, another deaf, a third dumb, one has a crooked neck, another is hunchback, one has no hands and the last, no legs. Yet each turns his or her seeming disability into an advantage. They all owe their success to their special disadvantage. As beggars, each knows that he or she has nothing in this material world and must depend on God for everything. The moral of the story: you must ask the Eternal to show you how to take advantage of even the worst of situations. Focus on the deeper meaning of your anguish.

Jewish sages ask us to see a life crisis, such as a terminal illness, as a wake up call, a challenge sent to us by God. Your torment may represent some sort of a test of your faith, a product of God's love and affection for you, however difficult for you to fathom. As the author of the Book of Proverbs reminds us: "For whom God loves, does God correct, as parents correct a child of whom they are proud." (Proverbs 3:12; see also Deuteronomy 8:5). The Holy One, in the Eternal's Wisdom, may be choosing you for an extra-difficult assignment involving considerable agony. But "Why me?" we continue to ask in a melancholy voice.

As difficult as it may be for you to contemplate, the chastisements you face may represent some type of Divine love. According to the prophet, the Second Isaiah, "And God was pleased to crush him or her by disease." (Isaiah 53:10). However, the Babylonian Talmud reminds us that suffering represents a gift from God, an expression of the Holy One's love for us, if only we can willingly accept it. (Berakhot 5a).[13]

Are you willing to accept God's challenge to develop your hidden potentials? Do you think you're being put to some sort of a test so that you can come to know and develop your innate qualities? Can you heighten your abilities to love and forgive? Only you can answer these questions.

Try to go beneath the surface of your anguish and extract something positive from your experience. You may be able to perceive a life crisis as enabling you to grow in wisdom and love. It's an opportunity for constructive change. Illness or disease may serve as a teacher, a source of spiritual insight and renewed strength; the worst can yield some benefit. Perhaps you need to learn the virtues of patience or faith in the Divine.

Your ailment may represent a piercing cry to shock you out of your complacency, out of your spiritual slumber: a heart closed to love or a refusal to accept the gift of life. The noted author, C. S. Lewis, a widely known defender of Christianity, writes, "God whispers to us in our pleasures, speaks in our conscience, but shouts in our pains: it is [the Divine] megaphone to rouse a deaf world."[14]

Your torment may contain a hidden meaning and an opportunity for personal growth and development. Ask yourself: What is it God is trying to get across to me? What does the Eternal want me to learn?

Two examples help illustrate that suffering may represent an opportunity for you to grow and develop, emotionally and spiritually. The poet and environmental activist, Gale Warner, was 30 years old when she went to the hospital for an investigation of a light but persistent cold. A chest x-ray revealed a mass in her lung the size of an avocado. A biopsy the next day confirmed the diagnosis: a rather aggressive form of fatal non-Hodgkins lymphoma.

Warner recorded her experience in a journal until her death nearly 13 months later. *Dancing at the Edge of Life*[15] the posthumously published memoir of her fight against cancer, records Warner's determination to carve meaning out of life. "I tell my friends that my first six months of cancer was my master's degree in love and life," she writes. "Now I'm in the doctoral program. I've got some intense research ahead and then I'll write my thesis. My brother said, 'Well, for heaven's sake, don't go for a postdoc!' He's right. But for me the essence of this journey remains learning." Even on her worst nights, when Warner starkly faced her most tormenting fears, she continued to seek out the lessons from her suffering. She continued to recount, "This is another teaching." News of a recurrence was followed by even greater dedication to her living with meaning. Like Gale Warner's, your pain and suffering can be turned into a source of profound insight, strength, and courage.

S. R., a sixty-three year old college teacher, experienced the terminal stages of metastatic lung cancer. He was afflicted with a highly malignant tumor and underwent surgery followed by radiation and chemotherapy. He lived for three and one half years following the initial diagnosis of the tumor.

The medical treatments slowed the cancer's progression. However, the treatments resulted in significant side effects, including pain, rashes, intestinal difficulties, and general physical weakness. S. R., at first, found these unpleasant and then awful. It was not clear whether the medical treatment he received improved the quality of his life or made it more distressing.

Yet the hospice care he received in the terminal stage of his life, enabled S. R. to die as he wished, at home, surrounded by his family members, sufficiently free from pain. He remained clearheaded and able to do what he highly valued -- reading, talking, observing nature -- until his final hours.

S. R. did not feel depressed during this final stage of his life. His terminal illness enabled him to confront his life and determine with greater clarity and certainty what mattered to him. Rather than feeling defeated, he felt invigorated. He experienced a sense of moral regeneration.

According to S. R., "I'm better than usual in one way. I don't feel so uncertain. I think our world is one where we are made to feel uncertain, to question everything. In some bizarre way, I don't feel that way now. Something has changed, for me. . . . I'm ever thinking maybe we live in a world where religion or faith only really counts when you're up against the end. Then everything is clear. Otherwise, it's pulling in all directions. Our world doesn't let you . . . doesn't let you . . . well, you just don't see, maybe can't see, what matters most of the time."[16]

Your illness or condition may open the pathways to self-examination, leading to the reestablishment of the wholeness of your mind-body-and spirit. What is your purpose in life? What are your values and priorities? What are your strategies for implementing your values and priorities and attaining your goals, in a life perhaps cut far too short? Where do you want to put your limited time and energies?

Through your illness or condition, you may begin to see what you truly believe in life. You may find new meaning and renewed reasons for living for as long as you can.

We all need a sense of meaning and direction in our lives. Ask yourself: What's my unique purpose? Why am I here?

Discovering this sense of meaning and purpose may give you the strength to endure your tragedy. Continue to ask yourself: What is it I'm here for, even in the remaining weeks or months? The spiritual awakening engendered by your suffering may enable you to focus on the nonmaterial dimensions of earthly life. You may perceive that the spiritual order transcends the physical order. From the perspective of Spiritual Judaism, contemplate your life's meaning and purpose in terms of contributing love to the world, expressing unconditional love to others, forgiving and experiencing forgiveness, and joining with God in perfecting the world.

Find your fulfillment in spiritual values and your interactions with others. Do you need to learn to open your heart in love in others, your family, friends, neighbors, colleagues, even to God? What about trying to forgive others? Ask yourself: what is preventing me from living the remaining days, weeks, months or years of my life with as much lovingkindness, compassion, and forgiveness as I possibly can?

You may need to become more dependent and accept help from others, to express thanks to your loved ones for their serving as your caregivers, and to attain a new sense of closeness with others and a heightened interest in their lives. You may begin to realize that agony and loss are a part of life and that change and impermanence are inevitable in human existence. You may finally be able to let go of some aspect of yourself. You may also come to perceive better the agony of other innocent people like yourself. As the author of the Book of Job tells us (24:4, 7, 8, 12): "All the poor of the land are forced into hiding. . . . They sleep at night without clothing. . . . They are drenched by the mountain rains. . . . People groan in the city. The souls of the dying cry out. . . ."

How you interpret and respond to the suffering you face may make you stronger than ever, at least from a spiritual and an emotional perspective. Naturally, this is quite difficult.

Finding meaning and purpose in your life always remains an option. You can choose your attitude in any situation. See the positive when others only perceive the negative. You can transform the dying process into a time of unparalleled spiritual and emotional growth -- of insight and serenity. You can, if you wish, optimistically move forward, affirming life and the Holy One.

Fever, exhaustion, and pain, of course, may make sustained introspection difficult, if not almost impossible. Yet, physical and emotional suffering can be conducive to deeper insight and self-understanding.

In view of medical advances prolonging the dying process and the prospect of massive numbers of elderly being afflicted with dementia, however, we need to ask: how much suffering as a learning experience and an opportunity for spiritual and emotional growth is sufficient? When is "enough, enough"? We'll return to these troubling questions in subsequent chapters.

Like Job, through your doubts, but not your faithlessness, you probably will not understand the reasons for what you are experiencing, your agony, and ultimately your death. As you are forced to come to terms with life, in all its rawness, try not to lose your trust in God in a time of seeming bleakness and despair. You can grow through your experience, respond with courage and hope, commit more fully to your spiritual development, and move to a new understanding and a deeper relationship with the Supreme Sovereign. As you build a bridge of hope, you'll encounter God, Who, in all of the Eternal's ambiguity, although omnipotent and good, does not always provide a physical or mental cure. Like Job, you will realize the answers to your questions cannot easily be attained, if at all. On your lifelong journey and at the end, keep faith with the Holy One, Who not only controls the world but also holds the key to all wisdom and knowledge. Someday, perhaps, you'll understand why your spiritual growth requires so much agony. Always remember: You are comforted by God, Who is with you, Who will not leave or abandon you (Joshua 1:5), even in your anguish and, ultimately, on your physical demise.

Having explored the meaning of suffering from the perspective of

Spiritual Judaism, let's next consider the contemporary quest to define "death."

Notes

1. Eric J. Cassell, M.D., "The Nature of Suffering and The Goals of Medicine," *New England Journal of Medicine* 306:11 (March 1982): 639-645; Eric J. Cassell, M.D., *The Nature of Suffering and the Goals of Medicine* (New York: Oxford University Press, 1991), 35-37.

2. Jane Brody, "Personal Health: When a Dying Patient Seeks Suicide Aid, It May Be a Signal to Fight Depression," *New York Times*, 18 June 1997, sec. C11; R.K. Portenoy et al., "Symptom Prevalence, Characteristics and Distress in a Cancer Populations," *Quality of Life Research* 3 (1994): 183-189; William Breitbart, M.D. et al, "Neuropsychiatric Syndromes and Psychological Symptoms in Patients with Advanced Cancer," *Journal of Pain and Symptom Management* 10:2 (February 1995): 131-141.

3. Arthur Kleinman, "'Everything that Really Matters:' Social Suffering, Subjectivity, and the Remaking of Human Experience in a Disordering World," *Harvard Theological Review* 90:3 (1997): 332.

4. Harold S. Kushner, *When Bad Things Happen to Good People* (New York: Avon Books, 1983).

5. Ibid., 127.

6. Shmuel Boteach, *Wrestling with the Divine: A Jewish Response to Suffering* (Northvale, N.J.: Jason Aronson, 1995), 116-121; Shmuel Boteach provides a penetrating critique of Kushner's "lesser" God as does Abraham Cohen, "Theology and Theodicy: On Reading Harold Kushner," *Modern Judaism* 16:3 (1996): 226-261.

7. Robert M. Seltzer, *Jewish People, Jewish Thought: The Jewish Experience in History* (New York: Macmillan, 1980), 462-467.

8. Elliot N. Dorff, "God and the Holocaust," *Judaism 26:1* (Winter 1977):27-34.

9. In trying to answer these questions, I have drawn on John Bowker, *Problems of Suffering in Religions of the World* (Cambridge: Cambridge University Press, 1970), 5-41 and David Birnbaum, *God and Evil: A Unified Theodicy/Theology/Philosophy* (Hoboken, N.J.: KTAV, 1989), 16-31. Looking to a number of religious traditions, Reynolds Price provides a helpful overview in *Letter to a Man in the Fire: Does God Exist and Does He Care*? (New York: Scribner, 1999).

10. Ibid., 69.

11. The soul's journey in the afterlife is developed in detail in Lewis D. Solomon, *The Jewish Book of Living and Dying* (Northvale, NJ: Jason Aronson, 1999), 125-247. See generally, Simcha Paull Raphael, *Jewish Views of the Afterlife* (Northvale, N.J.: Jason Aronson, 1994).

12. *The Tales of Rabbi Nachman of Bratslav*, retold with commentary by Adin Steinsalz (Northvale, N.J.: Jason Aronson, 1993), 217-251.

13. David Kraemer, *Responses to Suffering in Classical Rabbinic Literature* (New York: Oxford University Press, 1995), 188-200; David Hartman, *A Living Covenant: The Innovative Spirit in Traditional Judaism* (New York: The Free Press, 1985), 197-198.

14. C.S. Lewis, *The Problem of Pain* (New York: MacMillan, 1962), 93.

15. Gale Warner with David Kreger, M.D., *Dancing at the Edge of Life: A Memoir* (New York: Hyperion, 1998), 77, 86.

16. Kleinman, "'Everything that Really Matters,'" 329.

Chapter 4

Our Immortal Soul and the Ebbing of Consciousness: The Quest to Define Death

Dying is a process. Not all of one's physical bodily parts cease functioning at the same time. Yet a line must be drawn separating those who are living human beings from those who are dead. Although modern medicine can extend the functioning of various organ systems, making the line demarcating the living from the dead more problematic, still a line must be drawn. A number of consequences follow the determination of death: removal of medical treatment, initiation of organ transplantation, disposition of the body, commencement of a time for mourning, and distribution of life insurance proceeds and other of the deceased's assets. Thus, we need to adapt criteria for when human life has ended. Is one, dead or alive, if one is in an irreversible condition apparently without awareness, thought, or feeling, but continuing to function vegetatively on multisystem life-support in a hospital?

In striving to draw the line between life-and-death, we also need to ask a series of other difficult questions: What does it mean to be alive? What is the essence of human life? What is lost in death that is essential to a human being?

In the past, is always seemed relatively easy to demarcate the end of life. Death came about when a person stopped breathing and one's heart ceased beating. The changes brought about by modern medicine, specifically, heart transplants, mechanical hearts, and breathing aids, enabling physicians to keep patients alive for months or even years, have resulted in a new definition of death. We will be examining the transformation of the definition of death in the American legal system and the contemporary Jewish tradition, marked by the general acceptance of the whole brain definition, as well as exploring the likely impact of the higher brain concept of death. But first this chapter will consider death moment visions, the process of dying, the death moment, and our immortal soul from the perspective of the Jewish mystical tradition. These are critical to Spiritual Judaism's approach to choices at the end of life.

Death Moment Visions in the Jewish Mystical Tradition

According to the Jewish mystical tradition, the dying generally experience four death moment visions -- internal, subjective visions -- immediately prior to, at, or shortly after the point of "death." With death imminent, we enjoy the ability to see elements in worlds generally otherwise unavailable to human beings. According to the mystical tradition:

> . . . [W]hen a man's [judgment] hour is near, [an angel] commences to call him, and no one knows [except] the patient himself, as we have [learned], that when a man is ill and his time is approaching to depart from the world, a new spirit enters into him from above, in virtue of which he sees things which he could not see before, and then he departs from the world. (Zohar II, 218b).

During the dying process, in addition to the dissolution of the elements of the physical body discussed later in this chapter, most individuals encounter four visionary experiences: first, seeing the clear light; second, encountering previously deceased relatives and friends as well as angels; third, undergoing a life review; and fourth, passing through a tunnel.[1] The order in which these visions occur varies from person to person, depending on the circumstances of death and extent of one's spiritual development. Even after physical death, the internal process of dissolution may continue.

Experiencing the Clear Light. During the dying process, an individual may experience a glimpse of the Clear Light, a beautiful and intense light, much brighter than anything seen on earth. The Clear Light represents the radiant light of the soul's higher spiritual aspects. This phenomenon generally occurs at or soon after the demise of one's physical body.

Jewish mystical sources describe how, at this time, a soul takes a dip in a River of Light and is cleansed from many of earthly life's defilements. The immersion in the River of Light also assists in restoring the soul to its initial radiance. The encounter with the River of Light not only assists someone who is dying to leave the physical world but also helps his or her soul to become more identified with the spiritual realms.

A dying person may also be blessed with a brief glimpse of God's presence -- the feminine aspect of the Divine -- appearing as a formless, glowing image. According to the Jewish mystical tradition: "No man dies before he sees the Shekhinah and because of its deep yearning for the Shekhinah, the soul departs in order to greet her." (Zohar III, 88a). Thus, the deceased's soul may fleetingly see the radiant image of God's luminescence.

Whether a soul will notice the radiant Clear Light, in one or more of its various forms and not be scared by its majestic intensity, may depend on an individual's spiritual attainment during his or her lifetime. The mystical tradition notes:

> When a man is on the point of leaving this world, his soul suffers many chastisements along with his body before they separate. Nor does the soul actually leave him until the Shekhinah shows herself to him, and then the soul goes out in joy and love to meet the Shekhinah. If he is righteous, he cleaves and attaches himself to her. But if not, then the Shekhinah departs, and the soul is left behind, mourning for its separation from the body, like a cat which is driven away from the fire. (Zohar V, 53a).

According to Jewish sages, some "righteous" individuals may recognize the River of Light, representing the upper levels of the soul's inner luminosity, and glory in its radiance. For others, the sight of the River of Light may engender fear. Many may be completely unaware of the vision of the Clear Light as their souls embark on their postdeath journeys.

Encountering Deceased Relatives and Angels. During the dying process, according to the Jewish tradition, each of us encounters beloved, deceased relatives, close friends, and wise teachers as well as angels. Prior to or at the death moment, the spirits of deceased relatives and friends, those who loved us the most, visit a dying person to offer a welcome and ease the transition from the world of the living to the postdeath World of the Souls.

The Jewish mystical tradition describes the deathbed vision of their deceased loved ones as follows:

> Rabbi Simeon then said to Rabbi Isaac: Have you seen today the image of your father? For so we have [learned] that at the hour of a man's departure from the world, his father and his relatives gather round him, and he sees them and recognizes them, and likewise all with whom he associated in this world, and they accompany his soul to the place where it is to abide. (Zohar II, 218a).

The elderly, terminally ill sometimes ramble and call out incoherently for a departed mother, now dead decades ago, a younger brother, deceased for ten or fifteen years, and perhaps an older sister, who may have died, unknown to him or her, one week ago. In retelling the death of her father-in-law, one modern writer described it this way: "It seems to me his dead were calling to him. They were waiting for him."[2]

In addition to previously deceased relatives and close friends, the dying sometimes encounter angels. In portraying various angels, Jewish sages often refer to a particularly vicious, destroying angel, the Angel of Death. This fiery angel, who is viewed as "all fire," is said to have the task of taking each soul from its physical body.

Undergoing a Life Review. Each of us undergoes a review of his or her immediate past life experiences and is held accountable for his or her thoughts, deeds, and words. According to the rabbinic literature, an individual receives an instantaneous, extraordinarily rapid, full color, three-dimensional, panoramic review of all of his or her life's thoughts, words, and deeds, good and bad.

During this flashback, all the details of one's life experiences are revealed. A person's entire life occurs at once. He or she knows every thought he or she ever had; every word ever spoken; every deed. According to the rabbis, "At the hour of a departure to his eternal home, all his deeds are enumerated before him, and the angels say to him: 'You did such and such in such and such a place on such and such a day.'" (Babylonian Talmud Ta'anit 11a).

At that point, each of us will understand the reasons for and the consequences of our thoughts, words, and actions. For each experience, events are put in perspective. We see how our actions and words affected others, including strangers. We perceive how everyone's life is intertwined with others. We become more sensitive regarding our treatment (or mistreatment) of others.

Because each of us has angels assigned to maintain records of our good and bad deeds, words, and thoughts, the balance of one's life experience is immediately apparent in the Divine data bank. Building on the notion of a just reward or retribution for each individual according to his or her earthly actions, words, and thoughts, the Jewish mystical tradition describes the life review as follows:

> Rabbi Eleazar said: On the day when a man's time arrives to depart from the world. . . . [t]hree messengers [the Angel of Love, who records a person's merits; the Angel of Judgment, who records a person's sins; and the Angel of Mercy, who notes the length of a person's life] stand over him and take an account of his life and of all that he has done in this world, and he admits all with his mouth and signs the account with his hand. . . . the whole account is signed with his hand so that he should be judged in the next world for his actions, earlier and later, old and new, not one of them is forgotten. . . . (Zohar I, 78b-79a).

The life review typically occurs at the time of death or shortly thereafter. However, in the case of a slow, lingering death, the life review may take place much more slowly, over many, many days.

Passing Through a Tunnel. At some point during the dying process, the soul passes through a tunnel, a celestial pathway, on its journey from the physical realm to the world beyond. This tunnel serves as the bridge between life-and-death. Once the soul crosses the boundary line -- death is irreversible. The "silver cord" linking the physical body and the soul is severed. (Ecclesiastes 12:6).

The Process of Dying in the Jewish Mystical Tradition

Dying involves a process consisting of the disintegration of one's physical body. It is manifest in the sequential demise first of organ systems, then individual organs, and finally, separate cells.

Near the end of the process of dying, the structural units of the physical body break down and separate. The Jewish mystical tradition teaches:

> We have [learned] that on the [dreaded] day when a man's time comes to depart from the world, the four quarters of the world indict him, and punishments rise up from all four quarters, and the four elements fall to quarreling and seek to depart each to its own side. (Zohar II, 218b).

Although this cryptic passage fails to describe the four elements, the author probably refers to the four essential elements of human existence:

earth (or flesh), water (or bodily fluids), fire (or bodily heat), and air (or breath). The quarreling may connote the tumultuous and rather upsetting process taking placing in the dying person's inner consciousness.[3]

On a physical level, the process of dying, from my observation, involves the gradual shutting down of different life functions. Someone close to death generally is drained of energy. Her body becomes heavy and she encounters difficulty in standing or even moving her legs or arms. Breathing changes, and nothing seems to work right. One part of body is hot, another cold. The body's metabolism is failing to work. She can't swallow. A dying individual often experiences dehydration and feels extremely thirsty, needing ice chips on her face, mouth, and lips to avoid becoming parched. Losing the ability to control bodily fluids, she typically becomes incontinent. Her body loses heat and her limbs become cold. The body is slowly shutting down.

One day or so before the end the skin starts to look mottled. Blood pressure drops. Circulation is cut back so the body can concentrate on getting blood to the brain and vital organs. Blood begins to pool in her back. Blotches are visible when she is turned over.

Near death, one is quiet, eyes are partially open, and breathing slows even more. Her jaw juts forward just slightly. Hearing is the last sense to go. She sleeps with her eyes and her mouth only partly open because it takes energy to keep her eyes and mouth fully open. She is losing energy.

Finally, it becomes harder and harder to breathe. Many dying persons develop very noisy breathing near death. The so-called death rattle results from the relaxation of the throat's muscles. In-breaths become shallower and out-breaths longer. Ultimately, her breath stops. The traditional moment of physical death has arrived.

The Death Moment in the Jewish Mystical Tradition

In the Jewish tradition, the exact moment of physical death is perceived as painless.[4] Death, at least for the "righteous," is effortless. "Like drawing a hair out of milk" (Midrash on Psalms 11:6), there is no resistance, only blissful peace, in death. Even cancer patients, ravaged by pain and suffering, at death typically manifest a peaceful radiance, a tranquil smile of comfort and quietude. Loved ones often describe their faces as "radiant, peaceful at long last."

However, a gentle death is not universal. The rabbinic literature, using a variety of metaphors, like "pulling a tangled rope through a narrow opening" (Midrash on Psalms 11:6), describes the moment of death for the "wicked" as a painful experience -- a time of considerable agitation. A wicked person departs, one sage, Rabbi Samuel stated: "Like a moist and inverted thorn [tearing its way] out of the throat." (Midrash Rabbah Ecclesiastes 6:6, 1).

For Jews steeped in the mystical tradition, death did not evoke anxiety. Rather, the Jewish mystics saw it as another phase in the soul's evolution. Death was viewed as a peaceful process transporting an individual from the material world to other realms of disembodied consciousness. With an awesome sense of calmness, the pious of old made the transition from earthly life without fear prior to their death.

The following description of the death in 1760 of the Baal Shem Tov, the founder of the Hasidic movement in Judaism, continues to serve as an ideal model for fully accepting death and living with the sense of the transcendent meaning of life. Note the Baal Shem Tov's inner confidence and peace, his control and connectedness with self, others, and God as well as his love and devotion for others:

> When the Baal Shem Tov fell ill shortly before his death, he would not take to his bed. His body grew weak, his voice faint, and he would sit alone in his room meditating. On the eve of [Jewish holiday of Shavuot], the last evening of his life, his [disciples] were gathered around him and he preached to them about the giving of the Torah. In the morning, he requested that all of them gather together in his room and he taught them how they should care for his body after death. Afterward he asked for a [prayer book], and said: "I wish to commune yet a while with [the Name, may God be blessed]."
>
> Afterward they heard him talking to someone and they inquired with whom he was speaking. He replied, "Do you not see the Angel of Death? He always flees from me, but now he has been given permission to come and flaps his wings and is full of joy." Afterward all the men of the city gathered together to greet him on the holiday and he spoke words of Torah to them. Afterward he said, "Until now I have treated you with [lovingkindness]. Now you must treat me with [lovingkindness]." [Burial is considered the truest act of lovingkindness, because there is no repayment.] He gave them a sign that at his death the two clocks in the house would stop.
>
> While he was washing his hands, the larger clock stopped and some of the men immediately stood in front of it so that the others should not see it. He said to them, "I am not worried about myself, for I know clearly that I shall go from this door and immediately I shall enter another door." He spoke

> words of Torah and ordered them to recite the verse -- "And let Your graciousness, O [Eternal] our God, be upon us; establish You also the work of our hands for us. . . ." He lay down and sat up many times and prayed with great devotion, until the syllables of his words could no longer be distinguished. He told them to cover him with blankets and began to shake and tremble as he used to do when he prayed the Silent Prayer. Then little by little he grew quiet. At that moment they saw that the small clock too had stopped. They waited and saw that he had died.[5]

The Hasidic rebbes strove to go through death, particularly the death moment, fully conscious and in contact with God. They made the transition from earthly life with calmness and equanimity. They accepted death as a means of affirming life. They did so because of their belief in the survival of each person's immortal soul. Thus, Jewish mystical writings focus on the soul: its various dimensions, its relationship to the physical body, and its capacity for transcendent awareness of the Divine.

Our Immortal Essence: The Soul in the Jewish Mystical Tradition

The soul, a one syllable word, conveys something primary, something beyond the physical. In the Jewish tradition, our soul, the essence of our humanity, lives on when our physical body dies and decays.

The Jewish mystical tradition portrays the soul as a unified whole, one totality consisting of interrelated fields of awareness and energy connecting each individual to God. Jewish mystics view the soul -- our unique inner substance, our essential spirit, our higher level of consciousness -- as consisting of four intertwined energy fields or levels: physical; emotional; intellectual; and spiritual.[6]

First, the physical level, a field of vital energy in each human being, attaches to, animates and preserves a human's body. It directs the functions of our organs and orders our vital processes. The physical level is sometimes described as a biological life force linking each human to the earthly world.

Second, the emotional level, a field of emotional energy, filling the heart with love, sympathy, tenderness and compassion, represents the locus of one's personality. This emotional level, sometimes characterized as emotional awareness, links the soul's physical level with its intellectual and spiritual aspects.

Third, the mental (or intellectual) level, a mental energy field as well as the energy of the transpersonal (nonphysical) self, connects each of us to the higher spiritual aspects of our existence. It is the invisible source of the mind's thoughts and inspirations, a channel through which our intellectual powers flow.

This mental level of awareness serves as a bridge between the human and the Divine realms. The development of an individual's mental level produces one's higher consciousness of God.

Fourth, each soul is characterized by a spiritual level consisting, in turn, of two spiritual or transcendental fields or levels. Within the soul's first spiritual level, each individual connects, consciously or unconsciously, with God and the Divine Life Force. Each of us experiences our separate self within the context of a larger whole. We strive to belong to this greater whole -- to the Soul of the Universe, in other words, to God -- and to find a context for our existence. We sense that somehow we can transcend our own existence, yet not lose our essence. This aspect of the soul represents the highest degree of awareness accessible to most humans.

But there is an even higher spiritual level, sometimes viewed as a transcendent field of light, in which the soul strives to unite and merge with God. It represents the part of the soul that is inseparable from the Eternal. This higher spiritual level constitutes the pure part of the soul.

During every human being's lifetime, the soul's four invisible and often rather difficult to fathom aspects are interconnected forming one seamless, unified, organic whole without any division. The interaction of these four levels characterizes a human's soul nature, one's soulfulness. The soul represents the essence of a human being; it comes from and is a part of God.

With this background on the Jewish mystical teachings relating to the dying process, the soul, and its survival in the afterlife (this last aspect was previously considered in Chapter 3), let us turn to and examine the transformation of the definition of death in both the American legal system and the Jewish tradition.

The American Legal System and the Transformation of the Definition of Death

Prior to heart transplants or heart-lung machines designed to pump blood and circulate oxygen, when someone's vital physical functions, one's respiration and pulsation ceased, he or she was dead. Thus, the criteria for death centered on the permanent cessation of the flow of vital bodily fluids. After breathing and circulation ended, then following some decent interval, physicians could be certain a patient was dead.

Yet over the past thirty years or so, the definition of death in the United States has changed in response to technological advances, rendering obsolete the traditional signs of death. Spurred on by the ability to maintain organ systems artificially through the use of respirators and cardiopulmonary bypass machines, and by organ transplantation programs requiring the procurement of organs, initially kidneys, then livers and hearts, and now others as well before they deteriorate, the legal definition of death was transformed. Throughout the United States, brain-based standards for death gained widespread acceptance.

In 1968, the Harvard Brain Death Committee (the Harvard Committee), an ad hoc committee consisting mostly of medical professionals, supplemented by an attorney, a historian, and a theologian, attempted to meet this need. Although lacking any legal weight, the committee defined an irreversible coma, a permanently nonfunctioning brain, as the criterion for death. The Harvard Committee's report specified that its recommendations applied only to those individuals who have "no discernible central nervous system activity."[7]

The Harvard Committee set forth four types of neurological examinations to establish brain death, the complete and irreversible loss of functioning of the whole brain. The four types of examinations are as follows: first, a lack of receptivity, awareness, and response to externally applied stimuli, a lack of awareness of internal needs, and a lack of response to pain; second, the absence of spontaneous breathing or movement or response to pain, touch, sound or light as observed by a physician over a period of at least one hour; third, the absence of reflexes, for example, one's pupil is fixed, dilated, and unresponsive to light, or on turning the patient's head there is no eye movement or blinking; fourth, a flat electroencephalogram confirming the first three criteria.

The report suggested that these examinations be repeated after an interval of twenty-four hours. Two types of patients were to be excluded from these tests: first, those with a body temperature below 90°F (that is, those suffering from hypothermia) and second, those with central nervous system depressants, such as drugs.

The Harvard Committee's report presented two reasons for the need for a new definition of death. First, the report reasoned that we should end medical treatment when it does no good. Maintaining patients in an irreversible coma constituted a great burden on their families and on hospitals. Thus, families would be spared the agony of watching a loved one undergo a prolonged death. Hospitals could also reallocate expensive medical resources by freeing up space in intensive care units for those who could benefit. Also, presumably very few patients would want to be maintained on a respirator if they clearly could never recover consciousness.

Second, the impetus for the definitional change also came from the well-publicized progress in organ transplantation, especially heart transplants. Once a heart stops, rapid tissue degeneration makes it unsuitable for transplantation. To increase the chances for a successful heart transplant, it must be removed as a quickly as possible after a donor's death. Thus, the new definition would make possible the salvaging of more organs and tissues and provide the gift of life to an ever greater number of recipients.

By 1981, after examining the issue, the U.S. President's Commission for the Study of Ethical Problems in Medicine and Biomedical and Behavioral Research (the President's Commission) wrote of "the emergence of a medical consensus" around whole brain criteria similar to those proposed by the Harvard Committee. The President's Commission focused on the brain's primacy in integrating body functions and its secondary function in its serving as the seat of consciousness. The whole brain criteria won out because they describe a case having many of the qualities which we usually associate with death: lack of spontaneous breathing and movement as well as any response to the environment.

At that time, agreement could not be reached on what portions of the brain were required for consciousness. The President's Commission also noted an inability to test reliably for these higher functions and assure irreversibility within reasonable limits.

Furthermore, the whole brain criteria had proven to be clinically reliable. As the President's Commission stated, "No case has yet been found that met [the Harvard Committee's] criteria and regained any brain functions despite the continuation of respirator support."[8]

The Uniform Determination of Death Act (the Act) approved by the National Conference of Commissioners on Uniform State Laws in 1980, gained widespread approval throughout the United States beginning in 1981. The Act, now adopted, in whole or in part, by legislatures and administrative agencies in forty-seven states and the District of Columbia, and by courts in three states, Arizona, Massachusetts, and Washington State, provides a legal articulation for the whole brain criterion of death as the irreversible cessation of all brain functions, including the brain stem.[9] The definitional portion of the Act reads as follows: "An individual who has sustained either (1) irreversible cessation of circulatory and respiratory functions, or (2) irreversible cessation of all functions of the entire brain, including the brain stem, is dead." A determination of death must be made in accordance with accepted medical standards. Thus, the Act provides a definition of death based on either the traditional cardiorespiratory criteria or the new whole brain standard.

In constructing its definition of death, the Act focuses on function, not activity, reflecting the view that bodily parts (and their subparts) are important for the functions they perform. Note that the Act also provides an alternative test following the traditional determination, specifying as dead one who has sustained total failure of the cardiorespiratory system. The Act does not specify the diagnostic tests or medical procedures required to determine death. Instead, the determination of death is made according to accepted medical standards. The medical profession is free to use new medical knowledge and diagnostic advances as they become available.

In short, medical technology has revolutionized the legal definition of death in the United States. It also has impacted the contemporary Jewish approach.

The Contemporary Jewish View of the Definition of Death

A system which takes seriously the sanctity of earthly life must carefully spell out its concept of death and the criteria used to determine when life has ended.[10] As we will see, liberal authorities and some traditionalists accept the whole brain definition. Other traditionalists firmly adhere to the cardiorespiratory test.

The traditional criteria for determining death in Jewish law focused on the cessation of respiration, generally recognized as the most reliable physical indicator of death, and to a lesser extent, on heart action, the maintenance of circulation, and one's pulse. These cardiorespiratory functions represent vital signs manifesting life.

Jewish traditionalists cite the Babylonian Talmud (Yoma 85a) as the focus for their definition of death. The cessation or absence of breathing with no bodily motion represents the key determinant of death. Dealing with a person trapped under a building, Yoma 85a states: How far does one search [to ascertain whether one is dead or alive after the debris of a collapsing building falls on him or her]. Until [one reaches] his or her nose. . . . [L]ife manifests itself primarily through the nose especially as it is written: "In whose nostrils is the breath of the spirit of life. . . ." (Genesis 7:22). Because Jewish sages concluded that one's spirit entered and departed through the nose, life is present as long as respiratory activity persists.

A feather is to be placed under a patient's nostrils. The movement of the feather, so placed, demonstrates life; conversely, the lack of the feather's movement indicates death.

A minority view in the Babylonian Talmud (Yoma 85a) maintains that you dig until you reach the chest in order to listen for the heartbeat. In other words, the cessation of heartbeat is also required to determine death.

A split exists today among Jewish traditionalists, however, giving rise to an intense, ongoing debate. According to one leading contemporary commentator, Rabbi Dr. J. David Bleich, Jewish sources define death as the irreversible cessation of both respiratory and cardiac activities long enough to make resuscitation impossible. At that moment, death occurs. He relies on the above-cited Yoma passage focusing on the absence of breathing as confirming a lack of bodily movement.[11] In other words, for Bleich and some other traditionalists, brain death represents an unacceptable criterion from the standpoint of Jewish law.

Bleich regards the establishment of the time of death as an ethical and religious issue, a moral and theological problem, not a medical or a scientific question.[12] According to Bleich, modern medical advances should not impact on Jewish teachings in this area.

An emerging majority of traditionally-oriented commentators, led by Rabbi Dr. Moshe Tendler and Fred Rosner, M.D., reach a different conclusion.[13] For Tendler and Rosner, the brain, including the brain stem, controls all bodily functions, including respiration and cardiac activity. If there is the irreversible and complete cessation of all brain functions, one is dead. A person who is brain dead, even if he or she exhibits transient, spontaneous cardiac activity, is no longer living. However, if a patient survives with a functioning brain stem, he or she is alive.

In reaching this conclusion, Tendler and Rosner question whether the passage from Yoma is relevant for establishing a Jewish definition of death as opposed to confirming the occurrence of death. The Talmud passage focuses on whether or not any sign of life exists in order to dig a person out and thereby desecrate the Sabbath. Today, when a patient is in an intensive care unit, for instance, and every bodily function is fully monitored, we are interested in the definition, not the confirmation, of death. In contrast to Bleich's strict construction of Jewish texts, using the principle of purposive interpretation and relying on modern medical technology, Tendler and Rosner construe the criterion for determining death in a broader way.

With decapitation traditionally providing a sufficient definition of death in Jewish law, Tendler and Rosner view the total cessation of all brain functions as the modern day equivalent of decapitation. A decapitated individual was viewed, according to Jewish sources, such as Mishnah Oholot (1:6), as dead immediately on the severance of the brain from the rest of the body, specifically, as a result of the separation of the brain from the spinal cord or the cessation of the blood supply to the brain, even if one's heart continued to beat for a period of time or he or she exhibited bodily movement. In an actual decapitation, the head ceases to function as part of an integrated human being; one's body becomes a residual life without ethical import. Similarly, the loss of brain functions, for Tendler and Rosner, removes the brain's central role in the integration of bodily functions and deprives a person of consciousness.

Tendler and Rosner also note, focusing strictly on the Talmudic text, that it says nothing, one way or the other, regarding the ancient rabbis' view of brain death as the definition of death. According to Tendler and Rosner, Jewish sages might not have rejected the brain death test if they had known about electroencephalograms and other modern technology.

More liberal Jewish commentators also accept the whole brain definition of death. Conservative Movement rabbis Daniel G. Goldfarb and Seymour Siegal suggested nearly twenty-five years ago that a flat electroencephalogram, indicating the cessation of brain functions, in conformity with modern medical practice, is sufficient to determine death.[14] The Conservative Movement's Committee on Jewish Law and Standards subsequently approved the responsa of Rabbis Elliot N. Dorff and Avram Israel Reisner, both of which accept the new definition.[15] Likewise one of many Reform responsa on this topic concludes: "We are satisfied that [the Harvard Committee's] criteria include those of the older tradition and comply with our concern that life has ended."[16]

Where Do We Go From Here?: The Higher Brain Definition of Death

I do not want to serve as a referee or judge between the starkly different conclusions offered by the traditionalists. Suffice it to say that if the Jewish definition of death requires the irreversible cessation of both cardiac and respiratory functioning, the use of this standard will generally prolong the dying process and reduce (if not end) the likelihood that hearts from Jews who adhere to this standard will be suitable for safe and successful transplantation, at least as we know the transplant process today. Unlike other cadaver transplants, the heart must be removed immediately after brain death if the procedure is to have any chance of success.

Rather, in this section I first want to reexamine the higher brain definition of death, which was rejected by the President's Commission, and then develop its relationship to the Jewish tradition's concept of the soul. I want to do this within the context of modern medicine's ability to sustain the physical bodies of individuals who are permanently and irreversibly unconscious. We will discover that several things are amiss with the American legal and the emerging Jewish consensus regarding the whole brain definition of death. Let's begin, however, with some scientific background on the human brain.

The human brain, roughly speaking, consists of both higher and lower parts. The higher brain, including the cerebral cortex, serves as the seat of consciousness and memory and performs most of our mental functions. The higher brain enables us to see, hear, feel pleasure or pain, form intentions and desires. It also controls various muscle functions.

The lower brain consists mainly, but not exclusively, of the brain stem. It controls our vegetative functions and unconscious acts -- our reflexes, our heartbeat, our respiration.

If our definition of death requires the whole brain to cease to function, then individuals with a functioning brain stem generally can exhibit spontaneous respiration and heartbeat. For example, Karen Ann Quinlan tragically remained in a persistent vegetative state for ten years; her heart and lungs functioned without mechanical assistance; her body was warm; her blood vessels pulsated. She was not considered dead under the whole brain standard because her vegetative functions, such as breathing, blood pressure, and temperature, continued. The lower portion of her brain performed these functions.

Today, however, tests conducted as a part of accepted medical practice to determine brain death do not focus on the cessation of all brain functions. A declaration of death is made on the basis of the irreversible cessation of most, but not all, brain functions. Patients diagnosed as "dead" on neurological grounds may show some cerebral electrical and hormonal activity as well as retain some evidence of being responsive to their environment. They may exhibit some spinal reflexes occasionally resulting in dramatic and disturbing limb movements.[17]

As one expert on medical ethics concludes, the whole brain definition of death, clearly requiring all functions of the entire brain be gone, has been construed to exclude certain functions. As so interpreted, the whole brain definition has come to mean that "function rather than structure is irreversibly destroyed and that not only certain cellular-level functions and microvolt-level electrical functions be ignored as 'insignificant,' but also certain 'nests of cells' and associated supercellular-level functions as well."[18]

Although defenders of the whole brain concept may insist that it is possible to consider cellular, electrical and supercellular functions as insignificant activities, not functions, or as functions not relevant to the brain's integrative role, we must focus on the basic question: What does it mean for a human being to be "alive?" Is it physiological integration or consciousness? If the latter, how does that concept relate to the departure of the immortal soul from one's physical body?

In coming years, we may see an ever greater acceptance of and focus on the higher brain to arrive at a legal definition of death in the United States and the criteria for one's demise. What is significant to our living as human beings, it seems to me, centers on our capacity for consciousness and cognition. Consciousness includes our self-awareness, our awareness of others and our environment, our capacity to feel and respond to stimulation, and our capability for sensory activity. Cognition denotes our capacity for imagination, for reason, and for thought. Our consciousness and cognition functions are basically located in the cerebrum, particularly the neocortex part of the brain, in other words, the higher brain.

The focus on consciousness and cognition has given rise to the higher brain-oriented definition of death.[19] The death of the higher brain marks the end of our consciousness. It eliminates any potential for self-awareness, for a purposeful existence, for plans, hopes, ambitions, and for future relationships. It removes any interest in controlling and shaping one's life, or in acting as an autonomous, moral agent. Thus, if there is an irreversible loss of all higher brain functions, specifically, the cessation of the capacity for consciousness and cognition, an individual is dead, even if he or she has not lost brain stem functions. What exists is merely a mindless organism. Conversely, if one has the capacity for consciousness and cognition, then he or she remains a living human being.

The higher brain definition of the test offers two major advantages. First, the use of this test would reduce the financial, social, and emotional costs entailed in the artificial extension of the life. If there is no reasonable possibility for a recovery of consciousness, there seems to be no point in maintaining the continued existence of one's physical body. Family members should carefully consider whether in the absence of a patient's written advance care directive (a topic considered in detail in Chapter 10) providing guidance on this question, they want to continue to support human "life," lacking any reasonable hope for the recovery of consciousness, where one cannot communicate or feel pain. What is the benefit of such a life? To the patient? To the patient's family? Perhaps for family members to learn compassion? But, at what cost -- financial, social, and emotional -- and for how long? Families should consider the burdens: the huge medical costs and the emotional drain.

Second, with a higher brain definition of death, which accelerates the time of death, more organs would also likely become available for transplantation as well as for medical research and education.

Not unexpectedly, objections exist to the higher brain, as opposed to the whole brain, definition of death. There are basically three objections.

First, critics assert that the higher brain definition of death is too vague.[20] They raise the question of whether physicians will not strictly adhere to what are the higher brain functions and what constitutes the irreversible cessation of the capacity for consciousness. They raise the specter that the higher brain definition of death will lead us down a slippery slope, namely, to declaring dead someone with only marginal consciousness, someone who lacks significant mental functions or is in some way functionally compromised. Also, what about someone experiencing extreme senility or dementia? Has he or she sufficiently lost the capacity for consciousness? What about someone who is severely retarded? However, serious, but not complete, mental impairment differs from the total and irreversible loss of consciousness.

Secondly, how can we be sufficiently certain that the capacity for consciousness cognition is lost? For the higher brain definition of death what are the operational criteria and are they reliable? Sophisticated scanning and imaging techniques enable us to obtain a picture of the brain. We can tell in what sections of the brain blood is flowing and where blood is not flowing. Thus, if blood is not flowing to the higher brain, the patient will never recover any form of consciousness, even if the brain stem is functioning.

Particular problems surround those patients, such as Karen Ann Quinlan, who existed in what is known as a persistent vegetative state. These individuals have completely lost consciousness but still breathe on their own and exhibit continuing cardiopulmonary activities. Although wakeful, opening their eyes and having sleep-awake cycles, they lack all conscious experience. They are unaware of themselves or their environment. They lack thoughts or feelings. Although they may yawn, smack their lips, or sigh, these responses are physiological reflexes. People in this state are mindless organisms.

Experts indicate that for patients in a persistent vegetative state, specifically, for longer than one month, who have lost consciousness as a result of a car accident, a stroke or near drowning, depriving the brain of blood for a sufficient period, we can know with a very high degree of accuracy when severe, irreversible destruction of the cerebral cortex -- the higher brain -- has occurred and consciousness is irreversibly lost. The American Medical Association's Councils on Scientific Affairs and on Ethical and Judicial Affairs concluded that with this diagnosis, the prognosis of cognitive recovery for such patients is less than one in one thousand (0.1%).[21]

Even greater certainty exists with respect to those in a permanent vegetative state, that is, a vegetative state lasting more than twelve months after a traumatic event or more than three months after a nontraumatic incident. The Multi-Society Task Force on the Persistent Vegetative State (the Task Force), consisting of representatives from five medical specialities, in consultation with an advisory panel of legal, ethical, and medical experts, concluded that sufficient data are available to make the diagnosis of a permanent vegetative state with a high degree of certainty and a low risk of prognosis error. An accurate diagnosis and prognosis rest on allowing sufficient time to pass and on objective testing.

Recovery by adults of consciousness from a posttraumatic, permanent vegetative state after twelve months is extremely unlikely. According to studies cited by the Task Force, only seven out of 434 adults in a permanent vegetative state from traumatic head injuries, for example, sustained in a motorcycle or car accident, regained consciousness after twelve months and most of these remained severely disabled with limited cognition, dependent on others for daily support. Also, recovery by adults from a nontraumatic persistent vegetative state, resulting, for example, from a brain tumor, a drug overdose, acute alcoholism, or diabetes, after only three months is exceedingly rare.[22] Thus, if reasonable care is taken, in the terms of following criteria for the diagnosis of a permanent or persistent vegetative state and observing its duration for a sufficient period of time to establish its irreversibility, physicians can diagnose the patient's condition and the resulting loss of consciousness with virtual certainty.

Third, even if we can make an accurate diagnosis and prognosis of a patient's vegetative state, what should we do with the physical body, the "living remains" of one who is brain dead under the higher brain definition but who continues to breathe? The patient, by advance directive, or in accordance with the wishes of his or her family, could opt to preserve biological existence at the expense of the patient's estate or his or her relatives.

In the absence of funding, through private or public sources, as emotionally difficult as it is for us to contemplate, two ways exist to dispose of the bodily remains prior to the cessation of cardiopulmonary functions of a patient who has permanently lost consciousness. First, we can withdraw life sustaining treatment and artificial support,[23] such as nutrition and hydration, as considered in the next chapter, and wait for respiration to cease, which may take days to several weeks, or we can use ever increasing doses of medication to stop a body's heartbeat and respiration more quickly. Second, because continuing bodily life cannot benefit such a person, it may be more humane to give a lethal chemical injection, as discussed in Chapter 6. This technique is, of course, exceedingly controversial and is, at present, illegal throughout the United States. In any event, we must of course, make certain that such patients lack any reasonable chance of recovery.

At The Frontier of Medicine and Spiritual Judaism: When Does Disensoulment Occur?

Even accepting the higher brain definition of death for American legal purposes, from the perspective of Spiritual Judaism, we must try to grapple with one more question: When does disensoulment occur? In other words, when does a physical body lose its spiritual essence? Although we cannot definitely answer this question (and may never be able to do so), let me offer some tentative suggestions.

On one level, a lack of consciousness, the loss of the sense of self and others, in other words, the absence of higher brain functions, may point to the departure of the soul and its emotional, mental and spiritual elements from one's physical body.[24] Only certain of the soul's physical level functions remain. Patients in a persistent or permanent vegetative state typically open and close their eyes; some may respond to noises or moving objects with eye movements or by turning their heads. Pupil size will change with the exposure to light. These remaining instinctive activities, as well as heartbeat and respiration, are performed by the lower brain. The soul may be gone if one lacks consciousness. At the very least, the irreversible loss of consciousness and presumably the departure of the soul from the body serve as some sort of transition between life-and-death. Simply put, human life may be over when higher brain death occurs marked by an irreversible loss of the capacity for consciousness. The physical remains of one lacking consciousness represent a soulless body.

We must ask whether one in a persistent (or permanent) vegetative state retains the ability to communicate his or her emotions and responses because of the survival of his or her essence -- spirit -- soul -- in some state of altered consciousness? These patients may have some sort of inner life not dependent on the higher brain function.[25]

For Spiritual Judaism, however, the ultimate value of each human being, and thus our concept of life, stems from the integration of our immortal soul and our physical body. Under the higher brain definition of death, life consists of a conscious state. Life-and-death turn on the existence (or absence of) consciousness manifested through the body. If consciousness is gone, so too is one's soul. Someone lacking higher brain functions is dead even if cardiorespiratory functions and vegetative responses continue.

The next chapter considers the difficult problem of withholding or withdrawing medical treatment, popularly known as passive euthanasia. Both the American legal and the Jewish traditions, with sharp dissents from some traditionalists, have increasingly come to accept the notion of "pulling the plug," at least in most situations.

Notes

1. Lewis D. Solomon, *The Jewish Book of Living and Dying* (Northvale, NJ: Jason Aronson, 1999), 98-110; Simcha Paull Raphael, *Jewish Views of the Afterlife* (Northvale, N.J.: Jason Aronson, 1994), 132-136, 288-291, 294, 342, 379-380.

2. Marcia Moskowitz, "Charlie and the Angel of Death" in *Jewish Insights on Death and Mourning*, ed. Jack Riemer (New York: Schocken, 1995), 43.

3. Solomon, *Living and Dying*, 65-66; Raphael, *Jewish Views of the Afterlife*, 295-296, 378-379.

4. Solomon, *Living and Dying*, 75-78.

5. Adapted from *Jewish Reflections on Death*, ed. Jack Riemer (New York: Schocken, 1974), 26-27.

6. My concept of the soul is further developed in Solomon, *Living and Dying*, 55-59.

7. Report of the Ad Hoc Committee of the Harvard Medical School to Examine the Definition of Brain Death, "A Definition of Irreversible Coma," *Journal of the American Medical Association* 205:6 (August 1968): 85-88.

8. President's Commission for the Study of Ethical Problems in Medicine and Biomedical and Behavioral Research, *Defining Death: A Report on the Medical, Legal and Ethical Issues in the Determination of Death* (Washington, D.C.: U.S. Government Printing Office, 1981), 24-25.

9. Uniform Laws Annotated, vol. 12A, *Civil Procedural and Remedial Laws*. The Act has been adopted by statute in Arkansas, California, Colorado, Delaware, District of Columbia, Georgia, Idaho, Indiana, Kansas, Maine, Maryland, Michigan, Minnesota, Mississippi, Missouri, Montana, Nebraska, Nevada, New Hampshire, New Mexico, North Dakota, Ohio, Oklahoma, Oregon, Pennsylvania, Rhode Island, South Carolina, South Dakota, Tennessee, Utah, Vermont, West Virginia, Wyoming. Furthermore, the Act is incorporated into the Illinois Health Care Surrogate Act, a New York State Department of Health Regulation, and a

Washington State judicial decision, *Matter of Bowman*, 617 P.2d 731 (Wash. 1980). Courts in Arizona have fashioned a definition of death in accordance with prevailing medical opinion and practices, which include brain death *State v. Fierro*, 603 P.2d 74 (Az. 1979). In *Commonwealth v. Golston*, 366 N.E. 2d 744 (Mass. 1977) the court used the whole brain death standard in determining whether a homicide had been committed. In addition, brain death is incorporated into the statutory definition of death in Alabama, Alaska, Connecticut, Florida, Hawaii, Iowa, Kentucky, Louisiana, New Jersey, North Carolina, Texas, Virginia, and Wisconsin.

10. David H. Ellenson, "How to Draw Guidance From a Heritage: Jewish Approaches to Mortal Choices," in *A Time to be Born and a Time to Die: The Ethics of Choice*, ed. Barry S. Kogan (New York: Aldine De Gruyter, 1991), reprinted in *Contemporary Jewish Ethics and Morality: A Reader*, ed. Elliot N. Dorff and Louis I. Newman, New York: Oxford University, 1995), 131-133. See generally, Fred Rosner, M.D., "The Definition of Death in Jewish Law" in *The Definition of Death: Contemporary Controversies*, ed. Stuart J. Younger, Robert M. Arnold, and Renie Schapiro (Baltimore: Johns Hopkins University Press, 1999), 210-221; Basil F. Herring, *Jewish Ethics and Halakhah For Our Time: Sources and Commentary*, vol. 2 (Hoboken, NJ: KTAV, 1989), 46-74, 80-83; Rabbi Yitzchak Breitowitz, "The Brain Death Controversy in Jewish Law," *Jewish Action: The Magazine of the Orthodox Union* 52:2 (Spring 1992): 61, 63-66.

11. J. David Bleich, *Judaism and Healing: Halakic Perspectives* (New York: KTAV, 1981), 146-157; J. David Bleich, *Contemporary Halakhic Problems*, vol. 3 (New York: KTAV, 1989), 161, 180-184; J. David Bleich, "Establishing Criteria for Death" in *Jewish Bioethics*, ed. J. David Bleich and Fred Rosner (New York: Hebrew Publishing, 1979), 277-295. See also Rabbi Ahron Soloveichik, "Death According to the Halacha," *Journal of Halacha and Contemporary Society*, no. 17 (Spring 1989): 41-48; Aaron Soloveichik, "The Halakhik Definition of Death" in *Jewish Bioethics*, 296-302; Rabbi Aaron Soloveichik, "Jewish Law and Time of Death," *Journal of American Medical Association* 240:2 (July 1978): 109; Dr. Immanuel Jakobovits, *Jewish Medical Ethics: A Comparative and Historical Study of the Jewish Religious Attitude To Medicine and Its Practice* (New York: Bloch, 1976), 277-278; Sir Immanuel Jakobovits, "Ethical Problems Regarding the Termination of Life," in *Jewish Values in Bioethics*, ed. Rabbi Levi Meier (New York: Human Sciences Press, 1986), 92.

12. J. David Bleich, *Contemporary Halakhic Problems*, vol. 1 (New York: KTAV, 1977) 372-393; J. David Bleich, "Establishing the Criteria for Death," 279.

13. Fred Rosner, M.D., *Modern Medicine and Jewish Ethics*, 2nd ed. (Hoboken, N.J.: KTAV, 1991), 269-275; Fred Rosner and Moshe David Tendler, "Definition of Death in Judaism," *The Journal of Halacha and Contemporary Society*, no. 17 (Spring 1989), reprinted in Fred Rosner and Moshe D. Tendler, *Practical Medical Halachah*, 3rd rev. ed. (Northvale, N.J.: Jason Aronson, 1997), 56-69; Fred Rosner, "Jewish Perspectives on Issues of Death and Dying," *The Journal of Halacha and Contemporary Society*, no. 11 (Fall 1985): 66; Moshe Dovid Tendler, *Responsa of Rav Moshe Feinstein: Translation and Commentary*, vol. 1 (Hoboken, N.J.: KTAV, 1996), 35-37.

14. Daniel G. Goldfarb, "The Definition Death: In the Common Law and Jewish Tradition," *Conservative Judaism* 30:2 (Winter 1976): 18, 22; Seymour Siegel, "Updating the Criteria for Death," *Conservative Judaism* 30:2 (Winter 1976): 23-30.

15. Elliot N. Dorff, "A Jewish Approach to End-Stage Medical Care," *Conservative Judaism* 43:3 (Spring 1991): 36-37; Avram Israel Reisner, "A Halakhic Ethic of Care of the Terminally Ill," *Conservative Judaism* 43:3 (Spring 1991): 80-82 n. 43; Elliot N. Dorff, *Matters of Life and Death: A Jewish Approach to Modern Medical Ethics* (Philadelphia: Jewish Publication Society, 1998), 229 n. 17, 380.

16. Central Conference of American Rabbis (CCAR), "Responsum 79. Euthanasia (1980)," *American Reform Responsa: Collected Responsa of the Central Conference of American Rabbis 1889-1983*, ed. Walter Jacob (New York: CCAR, 1983), 273; See also CCAR, "Responsum 78. Banks for Human Organs (1986)," in Walter Jacobs, *Contemporary American Reform Responsa* (New York: CCAR, 1987), 131; CCAR, "Responsum 156. Living Will (1989)," in Walter Jacob, *Questions and Reform Jewish Answers: New American Reform Responsa* (New York: CCAR, 1992), 257-258.

17. Robert D. Truog and James C. Fackler, "Rethinking Brain Death," *Critical Care Medicine* 20:12 (December 1992): 1705-1713.

18. Robert M. Veatch, "The Impending Collapse of the Whole-Brain Definition of Death," *Hastings Center Report* 23:4 (July-August 1993): 19.

19. Ibid., 18-24; Truog and Fackler, "Rethinking Brain Death;" Robert M. Veatch, "Whole-Brain, Neocortical, and Higher Brain Related Concepts" in *Death: Beyond Whole-Brain Criteria*, ed. Richard M. Zaner (Boston: Kluwer Academic Publishers, 1988), 171-186; Joseph Fletcher, "Indicators of Humanhood: A Tentative Profile of Man," *The Hastings Center Report* 2:5

(November 1972): 1-4.

20. James L. Bernat, "How Much of the Brain Must Die in Brain Death?" *The Journal of Clinical Ethics* 3:1 (Spring 1992): 21-26.

21. Council on Scientific Affairs and Council on Ethical and Judicial Affairs, "Persistent Vegetative State and the Decision to Withdraw or Withhold Life Support," *Journal of the American Medical Association* 263:3 (January 1990): 428.

22. The Multi-Society Task Force on PVS, "Medical Aspects of the Persistent Vegetative State," *New England Journal of Medicine* 330:22 (June 1994): 1572-1579. There are case reports of patients, particularly those younger than age 25, who met the permanent vegetative state criteria for twelve months and then recover some neurological functioning typically with continued, severe physical disability. These reports lead critics of the higher brain definition to assert that the requisite degree of diagnostic "certainty" is lacking. Nancy L. Childs and Walter N. Mercer, "Brief Report: Late Improvement in Consciousness after Post-Traumatic Vegetative State," *New England Journal of Medicine* 334:1 (January 1996): 24-25; W.F.M. Arts et al, "Unexpected Improvement After Prolonged Posttraumatic Vegetative State," *Journal of Neurology Neurosurgery and Psychiatry* 48:12 (December 1985): 1300-1303; Gary A. Rosenberg, Stephen F. Johnson, Richard P. Brenner, "Recovery of Cognition After Prolonged Vegetative State," *Annals of Neurology* 2:2 (August 1977): 167-168. In one study, 11 of 43 patients in a persistent vegetative state regained awareness four or more months after suffering brain damage. Keith Andrews, "Recovery of Patients After Four Months or More in a Persistent Vegetative State," *British Medical Journal* 306:6892 (June 1993): 1597-1600.

23. In *Matters of Life and Death*, 378 n. 72, Conservative Rabbi Elliot N. Dorff agrees, stating, "I cannot say that I am thrilled to permit removal of nutrition and hydration tubes from [persistent vegetative state] and advanced Alzheimer's patients - such cases are always tragic, no matter what you do - but I do think that, after trying to revive such patients for some time, it is permissible and probably appropriate to do so." For Rabbi Reisner, modern medicine cannot provide absolute certainty that a persistently vegetative patient has no "life." We are thus left with a presumption of life under Jewish law. Reisner, "A Halakhic Ethic of Care," 68-69.

24. Mark N. Staitman, "Withdrawing or Withholding Nutrition, Hydration or Oxygen from Patients" in *Death and Euthanasia in Jewish Law: Essays and Responsa*, ed. Walter Jacob and Moshe Zemer (Pittsburgh: Rodef Shalom Press, 1995), 9-10.

25. In *Coma: Key to Awakening* (Boston: Shambhala, 1989), Arnold Mindell, a therapist, provides anecdotal examples, detailing his ability to communicate with seemingly unconscious patients by touching and speaking to them. Because of the rudimentary nature of Mindell's evidence, researchers must undertake further studies to determine whether it is possible to communicate with someone in a coma or a persistent (or permanent) vegetative state. See also Arthur S. Berger, "The Role of Parapsychology in Life-Death Decisions," *The Journal of the American Society for Psychical Research* 89:3 (July 1995): 199-214; Brad Lemley, "Back From Coma," *New Age Journal* 11:5 (September/October 1994): 80-83, 150, 152-154; Richard Leviton, "Mysteries of the Coma: Modern Medicine Views Coma as a Total Absence of Consciousness, But Radical Therapists are Exploring Its Links to Creativity and Awareness," *East West* 20:9 (September 1990): 64-69, 116. Amy Mindell provides intensive training for helpers in her book, *Coma, A Healing Journey: A Guide for Family, Friends and Helpers* (Portland, Oreg.: Lao Tse Press, 1999).

Chapter 5

The Jewish Tradition and Pulling the Plug: Withholding or Withdrawing Medical Treatment and the Use of Pain Medication

In an era marked by the heroic efforts to keep people alive, through high tech interventions, invasive surgeries, and aggressive treatments, patients and loved ones must consider at what point medical care, rather than less prolonging acceptable life, extends a miserable dying process. When may we "pull the plug" and engage in passive euthanasia?

When can a patient refuse or stop cancer treatments by saying "No" to more radiation or chemo? Consider Sally, a woman with ovarian cancer who initially responded to chemotherapy but whose cancer is now impervious to medical treatment. In addition, she has developed bowel obstructions. A cancer specialist might recommend an operation to remove the obstructions. Assume, however, that it would probably do no good. The alternative is to put in a tube to drain her stomach so she does not throw up. Sally asks, "Is that what I really want, to live with that tube in me for the rest of my life?" Absent the tube, Sally knows there's no hope. She is going to die.

Or, consider Marge, who has been wired in every way in a hospital bed for weeks. Physicians are using a feeding tube to supply nutrition and hydration and a breathing machine because it is expected Marge will recover from a "temporary" setback. However, should we extend life to the absolute limit to the capabilities of modern medicine? Should we have initiated these means of artificial life-support? When is it permissible to stop trying to help a human being live? Once begun, when may we terminate the use of these procedures? When is it reasonable to remove a feeding tube? When can we take a person off a ventilator, a mechanical pump pushing oxygen into a patient's lungs at set intervals? When can we disconnect IVs and move Marge from an intensive care unit marked by invasive monitoring and treatment as well as round-the-clock medical activity to a private or semi-private room so that she may die?

Hal, a fragile eighty-three year old faces multiple medical problems, including a paralyzing and brain-damaging stroke. His physician has discharged him from the hospital and sent him home to his family, a decision to let death come soon. If Hal develops a fever, the family will do nothing. Hal will die.

In other cases, physicians may discharge patients, such as Jack, from hospitals with the implicit understanding that they are going home to die, with just a morphine drip to ease their pain which will depress and may ultimately stop their breathing. When may physicians increase the dosages of pain medication and even terminally sedate patients to unconsciousness?

The situations facing Sally, Marge, Hal and Jack force us to consider when can we embark on a course of conduct aiming at stopping the process of dying and bring about the death of a human being? Before we try to answer this difficult question, from the perspective of American law, medical ethics, the Jewish tradition, and Spiritual Judaism, let's start by considering modern terminal healthcare decision-making.

Medical Care Decision-Making at the End of Life

The overwhelming majority of patients dying in hospitals succumb after forgoing life sustaining treatment. Today, patients can be supported for days, weeks, or even months without fatality. Thus, the withholding or withdrawal of life sustaining interventions has become commonplace.

Death happens after physicians withhold or withdraw treatment -- antibiotics or a respirator -- and let nature take its course. Experts estimate that some 70% of all in-hospital deaths, about 1.3 million per year in the United States, are somehow negotiated or timed, marking a dramatic transformation of the dying process.[1]

In one study of patients in intensive care units in two hospitals affiliated with the University of California, San Francisco, physician-initiated recommendations to withhold or withdraw life-support treatments were made in 90% of the deaths, 179 recommendations out of 200 deaths.[2] Only 4% of the recommendations to limit life-support were rejected. Furthermore, 90% of patients or their surrogates accepted these recommendations within five days; the vast majority did so within 48 hours. The overwhelming percentage of deaths preceded by the withholding or withdrawal of life-support in this study of patients in 1992 and 1993 represents a significant change from data collected only five years earlier in 1987 and 1988 at these same two hospitals. Then, only about half of the deaths in these same two intensive care units were preceded by physicians' recommendations to withhold or withdraw life-support.[3]

The parties involved, the patient, if capable of medical care decision-making (otherwise, his or her designated surrogate), his or her family and physicians often take concrete steps to limit life sustaining treatments. They carefully negotiate the end of life decision. Although sometimes these choices are made without the consent or even the knowledge of the patient or his or her family or in some cases, over their objections,[4] (in Chapter 10 I will discuss how to make certain it cannot happen),from my experience, patients and their families generally are actively involved in the decision to limit life sustaining interventions. They typically concur in the withdrawal of death-delaying medical interventions, often after the implementation of highly aggressive treatments, or they choose not even to start such interventions. As discussed later in this chapter, to minimize pain and suffering, physicians typically provide patients with palliative (comfort) care or prescribe increased dosages of painkillers sometimes resulting in terminal sedation during the withholding or withdrawal process.

Part of the shift to the far greater incidence of withholding or the removal of medical treatment, as well as the use of extensive use of pain medication, results from the growing recognition that modern technology and pharmacology can increase the likelihood of a "poor" death, but not improve a patient's quality of life. Medical interventions may keep sufferers alive, but not restore their health. The transformation was also brought about by the well-publicized activities of Dr. Jack Kevorkian and ballot initiatives to legalize physician-assisted suicide and active euthanasia in several states. In addition, cost considerations play a significant role in choices to offer less treatment. Third party healthcare payers do not view all end of life care as necessary. The growth of health maintenance organizations with their emphasis on cost containment, as well as cutbacks in public sector programs, Medicare and Medicaid, have focused attention on reducing expenditures for patients who will not survive their illnesses. The shift has also resulted from a sea change in judicial decisions and medical ethics allowing patients to refuse or stop life sustaining medical treatments, thereby leading physicians to do only as much as is reasonable for their patients. Patients (or their surrogates) came to realize that they could say "no" to treatments extending the process of dying but making life a torture. In short, the foundations of the sanctity of biological life principle have begun to crumble.

Building on the notions of our Godlike nature as well as the values of patient autonomy and freedom of choice, developed in Chapter 2, sufferers, family members, and physicians typically engage in a decision-making process involving the balancing of the benefits and burdens of any type of medical intervention. Because each patient is unique, the balance varies. We have entered an era of planned deaths and the consideration, explicitly or implicitly, of quality of life factors, to the consternation of nearly all contemporary Jewish commentators.

The Impact of Judicial Decisions and the Transformation of Medical Ethics Standards

Changes in critical care medicine stem, in part, from modern judicial decisions and the revision of medical ethics standards. Patients now have a legal right to refuse or to stop medical treatments once started. Physicians are required to forego or withdraw interventions at the request of a competent patient, even if the withholding or withdrawal will cause a sufferer's death. In refusing or stopping medical treatments, patients exercise their right of self-determination. By protecting their physical integrity, patients have come to possess authority over what happens to their bodies.

If a patient is unable to express his or her wishes regarding the refusal or the stopping of treatments once started, physicians generally follow clearly stated preferences in the form of advance care directives, popularly known as living wills, discussed in Chapter 10. If a patient, who lacks medical care decision-making capability, has not executed an advance care directive, physicians look to a patient's surrogate (or proxy) to make these end of life choices.

The *Quinlan* case,[5] decided in 1976, marked the beginning of the transformation of the legal landscape and medical practice. The New Jersey Supreme Court held that a patient had a right to refuse medical treatment even if this choice may lead to his or her death. The court based this right on the implied right of privacy under the Fourteenth Amendment to the United States Constitution. The *Quinlan* decision reaffirmed this right of privacy in a medical context.

The case involved Karen Ann Quinlan, a young woman in a persistent vegetative state. She was kept alive on a respirator. Her parents petitioned a state court to have the respirator removed. The New Jersey Supreme Court held that a right of privacy existed, including the right to refuse life sustaining treatment. The right was not, however, absolute. It had to be balanced against the state's interest in the preservation and the sanctity of biological life.

According to the court, decisions about the end of life care must take into consideration the invasiveness of the treatment and the patient's likelihood of recovery. The state's interest against the removal of treatment weakens and the individual's right of privacy grows as the degree of bodily invasion increases and one's prognosis decreases. Quinlan's physicians assumed, incorrectly as it turned out, that she would soon die if her respirator were removed. She faced an extremely poor prognosis. She would never resume cognitive life. Also, the bodily invasion, including twenty-four hour intensive nursing care, the use of antibiotics, the assistance of a respirator, a feeding tube, and a catheter, was very great. In balancing these interests, the *Quinlan* court granted the parents' request to turn off Karen Ann's respirator; however, the artificial administration of food and water kept her alive in a persistent vegetative state for about ten years after her respirator was disconnected.

Thus, in the *Quinlan* case, an American court, for the first time, allowed the discontinuation of a respirator from a patient who was not dead under the whole brain definition of death, discussed in Chapter 4, and who in fact lived for years after its removal. In this case, the court resolved an issue that previously had been decided by the medical profession.

The *Quinlan* case opened a debate, more than a quarter century ago, over the "right to die." During the fifteen year period after the *Quinlan* decision, courts in the United States repeatedly upheld the right of patients to refuse or stop life sustaining treatment. Competent patients as well as those lacking medical care decision-making capacity, whether through a designated surrogate or by means of an advance care directive, received the right to refuse therapies ranging from respirators to nutrition and hydration. Courts also explicitly recognized that a patient's right to refuse medical interventions encompassed his or her right to be free from pain or, perhaps more realistically, to face as little pain and other physical symptoms as possible.

In the 1990 *Cruzan* case,[6] the United States Supreme Court weighed in recognized the constitutional right of competent individuals, even if not in a terminal condition, to refuse or stop life sustaining medical treatment. The source of this right rested, the Court reasoned, on the United States Constitution's Fourteenth Amendment liberty interest. The Court assumed that this constitutionally protected right encompassed the refusal of lifesaving hydration and nutrition. Thus, the Court considered feeding tubes, providing artificial nutrition and hydration, like any other medical treatment a patient (or his or her surrogate) may refuse. Also, life prolonging interventions could be withdrawn from unconscious patients in a persistent vegetative state if they had previously expressed their wishes in an advance care directive. In short, voluntary starvation and dehydration became legally acceptable beginning in the 1990's.

Simultaneously with these judicial developments, the American Medical Association (AMA) reached similar, permissive conclusions. The AMA indicated that even if death is not imminent, "it is not unethical to discontinue all means of life prolonging medical treatment" for patients who are "beyond doubt" permanently unconscious.[7] Artificial nutrition and hydration were included in the interventions that could be withdrawn. Thus, consonant with medical ethics, physicians could withdraw artificial feeding and hydration from permanently or persistently vegetative patients provided the diagnosis is reasonably accurate and the patient's wishes are known.

The AMA also recognized that the use of large dosages of medication that free a patient from pain may inadvertently end his or her life. A physician's obligation to relieve the pain of the dying includes providing optimal palliative care even though such care "may also have the effect of shortening the patient's life."[8]

Thus, judicial decisions and principles of medical ethics conclude that it is acceptable for a patient to refuse or discontinue life sustaining treatments, such as a respirator or artificial feeding, provided it is an informed decision, made by: (1) a patient possessing decision-making capacity; (2) through either a patient's advance care directive; (3) in the absence of a directive, by his or her surrogate. Also, medication may be administered with the primary purpose of relieving pain even if it indirectly hastens death.

Against this American legal and medical ethical background, let's consider how the Jewish tradition views the withholding or withdrawal of medical care as well as the use of pain control medication.

The Jewish Approach: An Overview

In our struggle with the question: "When is enough, enough?" the Jewish tradition provides some answers. Although Jewish law prohibits any act hastening death, the removal of impediments to facilitate a peaceful death is permitted, if not required. Intervention is also forbidden for a moribund patient, a *goses* in Hebrew, one whose death is imminent.

The Jewish tradition has long taught that we need not use measures that prolong the dying process. Perhaps the oldest example of this principle comes from the Babylonian Talmud, some fifteen hundred years old. The Babylonian Talmud (Avodah Zarah 18a) tells us that when the Romans burned Rabbi Hanina ben Teradyon at the stake, in the second century C.E., for teaching Torah, he refused to open his mouth and let the hot flames bring about his death more quickly. He stated, "Better that God Who gave me life should take it away; however, one should not injure himself or herself." The Romans, however, attached wool rags soaked with water to his chest to make his dying slower and more painful. Facing certain death and experiencing terrible pain, Rabbi Hanina changed his mind. In response to his executioner's question, "Rabbi, if I raise the flame and take away the rags from over your heart, will you cause me to enter the World to Come?", Rabbi Hanina not only answered "Yes," but also swore it to him. Thus, he permitted his executioner to remove the rags thereby shortening the dying process and accelerating his death.

Although set in a nonmedical context, this text provides the basis for modern Jewish analysis. It supports the position that one may remove or withdraw an artificial impediment to the natural process of dying.

Later sources focused on doing nothing to delay the departure of the soul from the body. One thirteenth century source, *Sefer Hasidim*, a collection of the teachings of a medieval Jewish pietist sect, prohibited any action lengthening a patient's distress by preventing his or her quick death. For instance, to bar any noise from restoring the soul to the deceased, thereby causing severe pain, this text prohibited those attending the death moment to cry.[9] Later authorities, building on this text, advise:

> It is forbidden to hasten death, for example, if a person is undergoing a prolonged death throes and his soul cannot depart, it is prohibited to remove the pillow or cushion from underneath him following the popular belief that feathers of certain birds contained in the pillow or cushion may prevent the soul from departing. . . . If, however, there is something that causes a delay in the exit of the soul, as, for example, if near to his house there is a sound of pounding as one who is chopping wood, or there is salt on his tongue, and these delay the soul's leaving the body, it is permitted to remove these because there is no direct act involved here, only the removal of an obstacle.[10]

Removing anything inhibiting the departure of the soul represents, according to Jewish sages, the elimination of an impediment to a patient's imminent death, not a direct effort to hasten one's demise. When there is no hope for recovery, medical care should not be used to hinder a soul's flight from the physical body; nature should be allowed to take its course. Much more recently, Lord Jakobovits, the late Chief Rabbi of the United Kingdom, in his pioneering book on Jewish medical ethics, concluded: ". . . Jewish law sanctions, and perhaps even demands, the withdrawal of any factor -- whether extraneous to the patient himself or not -- which may artificially delay his demise in the final phase. . . . in which death is expected to be imminent."[11]

In the twenty-first century, given modern medical developments, it is, however, difficult to draw the line between precipitating death and removing an impediment to one's demise. We are generally no longer dealing with a dying individual, in his or her bedroom, surrounded by relatives and friends, who faces a quick death. Rather we face the more typical situation of a hospitalized patient, suffering from an incurable and inexorably fatal disease with sophisticated technology, such as a respirator and artificial feeding, maintaining his or her life.

The Traditional Jewish Principle of *Goses*

Aggressive medical intervention is not required, in the Jewish tradition, when a patient enters the state of *gesisah*. Medical efforts to save a patient, but not to relieve pain, may be suspended once the person becomes moribund, a *goses*. Although a *goses* is regarded as a living being and is to be accorded all the respect due a living person (Jerusalum Talmud Semachot 1:1-4), no obligation exists to perform any action which will lengthen the life of one in this state. However, the death of a *goses* may not be hastened.

Who is a *goses*? A person becomes a *goses* when the dying process has set in and his or her demise is imminent and irreversible. One enters this state when death, with a reasonable degree of certainty, will occur within seventy-two hours, despite the use of all possible medical means up to that point to save his or her life. Simply put, it is no longer medically feasible to prolong his or her life.[12]

A mortally ill person, a *goses*, who has lost control of his or her bodily functions, may not be disturbed at all and must be allowed to die. Positive actions to hasten death may not be taken. Except for comfort measures, a *goses* may not be touched, moved or jostled for fear of extinguishing his or her life, barely enduring as a "flickering candle." One may not take his or her temperature, measure his or her pulse or blood pressure, or draw blood unless pain relief measures will be undertaken based on the test results. According to Jewish sages, the slightest of movements may hasten a soul's departure. As Jerusalem Talmud (Semachot 1:4) states, "One may not close the eyes of the dying person. Whoever touches them or moves them sheds blood. Rabbi Meir used to say: 'This can be compared to a flickering flame. As soon as one touches it, it becomes extinguished. So too, whoever closes the eyes of the dying is considered to have taken his or her soul.'" (Also, Babylonian Talmud Shabbat 151b). However, medical treatment may be withheld or withdrawn from a *goses* in order to provide for an unimpeded death.

Linking the notion of a *goses* to the permitted removal of any impediments to dying, Orthodox Rabbi J. David Bleich offers the following metaphorical observation:

> Man has the right -- and indeed the obligation -- to rescue his fellow but man, unless he can prevail, ought not to interfere with, or hinder, the Angel of Death in the latter's discharge of his duties. The Angel of Death may take as long as three days to complete his assigned task. During that period man ought not to interfere and thereby prolong the time the Angel of Death must devote to discharging his duty unless he anticipates being able to take the

> Angel of Death by the scruff of the neck and eject him from the sick room, thereby canceling his mission.[13]

In the twenty-first century, the application of the principle of *goses*, particularly the traditional seventy-two hour rule, faces several difficulties. As a result of modern medical technology, a person at the "last stages" of life, a ventilating corpse if you will, may be on his or her hospital deathbed for weeks or months. It is difficult to know ahead of time how many hours or days a patient has to live. More importantly, because a *goses* is described in the Jewish tradition as a living person in every respect, the withholding or withdrawing treatment may lead to guilt and anxiety on the part of surviving family members.

Although advocating a seventy-two hour rule to define one who is a *goses*, Rabbi Bleich, for instance, severely limits the applicability of this category. Based on the twin notions of the sanctity of biological life (discussed in Chapter 2) and our obligation to save lives (considered later in this chapter), Bleich's teaching is that if a *goses* can be restored to good health, if the state of *gesisah* is reversible, or even if it is medically feasible to prolong life, then aggressive medical intervention must be continued. By elevating the importance of the prohibition against hastening death and focusing on the need to preserve earthly life, Bleich reduces the significance of the permissibility of removing impediments to death for one whose demise is imminent. Anything less than the most aggressive marshaling of available medical knowledge and technology for the longest possible time period constitutes, for Bleich, the impermissible sacrifice of human life. Thus, Bleich concludes that the classification of one as *goses* is "relative and will vary with the state of medical knowledge and technology."[14]

Many Conservative rabbis and the Reform Movement continue to use *goses* as an operative, albeit modified, category to delineate when actions to lengthen a patient's life need not be performed. For example, Conservative Rabbi Avram Israel Reisner, a member of the Conservative Movement's Committee on Jewish Law and Standards, defines the state of *gesisah* more flexibly than the traditional seventy-two hour rule to include those diagnosed as "imminently dying."[15]

In one Reform responsum, the authors focus on whether a patient's independent life has ceased. In other words, they ask: is the patient capable of independent life without artificial means? As long as "some form of independent life persists, nothing should be done to hasten death and all medicines which may be helpful must be used."[16] This responsum, as noted in Chapter 4, adopts the whole brain death criteria developed by the Ad Hoc Committee of the Harvard Medical School, to define the absence of independent life or the state of *goses*. Thus, the presence of four criteria, namely, the lack of response to stimuli, the absence of movement or breathing, the absence of reflexes, and the verifying electroencephalogram results, show that nothing more can and need be done for this moribund patient. Medical treatments, apart from comfort care, need not be continued. Also, another Reform responsum concludes that Cardiopulmonary Resuscitation (CPR) need not be given to a *goses*.[17]

Conservative Rabbi Elliot N. Dorff takes a different stance to the consternation of traditionalists who wish to maintain *goses* as the operative category. Dorff looks to another long-standing category, *terefah*,[18] an imperiled life, that is, one diagnosed with a terminal illness, to delineate when medical interventions may be withheld or withdrawn. An estimated life span of twelve months represents an important, but not a determinative, element in establishing inevitability. Unlike a patient who is a *goses* and, as previously discussed, is considered a fully living individual, a *terefah* is analogous to a dead person. Because a *terefah's* blood is "less red," he or she is not equivalent to a healthy human being. Dorff sees the life of one under the siege of a terminal illness as an imperiled life. Thus, healthcare professionals may stop aggressive medical treatments and concentrate on pain relief and comfort care. There is no need to try to do everything medically possible for someone who cannot be cured.

As with the ongoing disputes regarding the definition of death, considered in Chapter 4, I will not serve as a referee or judge regarding these two categories -- *goses* or *terefah*. I only want to point out that even among the strictest of traditionalists, the sanctity of biological life principle has some degree of flexibility.

Medical Futility and the Jewish Tradition

Jewish law implicitly recognizes the concept of medical futility. As Rabbi Bleich puts it, "If you can't vanquish the angel of death, leave him alone."[19]

Generally speaking, medical futility represents a slippery concept with both a quantitative and a qualitative aspect.[20] From a quantitative viewpoint, futility connotes the probability that a particular procedure or treatment will not be medically effective for a patient. He or she will not be cured or even sustained in any medically significant way. Within the range of futility, probability estimates vary. Basically, there is no benefit or almost none -- perhaps one in one hundred -- that any benefit can be achieved from an intervention. There is an inability to stop more than temporarily, perhaps, by days or weeks, a downward physical and/or mental deterioration. Quantitatively, futility connotes a procedure or a treatment having no or a very low probability of achieving its desired goals or an intervention that may achieve its objective but with unacceptable consequences, such as mutilation or loss of function. In either event, it is useless or nearly so.

From a qualitative standpoint, futility characterizes a procedure or a treatment which, even if successful, is unable to produce a reasonably meaningful quality of life for a patient. For instance, the procedure or treatment will still leave a sufferer in an irreversible, persistent vegetative state; he or she will remain totally medically dependent or unable to leave an intensive care unit. The qualitative aspect of medical futility involves a weighing of the expected benefits gained and burdens imposed from any medical intervention, particularly where the procedure or treatment is capable only of maintaining a patient's "poor" quality of life.

The mainstream of the Jewish tradition defines futility narrowly to protect the widely accepted sanctity of biological life principle, focusing on the quantitative aspect and disregarding the qualitative element. For example, one is not obligated to initiate resuscitative efforts if a patient is terminally ill without any chance of recovery. Thus, performing CPR on a terminally ill patient whose heart has stopped, because he or she has reached the point at which his or her body can no longer support life, not because of a cardiac abnormality, may be foregone. Although the patient may be revived, cardiac arrest will certainly occur very shortly. The procedure is futile because it lacks therapeutic value and merely prolongs the inevitable.[21] Independent of the concept of futility, Jewish law may also dictate nonintervention under the principle of *goses*, that is, if no cure is possible and death will inevitably occur within seventy-two hours.

With the Jewish tradition's general concepts in mind, let's examine their applicability to three specific situations: first, the withholding or withdrawal of machines, medications, and other medical treatments;

second, the withholding or withdrawal of artificial food and water; and third, the use of pain medication. When do the sophisticated medical interventions become like "salt on the tongue," techniques maintaining vital life signs without a hope of recovery? When do these modern medical efforts become counterproductive, only delaying the inevitability of death?

Withholding or Withdrawing Machines, Medications and Other Medical Treatments

In considering the withholding or withdrawal of medical treatments, the sanctity of biological life concept generally prevails for Jewish traditionalists. God is said to provide for all of humanity's needs, including medical machinery and medication. The artificiality of modern machines, such as respirators, does not diminish their role as Divine instruments in implementing our obligation to save human lives. Thus, if a patient is not a *goses*, traditionalists require the aggressive use of every type of nonhazardous, nonexperimental life prolonging measure, except for those who suffer from severe, unremitting pain and suffering. According to Rabbi Bleich, "life-prolonging therapy may be withheld only to avoid excruciating pain. However, when pain can be controlled, the obligation to preserve and prolong life remains in full force."[22]

Furthermore, a life-support machine, such as a respirator, maintaining the flow of oxygen to nonfunctioning lungs, may be removed, traditionalists maintain, only if no chance exists of curing a patient. In other words, before removal we need to ask: does a life-support apparatus only prolong the process of dying? More strict traditional authorities would permit the withdrawal of a respirator, even from an incurable sufferer, only when it has been definitely established that he or she is dead.[23] As noted in Chapter 4, the definition of death continues to divide Orthodox authorities. However, according to some traditionalists, if a respirator needs to be turned off, for instance, to allow a patient to be suctioned, and while disconnected, he or she shows no signs of life, the machine need not be reconnected.

Orthodox rabbis also differ with respect to the use of medication. Invoking the concept of futility, some traditionalists conclude that if medication will only prolong the life of a patient, who cannot live much longer, but offers no hope for a cure, it need not be administered. There is no need to perpetuate artificially one's pain and suffering. Rather, "nature may be allowed to take its course."[24] Others maintain, based on the long-standing obligation to save lives, that medication must be given to someone who is terminally ill until the very end.[25] In other words, physicians must continue to provide every means to enable incurable patients to survive.

The Conservative Movement permits the withholding or withdrawal of machines if reasonable certainty exists that such a strategy will only shorten the process of dying, but not interrupt life; however, Conservative rabbis divide on the question of medication. Rabbi Reisner views machines as trying to circumvent natural biological functions. They generally have no curative potential for the terminally ill. Rather, machines, such as respirators, serve as barriers to death. Reisner, however, emphasizes caution in classifying any medical intervention as an impediment to death. He suggests looking at the medical utility of any procedure or treatment, the medical situation in which it is applied, and the medical diagnosis and prognosis for each individual patient.[26]

Rabbi Reisner is far more restrictive with respect to medication than he is with machines. He does not view organic treatments, such as providing medicine, as impediments to death. According to Reisner, the effectiveness of medication in sustaining life is well established. Furthermore, the taking of medication generally does not pose any significant risks. Where the risk is more than minimal or the patient has an option for a different mode of treatment, according to Reisner, a patient (or his or her surrogate) may opt not to take the medication. Only in these limited circumstances, the patient may select the mode of treatment.[27]

Rabbi Dorff concludes that machines may be removed from patients suffering from terminal illnesses who fall within his preferred category of a *terefah*, an imperiled life, discussed earlier in this chapter.[28] Justifying the removal of medical apparatus on two grounds, first, as serving a patient's best interests, and second, as avoiding a lengthy dying process, Dorff emphasizes the need to back away from the American "can do" attitude leading to prolonging life even at a terrible cost to a patient, his or her family, and the greater community.

Dorff would also permit the withholding or removal of medication from a terminally ill patient based on an assessment of a sufferer's best interests and the possible benefits and burdens to him or her.[29] A patient (or his or her designated proxy) needs to consider whether the medication sustains life or merely prolongs the dying process. One may forego medication merely extending life without offering any hope for a cure. Thus, Dorff advocates withholding antibiotics from a terminally ill patient who develops pneumonia, thereby allowing death to come more quickly.

In a series of responsa, the Reform authorities permit the withholding or withdrawal of machines and medication under certain conditions.[30] Machines may be removed when the patient is "clearly and irrevocably" unable to sustain independent heartbeat and respiration. At this point, when circulation and respiration only continue by mechanical means, the machines cease to serve any therapeutic function and merely lengthen, the process of dying in an artificial manner. The patient, when disconnected from the machine, is left in his or her "natural state." Additional moments of life need not be attained through useless means, the Reform rabbis conclude.

Emphasizing the healing effects of medication, the Reform responsa advocate the continued use of medicine provided it is helpful in curing, reversing or controlling an illness or a condition. However, when medication ceases to be "effective and beneficial," merely preserving a patient for a continued period of suffering, it may be withheld. At that point, the medication serves as an impediment to the dying process; it hinders the soul's departure from one's physical body.

To support its conclusion, based in part on the concept of medical futility, one Reform responsum[31] cited the work of Orthodox Rabbi Moshe Feinstein, one of the twentieth century's most noted medical halakists. Rabbi Feinstein ruled that when a patient cannot recover from his or her illness and only continues to suffer, a physician need not continue to administer the treatments which prolong the pain and suffering. In addition, this responsum also cited the opinion of Lord Jakobovits who concluded that a diabetic patient with incurable cancer need not continue to take insulin.

Thus, this Reform responsum concluded that antibiotics need not be administered to an elderly patient, suffering from Alzheimer's disease who does not recognize her family, where she is terminally ill and death is "relatively near." In this situation the antibiotics serve as useless obstacles to death, performing no reasonable therapeutic function.

A Reality Check

In assessing the efficacy of medications and machines, a degree of realism is in order. Despite the rather blithe assumption that medications are always beneficial, it is important to be mindful of some of their burdens. Repeated injections and the increasingly difficult search for suitable injection sites may create considerable pain and suffering for some patients.

Antibiotics are not invariably beneficial. The use of antibiotics may lead to complications and substantial risks for some sufferers. Giving antibiotics may prolong a patient's pain and suffering and ultimately prove futile in fighting infections. Even with antibiotics, some patients may experience a series of more serious and painful infections resulting a severe deterioration of their condition.

Respirators exemplify many of the dilemmas brought about by machines. As noted earlier in this chapter, a ventilator pushes air and thus oxygen into the lungs. The use of a ventilator involves one of two techniques. First, a physician may insert a tube in the windpipe via a patient's nose or mouth. The uncomfortable nature of the tube results in patient anxiety. It also prevents one from speaking, swallowing and eating, and often triggers a gagging reflex. Or, a physician may perform a tracheotomy, cutting a hole in the windpipe in the front of a patient's neck. A tracheotomy requires surgery, but eventually allows one to take food by mouth and to speak for short periods.

Respirators do not reverse the underlying disease process and may also require extra sedation. Blood tests and x-rays may be needed to monitor a patient's condition. If a patient is very ill, it may be hard for him or her to ever recover sufficiently to come off a ventilator.

It is often recommended that patients engage in a time-limited trial of any medical apparatus with a planned withdrawal.[32] Patients may want to try a machine, such as a ventilator, for a reasonable, but limited, time period to see its benefits. Patients (or their surrogates) need to ask: Will the machine improve one's quality of life, for instance, his or her energy, alertness, or comfort? However, before commencing the use of a machine for a limited trial period, patients (or their proxies) must set a time limit when a reassessment will be undertaken. They also need to determine in advance what they and their physicians hope the intervention will accomplish. Using a benefits-burdens test, a patient (or his or her surrogate) may want to discontinue the intervention if it does not improve one's quality of life. Time trials also provide an opportunity for loved ones to let go emotionally of a patient.

Withholding or Withdrawing Artificial Nutrition and Hydration

Patients who are unable to eat or drink when their digestive system is impaired as a result of disease, trauma, or bodily deterioration, such as those in the last stages of throat cancer or Alzheimer's disease, may be fed through tubes. A physician inserts the least intrusive type of tubal feeding, the naso-gastric (esophageal) tube, into a patient's nose and down one's throat. If a patient tries to remove the naso-gastric tube or cough it up, his or her hands must be tied or physicians use a more invasive type of tubing, an intravenous (IV) feeding. As a last resort, physicians insert a gastrointestinal tube directly into a patient's stomach. The feeding tube is surgically placed through the abdominal wall.

Most Jewish traditionalists conclude, not unexpectedly, that artificial nutrition and hydration must be provided and cannot be withdrawn until death has occurred.[33] They reason that God provides all creatures with food and water to maintain life and ward off hunger and thirst. Food and water are universal, life sustaining human needs, not impediments to death. Everyone needs these to exist. They constitute general, supportive, not medical, care; they symbolize a caring, nurturing human community. When a person is unable to eat or drink independently, the Eternal provides artificial means to prolong life. We must, therefore, recognize the Divine presence in these techniques of sustenance.

For the traditionalist, denying food and water is not the same as withholding medicine. The failure to provide food and water will "certainly and directly lead to the patient's death, since survival without food and fluids is impossible, whereas life can continue without medication." Food is "not transformed into an exotic medical substance by the simple act of pouring it into a gastrostomy tube."[34]

Thus, most traditionalists assert that nutrition and hydration must be provided to a terminally ill patient regardless of how administered, even if they only prolong a life of pain and suffering. Depriving one of artificial nutrition and hydration represents an impermissible, positive action, the killing of another human being.

Viewing artificial nutrition and hydration as medical therapy, a minority of traditionalists permit these techniques to be withheld from or refused by a terminal patient (or his or her surrogate).[35] These more flexibly-minded traditionalists focus on each patient's circumstances, asking whether the artificial feeding and hydration of a terminally ill patient: first, provides a benefit without any anticipated harm, or second, may trigger potentially severe complications?[36]

Once initiated, traditionalists generally maintain that patients must continue to receive artificial nutrition and fluids. In other words, they oppose discontinuance until the very end, or at least, until the patient becomes a *goses*.

Conservative authorities differ among themselves markedly. Taking a restrictive position, Rabbi Reisner maintains that physicians must initiate the use of the IV tubes, especially for fluids. Generally, these tubes cannot be withdrawn. Reisner sees their withdrawal as shortening a patient's God-given, purposeful life. Even if the placement of an IV for fluids requires surgery, he would make it subject to a patient's (or proxy's) choice only in limited circumstances, namely, if the difficulties were significant and the sufferer were quite deteriorated. Because of the risk of significant difficulties in breathing and the high degree of discomfort, Reisner places the naso-gastric and gastrointestinal feeding tubes, the latter requiring a surgical insertion, within the ambit of a patient's (or his or her surrogate's) choice. Reisner concludes, "We may cajole, but should not resort to forcible tube feeding."[37]

Rabbi Dorff provides a quite different perspective on this matter.[38] Because artificial nutrition and hydration require the insertion of some type of tube into a patient, Dorff classifies these techniques as medication, not as normal food and water. The decision to administer or withdraw artificial nutrition and hydration becomes a medical one based on an assessment of the benefits to and burdens imposed on a patient. Dorff emphasizes the need to assess the risks, particularly, the increased likelihood of infection, as part of a benefit-burden analysis. In other words, we must ask: what reasonable benefits does the patient derive from exposure to the heightened risks? Furthermore, if intubation does not cure a patient but merely prolongs his or her process of dying, it is permissible, if not mandatory, according to Dorff, to remove the tube thereby enabling the patient to die within a natural time.

In reaching his conclusion, Dorff focuses on the principle of causation, particularly with respect to patients in a persistent vegetative state or with advanced Alzheimer's disease. Dorff views the cause of death in such a situation as the underlying illness or condition, not the withholding or withdrawal of treatment. If a dying person lacks any reasonable prospect of recovery, there is no need to delay the inevitable. He recommends maintaining a patient on artificial nutrition and hydration for a reasonable time period to protect against misdiagnosis and give family members time to begin to grieve their beloved's demise. Ultimately, Dorff would allow the removal of artificial nutrition and hydration when they lack any curative potential.

One recent Reform responsum follows a rather traditional line of reasoning. According to the Reform rabbis, food and water provide essential nutrients. We require food and water to survive. Eating food and drinking water represent human necessities. They are not ingested to treat a patient. The fact that tubes or machines supply nourishment does not transform them into "exotic" medical treatments.[39]

However, the responsum notes that a split exists among Reform authorities with respect to this subject. It cites an earlier responsum prohibiting the removal of a feeding tube providing essentials to sustain life, even if a patient's condition is hopeless.[40] The removal is seen as taking a positive step to hasten death.

However, several other responsa permit the withdrawal, analogizing the removal of a feeding tube to the wiping salt from a patient's tongue.[41] In other words, a feeding tube may be removed when it no longer provides any therapeutic benefit to a patient, merely prolonging the dying process. As the Reform proponents of removal reason: "Such feeding does not help the patient and at best must be debilitating, uncomfortable, if not painful. We should also realize that diminished interest by those patients normally capable of eating is another sign that life is ebbing and that the last stages have been reached."[42]

Returning to the most recent responsum dealing with this topic, the Reform authorities conclude that the "Jewish tradition does not categorically prohibit the withdrawal of artificial food and water from dying patients."[43] As noted above, this responsum stresses that food and water, no matter how delivered, comprise the very "staff of life" for humans. Also, the moral stakes are higher in withholding or withdrawing artificial nutrition and hydration than with machines or medication. In so doing, we starve or dehydrate humans to death. Thus, the responsum maintains that it is preferable to continue the artificial nutrition and hydration to preclude any possibility of causing death by starvation or dehydration. However, because the removal is not categorically forbidden in the eyes of Reform rabbis, patients, their surrogates, or their family members must allow their conscience to dictate their decision.

Another Reality Check

Feeding and hydration by a naso-gastric tube or IV are, in my view, medical procedures, implemented by healthcare professionals, with inherent risks and possible negative side effects. They are not the same as eating or drinking naturally. A physician (or someone under his or her direction) inserts a tube or a needle or performs surgery in the case of the gastrointestinal tube. In addition to requiring the efforts of healthcare professionals, these techniques require bodily interventions offering benefits and imposing burdens.

A mechanism for furnishing nutrition and water may help a patient get through an illness enabling him or her to recover from or live with what otherwise would be fatal. For instance, sometimes stroke victims initially cannot swallow. A tube provides artificial nutrition and hydration. When the patient learns to eat and drink again, physicians remove the tube. Even after a successful treatment, a patient with throat cancer may be unable to swallow. A feeding tube is appropriate and quite beneficial. The initial use and continuation of artificial feeding and fluids makes sense if the underlying disease will allow the patient a substantial period with a desirable quality of life.

Let's turn and focus on a variety of burdens artificial nutrition and hydration bring about,[44] especially for those who are terminally ill. The insertion of a naso-gastric tube is uncomfortable; its retention irritates the nose. In addition to the difficulty in breathing and a shortness of breath resulting from fluid buildup in one's lungs and throat requiring suctioning, the use of a naso-gastric tube may lead to serious side effects, such as pneumonia and nausea. Diarrhea may result from liquid feedings the stomach and intestines can no longer tolerate. The tube may irritate the surfaces in the inside of the nose, sometimes causing severe bleeding. Because restraints may be used to prevent patients from removing the tubes, these sufferers may develop pneumonia and serious bedsores from a lack of activity and their fixed position.

Use of IVs pose the risks of infection or inflamation. Because human veins are not designed to carry a continuous flow of IV nutrition and hydration, they may develop infections at the tube's entry point or collapse at some point. Because a tube's entry point is an open wound, gastrointestinal tubes present rare, but possible complications, especially for severely debilitated patients, from the procedure, including the risk of infection and bleeding.

The inexorable result of stopping artificial nutrition and hydration is death. There's no way to "sugar coat" it. If denied food and water, people die of starvation or dehydration usually within ten to fourteen days, although the process may take as long as three or four weeks. They become gaunt in the face, then they develop cold hands and feet, followed by fast and hard breathing that eventually stops. During this period, a patient retains an opportunity to change his or her mind. However, because the process is not swift, the vigil for loved ones often becomes burdensome and stressful.

In the interval before death, the deprivation of food and water may prove beneficial. The body's normal way to die is by starvation and dehydration. It is the natural way of shutting down. It is part of the last phase of a terminal condition. It is often quite comfortable. Refusing nourishment also serves as an opportunity to explore altered states of consciousness. Thus, fasting may facilitate the perception and exploration of death moment visions, considered in Chapter 4.

A physician, writing regarding the progressive illness and dying of his eighty-four year old mother, Virginia, the proverbial "little old lady in sneakers," described her last few days after she stopped eating and drinking as follows:

> Over the next four days, my mother greeted her visitors with the first smiles she had shown for months. She energetically reminisced about the great times she had had and about the things she was proud of. . . . She also found a calming self-acceptance in describing the things of which she was not proud. She slept between visits but woke up brightly whenever we touched her to share more memories and say a few more things she wanted us to know. On the fifth day it was more difficult to wake her. When we would take her hand she would open her eyes and smile, but she was too drowsy and weak to talk very much. On the sixth day, we could not wake her. Her face was relaxed in her natural smile, she was breathing unevenly, but peacefully. We held her hands for another two hours, until she died.[45]

In their last days prior to their demise, patients may spontaneously reduce their intake of hydration and nutrition without experiencing thirst or hunger.[46] The electrolyte imbalance builds up allowing a dying patient to drift off into a painless sleep rather than fighting for breath as the lungs otherwise fill up with fluids or having excess fluids collect throughout the body as one's kidneys are unable to process fluids adequately. Thus, without artificial hydration and nutrition, many patients die more comfortably.

If properly treated, it is often more comfortable near the end for a dying person to go without artificial fluids. Although dry mouth naturally results from dehydration at the end of life, to deal with this discomfort, healthcare professionals use ice chips, moistened sponge swabs, or if feasible, they provide sips of water. The beneficial effects of fluid deprivation on the terminally ill include: decreased awareness of suffering; reduced urinary output resulting in less need for a urinary catheter; diminished pulmonary secretions necessitating less need for suctioning; decreased likelihood of nausea and vomiting; and lessening of a predisposition for pressure sores.[47] Thus, two medical experts conclude, "The truth is, for those who are dying, the time comes when it might be more compassionate, caring, even natural, to allow dehydration to occur. Forcing tube feedings and IVs on dying patients can make the last days of their lives more uncomfortable."[48]

Facing death, a decrease in appetite is also natural. It is not letting someone "starve to death." Eating less may actually increase a patient's comfort and lead to a more peaceful death.[49] As the body shuts down, the withdrawal of artificial nutrition may have an analgesic effect resulting from an increase in the body's natural pain-relieving hormones. Conversely, artificial feeding until death often increases a patient's discomfort, especially for those with high fevers.

As death approaches, a patient does not keep up his or her strength by being forced to eat if it makes him or her uncomfortable. The loss of appetite may be distressing, especially if eating represents a social event or if care, comfort, compassion, and love have been expressed through food in the sufferer's family.

Family members, often even more than a patient, must deal with the symbolic and psychosocial meanings of eating and drinking. In other words, do the beloved feel that food is life? For some, food serves as the central mode of nurture and comfort. Eating is also associated with social interchange. Given their food fixation, family members may see the withholding of food and water as a form of abandonment resulting in death by starvation and dehydration. They need to reflect on their conscious and unconscious values. Also, loved ones should consider providing spiritual forms of nurturing, as an alternative to food, such as enhancing the atmosphere with music or special sounds, for instance, water or wind.

The Use of Pain Medication and the Jewish Tradition

Modern medicine provides the means to relieve the painful agonies of most dying patients. At least in theory, physicians are able to palliate discomforting symptoms so that substantial pain and suffering do not mark the dying process, for instance, after the forgoing of artificial nutrition and hydration. Physicians can blunt the most savage pain in 90 to 95% of terminal cancer patients.[50] Other experts indicate that physicians can achieve effective pain relief for upwards of 98% of all dying patients.[51]

The withdrawal of a respirator generally results in a sudden feeling of suffocation leading to a visceral panic. In removing a ventilator, physicians strive to keep patients comfortable. Doctors medicate patients so they will not be short of breath, characterized by noisy or gasping respiration and some degree of struggling.

Thus, after turning off a respirator for a terminally ill cancer patient, whose breathing has been assisted by the ventilator, physicians typically use a sedative (notably morphine) to relieve the accompanying distress. By depressing respiration, sedation may accelerate death by some measure of time.

Physicians may legally and ethically treat pain and other physical symptoms knowing that the therapy expedites death so long as they do not primarily intend to hasten one's end. When someone is in terrible pain, unresponsive to analgesics, a doctor may increase the amounts of morphine until death occurs from the suppression of respiration. This is called the principle of "double effect" in the guise of pain control.[52] It is ethically and emotionally helpful because physicians avoid feeling they are directly causing someone's death.

The stated, primary intent centers on treating pain, the severe distress brought about by the removal of a respirator, a "good" primary purpose, not the hastening of death. The pain relief has the side effect of respiratory depression typically shortening a patient's life to the point where death results. To be legally and ethically acceptable, the secondary consequences are foreseen but not intended. Neither the patient nor the physician intends to accelerate the demise but they both accept the risk of hastening death to relieve pain.

The double effect principle thus allows physicians to perform actions with foreseeable consequences that would be "wrong" to intend. A doctor's action is acceptable if death comes unintentionally as a result of an otherwise well-intentioned intervention, an effort to relieve pain, even if death is foreseen as a high probability. Thus, doing something foreseeable, but unintentional, is permissible.

The double effect principle has its limitations. For instance, patients with multiple sclerosis or Lou Gehrig's disease suffer severely but do not have the kind of pain requiring morphine. Thus, for these patients physicians cannot use the double effect principle to administer narcotics.

In the Jewish tradition, the elimination of pain comprises part of the general obligation to heal. In Leviticus 19:18, the Hebrew Bible mandates us to eliminate pain with the commandment: "And you shall love your neighbor as yourself." The lessening or eliminating pain is incorporated within the general obligation to save endangered life. Furthermore, the Jewish tradition does not see suffering as an independent good. Suffering need not be borne, as one contemporary commentator puts it, "as part of a divinely willed scheme of things. . . ."[53] Disagreements arise, however, regarding what happens when the treatment of pain conflicts with the goal of preserving life.

Traditionalists generally conclude that if the duty to preserve life conflicts with the palliation of pain, priority goes to preserving life. Rabbi Bleich maintains that the preservation of life always comes before other concerns, including pain therapy.[54] Although asserting, "Life accompanied by pain is . . . preferable to death,"[55] Bleich would permit the administration of medication to relieve pain and suffering provided it does not shorten one's life. He even goes so far as to approve of a physician giving someone who is terminally ill high doses of morphine as long as the dosage is not lethal and it is not administered for the direct purpose of terminating one's life.

Conservative authorities favor the remediation of pain but differ as to some details. Rabbi Reisner advocates pain treatment, but prohibits its administration if a probability exists that it will indirectly shorten a patient's life.[56] Reisner notes that the probability of death defeats any apparent benefit from the pain therapy. Like Bleich, Reisner puts pain treatment second to the preservation of life. Reisner allows, however, the use of large doses of medication to relieve pain but below an amount posing a significant threat to one's life.

Rabbi Dorff goes further than Reisner in defending the use of pain medication at the expense of a sufferer's life. Dorff explains that if a terminally ill patient is in severe pain, he or she may take any amount of pain medication even if that amount will simultaneously hasten his or her death.[57] If a patient (or surrogate) and his or her physician agree on a pain treatment plan that may hasten death, they are not engaged in physician-assisted suicide or voluntary active euthanasia, which as we will see in Chapter 6, the Jewish tradition nearly unanimously opposes. Adopting the double effect principle, Dorff notes that the essential factor is the primary intent to alleviate the pain rather than ending a sufferer's life. He bases his argument on a physician primarily intending to provide a benefit to a patient. Because suffering is not an "independent good" under Jewish law, its diminution serves as the key element in setting aside the traditional policy of preserving life. Dorff would, however, prohibit the giving of a lethal dose of pain medication if a physician primarily intends to cause a patient's death, for example, by administering a dosage that beyond all reasonable doubt would kill a patient.

In one responsum, Reform rabbis likewise agree with their Conservative counterparts, viewing pain relief as a proper medical objective. The Reform authorities conclude that a patient may take pain medication even though the therapy may "slightly" hasten death.[58] They view the treatment of pain as a long-term process. Over an extended period proper dosages of pain medication do not actually cause a patient's death; the underlying disease or condition leads to one's demise. The responsum notes, however, that the primary intent of the medication must be to relieve pain, not to hasten death.

Because of the technical capabilities of modern medicine, patients, in theory, need not suffer a painful dying process. If a patient forgoes life sustaining care, a treatment team may provide palliative care, designed to make one as comfortable as possible, including pain and symptom control, skin care, turning, and positioning. Palliative care can relieve most, but not all, of one's terminal pain and suffering.

Studies indicate, however, that pain and other physical symptoms often go untreated or insufficiently treated as a result of inadequate medical training, exaggerated fears about addiction to medication, or poor communication. In the largest study of how patients die in American hospitals, one half of the severely ill, but conscious, sufferers in five major hospitals experienced moderate or severe pain at least half of the time during the last three days of their life.[59] Between 10 and 50% of patients in programs devoted to palliative care still report significant pain, according to other experts, one week before death.[60]

Other physical symptoms, such as shortness of breath, difficulty in swallowing, incessant itching, nausea, vomiting, diarrhea, or constipation, are often less amenable to treatment than pain. Weakness and fatigue as well as the accompanying emotional and spiritual suffering may even be more intractable than pain and other physical syptoms.

Spiritual Judaism and the Dilemmas Posed by Aggressive Pain Relief Techniques

For patients experiencing extreme pain and suffering, those contorted to be barely recognizable and tormented in various physical, emotional, and spiritual dimensions, physicians may administer ever greater dosages of pain medication. Day-after-day, throughout the United States, the terminally ill receive heavier and heavier doses of painkillers. For example, cancer may metastasize to the brain resulting in severe pain and suffering. Physicians may sedate these terminal sufferers to unconsciousness, by inducing a drug coma to control extreme, otherwise unbearable and unrelievable pain and suffering. Also, disconnecting a patient from a ventilator typically results in discomfort and acute breathlessness, requiring extensive sedation, sometimes to the point that a patient becomes unconscious.

To deal with pain and other physical symptoms, physicians openly use a pharmacologically-induced sleep, known as terminal sedation. The extent to which physicians utilize terminal sedation to deal with pain varies widely, but it is quite extensive. In one study, physicians sedated to unconsciousness 50% of their advanced cancer patients prior to death to ensure adequate control of pain and other physical symptoms.[61]

Death by terminal sedation may take days. The time delay permits second guessing and a reassessment of the situation. However, when terminally sedated a patient cannot engage in the life closure tasks, as developed in Chapters 7 and 11, that are so vital from the perspective of

Spiritual Judaism. Although physically existing for a few more days, those who are terminally sedated cannot consciously benefit from this additional time. Similar to death by starvation or dehydration, the beloved may also suffer needlessly while waiting for sedated patients to die. These deaths are unlikely to be dignified or viewed as peaceful by loved ones. Those wishing to die at home may be unable to arrange for terminal sedation because this technique generally requires admission to a healthcare facility.

Patients, surrogates, and physicians contemplating the use of greater and greater dosages of pain medication should take into account the reality of the death moment visions and the search for closure in life. Increased dosages of pain medication generally leave patients in a zombielike state.

As detailed in Chapter 4, at or near the death moment, an individual undergoes significant internal, subjective changes. Death moment visions help one exit the earthly world and enter the postmortem realms as a disembodied soul. Many patients also want to complete their emotional and spiritual work as part of the dying process. Although sedatives quiet delirium and calm a patient, allowing loved ones to hold a dying person's hand or stroke his or her brow, these medications may take way the patient's chance to finish life emotionally and spiritually whole.

For those wanting a conscious death, the use of pain medication presents a dilemma. Unrelenting, uncontrolled pain distracts from one's spiritual practices, such as meditation or prayer, or the chance to extend or receive forgiveness. If you are in so much pain, request sufficient medication to take the edge off your discomfort, with the dosage allowing you to continue your spiritual practices, glimpse the death moment visions, and use the remainder of your life as well as meaningfully as possible. Strive to go through the death process, as the Baal Shem Tov did, fully lucid.

From the perspective of Spiritual Judaism, try not to leave this life in a haze or an unconscious state induced by large doses of pain-relieving drugs. Ask your doctor to administer pain medication to minimize (or hopefully, eliminate) your physical pain and suffering but allow you, if at all possible, to remain conscious, aware and able to connect with your inner experiences. A skillful physician can use a combination of drugs to diminish the pain and other physical symptoms without dulling the mind.

If you are terminally ill and have less than six months to live, consider hospice care at home. Providing only comfort care and pain relief, not medical interventions designed to cure, hospice care aims to keep sufferers alert, able to enjoy their family, visitors, and surroundings. Generally, hospice patients administer their own pain relief measures based on their own personal needs. From the perspective of Spiritual Judaism, they are better able to perceive and deal with their death moment visions and achieve closure at the end of life.

Whether a sufferer is at home or in a medical facility, his or her loved ones should insist that healthcare professionals try to use, as an alternative to (or in conjunction with) pain medication, nonchemical means, such as breathing exercises or some form of meditation or biofeedback, to work with and control pain and suffering. These nonchemical techniques do not cloud consciousness thereby facilitating the contemplation of the death moment visions and permitting the resolution of emotional and spiritual matters.

Learning about the Jewish tradition's views regarding the cessation of medical interventions and the use of pain medication may help patients and their beloved absolve their guilt and bring about peace of mind. Stopping treatment and allowing death to occur is quite compatible with the Jewish tradition's respect for life.

Ideally, patients, their families, and physicians need to talk ahead of time about when "enough's enough" and then what happens. This dialogue, as discussed in Chapter 10, forms the basis for the execution of an advance care directive and the preparation of a values statement.

Some sufferers and their loved ones may, however, want their physicians to go beyond withdrawing treatments and stopping the aggressive use of pain control medication. Passive euthanasia may invoke unnecessary distress for a patient and his or her beloved, who witness a gradually fading way over endless days and weeks, when everyone hopes for a much speedier end. To avoid a lingering dying process, which may turn into a terrible ordeal, consideration may turn to other alternatives: suicide, physician-assisted suicide, or voluntary active euthanasia. The use of palliative measures, increased dosages of painkillers, or the participation in a hospice program, may not obviate the desire on the part of some for physician-aid-in-dying.

Notes

1. Alan Meisel, "The Legal Consensus About Forgoing Life Sustaining Treatment: Its Status and Prospects," *Kennedy Institute of Ethics Journal* 2:4 (1993): 334-335 n. 6; Gina Kolata, "'Passive Euthanasia' is the Norm in Today's Hospitals, Doctors Say," *New York Times*, 28 June 1997, sec. A1; Kathryn A. Koch, Henry D. Rodeffer, and Robert L. Wears, "Changing Patterns of Terminal Care Management in an Intensive Care Unit," *Critical Care Medicine* 22:2 (February 1994): 233-243.

2. Thomas J. Prendergast and John M. Luce, "Increasing Incidence of Withholding and Withdrawal of Life Support from the Critically Ill," *American Journal of Respiratory & Critical Care Medicine* 155:1 (January 1997): 15-20.

3. Nicholas G. Smedira et al, "Withholding and Withdrawal of Life Support from the Critically Ill," *New England Journal of Medicine* 332:5 (February 1990): 309-315.

4. David A. Asch, John Hansen-Flaschen and Paul N. Lanken, "Decisions to Limit or Continue Life-Sustaining Treatment by Critical Care Physicians in the United States: Conflicts Between Physicians' Practices and Patients' Wishes," *American Journal of Respiratory & Critical Care Medicine* 151:2, part 1 (February 1995): 288-292.

5. In the *Matter of Quinlan*, 70 N.J. 10, 355 A.2d 647 (1976), cert. denied.

6. *Cruzan* v. *Director*, *Missouri Department of Health*, 497 U.S. 261 (1990).

7. Council on Ethical and Judicial Affairs, American Medical Association and Southern Illinois University Schools of Medicine and Law, *Code of Medical Ethics: Annotated Current Opinions*, annotated by E2.20 *Withholding or Withdrawing Life-Prolonging Medical Treatment* (Chicago: American Medical Association, 1992), 18-19.

8. Council on Ethical and Judicial Affairs, American Medical Association, "Decisions Near the End of Life," *Journal of the American Medical Association* 267:16 (April 1992): 2231.

9. Elliot N. Dorff, *Matters of Life and Death: A Jewish Approach to Modern Medical Ethics* (Philadelphia: Jewish Publication Society, 1998), 199, 376 n. 52. See also Rabbi Yehudah HeChasid, *Sefer Chasidim: The Book of the Pious*, trans. Avraham Yaakov Finkel (Northvale, NJ: Jason Aronson, 1997), 335.

10. Daniel B. Sinclair, *Tradition and the Biological Revolution: The Application of Jewish Law to the Treatment of the Critically Ill* (Edinburgh: Edinburgh University Press, 1989), 11-12. See also Central Conference of American Rabbis (CCAR), "Responsum 156. Living Will (1989)," in Walter Jacob, *Questions and Reform Jewish Answers: New American Reform Responsa* (New York: CCAR, 1992), 256.

11. Dr. Immanuel Jakobovits, *Jewish Medical Ethics: A Comparative and Historical Study of the Jewish Religious Attitude To Medicine and Its Practice* (New York: Bloch, 1975), 124.

12. J. David Bleich, *Bioethical Dilemmas: A Jewish Perspective* (Hoboken, NJ: KTAV, 1998), 77-80; J. David Bleich, "Treatment of The Terminally Ill," *Tradition* 30:3 (1996): 63-70; J. David Bleich, *Judaism and Healing: Halakhic Perspectives* (New York: KTAV, 1981), 137, 140-142; J. David Bleich, "The Obligation to Heal in the Judaic Tradition: A Comparative Analysis" in *Jewish Bioethics*, ed. J. David Bleich and Fred Rosner (New York: Hebrew Publishing, 1979), 33-35.

13. Bleich, *Bioethical Dilemmas*, 84. See also Bleich, "Treatment," 68.

14. Bleich, *Bioethical Dilemmas*, 83.

15. Avram Israel Reisner, "A Halakhic Ethic of Care for the Terminally Ill," *Conservative Judaism* 43:3 (Spring 1991): 57, 64.

16. CCAR, "Responsum 79. Euthanasia (1980)," in *American Reform Responsa: Collected Responsa of the Central Conference of American Rabbis* 1889-1983, ed. Walter Jacob (New York: CCAR, 1983) 272. See also CCAR, "Responsum 156. Living Will (1989)," *Questions and Reform Jewish Answers*, 256-258; CCAR, "Responsum 5754.14. On the Treatment of the Terminally Ill," in *Teshuvot for the Nineties: Reform Judaism's Answer to Today's Dilemmas*, ed. W. Gunther Plaut and Mark Washofsky (New York: CCAR, 1997), 343-346.

17. CCAR, "Responsum 160. CPR and The Frail Elderly (1989)," *Questions and Reform Jewish Answers*, 267.

18. Dorff, *Matters of Life and Death*, 200, 232; Elliot N. Dorff, "A Jewish Approach to End-Stage Medical Care," *Conservative Judaism* 43:3 (Spring 1991): 19-26. See also Sinclair, *Tradition and the Biological Revolution*, 20-23, 71-75.

19. J. David Bleich, "Care of the Terminally Ill," in *Jewish Values in Health and Medicine*, ed. Rabbi Levi Meier (Lanham, MD: University Press of America, 1991), 155.

20. Because of the difficulty of achieving a consensus on the definition of futile care, the American Medical Association Council on Ethical and Judicial Affairs recommends a process approach to futility determination. Council on Ethical and Judicial Affairs, American Medical Association, "Medical Futility in End-of-Life Care: Report of the Council on Ethical and Judicial Affairs," *Journal of the American Medical Association* 281:10 (March 1999): 937-941.

21. Fred Rosner, *Modern Medicine and Jewish Ethics*, 2nd ed. (Hoboken, NJ: KTAV, 1991), 209, 246 n. 41.

22. Bleich, *Bioethical Dilemmas*, 95.

23. Rosner, *Modern Medicine*, 208-209, 241; Bleich, *Bioethical Dilemmas*, 72-74; Bleich, *Judaism and Healing*, 138; Fred Rosner and Moshe D. Tendler, *Practical Medical Halachah* (Northvale, N.J.: Jason Aronson, 1997), 54.

24. Rosner, *Modern Medicine*, 237-240.

25. Rosner, *Modern Medicine*, 246 n. 41; Bleich, *Bioethical Dilemmas*, 72, 74; Bleich, *Judaism and Healing*, 137-139.

26. Reisner, "A Halakhic Ethic," 59, 64.

27. Ibid., 62-63.

28. Dorff, *Matters of Life and Death*, 206-207; Dorff, "End-Stage Medical Care," 27, 30.

29. Dorff, *Matters of Life and Death*, 206-208; Dorff, "End-Stage Medical Care," 27-30.

30. CCAR, "Responsum 5754.14. On the Treatment of the Terminally Ill," *Teshuvot for the Nineties*, 343-346, 348-349. See also CCAR, "Responsum 156. Living Will (1989)," *Questions and Reform Jewish Answers*, 257-258; CCAR, "Responsum 79. Euthanasia (1980)," *American Reform Responsa*, 272-274.

31. CCAR, "Responsum 5754.14. On the Treatment of the Terminally Ill," *Teshuvot for the Nineties*, 349, 352-353.

32. Joanne Lynn, M.D. and Joan Harrold, M.D., *Handbook for Mortals: Guidance for People Facing Serious Illness* (New York: Oxford, 1999), 130.

33. Rosner, *Modern Medicine*, 240, 242.

34. Ibid., 234.

35. Rabbi Zev Schostak, "Jewish Ethical Guidelines for Resuscitation and Artificial Nutrition and Hydration of the Dying Elderly," *Journal of Medical Ethics* 20:3 (June 1994): 97-98; Rabbi Zev Schostak, "Ethical Guidelines for Treatment of the Dying Elderly," *The Journal of Halacha and Contemporary Society*, no. 22 (1991): 83-84.

36. Daniel Eisenberg, M.D., "Halachic Issues Regarding the Futility of Medical Treatment: Applications to Nutrition and Hydration in The Terminally Ill Patient," available from the website of The Institute for Jewish Medical Ethics (http://wwv.ijme.org).

37. Reisner, "A Halakhic Ethic," 63.

38. Dorff, *Matters of Life and Death*, 208-217; Dorff, "A Jewish Approach," 34-39.

39. CCAR "Responsum 5754.14. On the Treatment of the Terminally Ill," *Teshuvot for the Nineties*, 353-354.

40. CCAR, "Responsum 5750.5. Hospital Patient Beyond Recovery," *Teshuvot for the Nineties*, 365-369. See also CCAR, "Responsa 78. Euthanasia (1950)," *American Reform Responsa*, 263.

41. CCAR, "Responsum 159. Nutrition and Incurable Cancer (1991)," *Questions and Reform Jewish Answers*, 263-264; CCAR, "Responsum 77. Allowing a Terminal Patient to Die (1969)," *American Reform Responsa*, 259-260.

42. CCAR, "Responsum 159. Nutrition and Incurable Cancer (1991)," *Questions and Reform Jewish Answers*, 264.

43. CCAR, "Responsum 5754.14. On the Treatment of the Terminally Ill," *Teshuvot for the Ninties*, 355.

44. David Major, M.D. "The Medical Procedures for Providing Food and Water: Indications and Effects," in *By No Extraordinary Means: The Choice to Forego Life-Sustaining Food and Water*, ed. Joanne Lynn, M.D. (Bloomington, Ind.: Indiana University, 1989) 24-26; Council on Ethical and Judicial Affairs, American Medical Association, "Decisions Near the End of Life," *Journal of the American Medical Association* 267:16 (April 1992): 2230-2231; Jerry O. Ciocon et al, "Tube Feedings in Elderly Patients: Indications, Benefits, and Complications," *Archives of Internal Medicine* 148:2 (February 1988): 429-433.

45. David Eddy, "A Conversation with My Mother," *Journal of American Medical Association* 272:3 (July 1994): 179-181.

46. The Hastings Center, *Guidelines on the Termination of Life-Sustaining Treatment and the Care of the Dying* (Bloomington, Ind.: Indiana University, 1987), 60.

47. Paul C. Rousseau, "How Fluid Deprivation Affects the Terminally Ill," *RN* 54:1 (January 1991): 73-76.

48. Lynn and Harrold, *Handbook for Mortals*, 133. See also Ira Byock, "Patient Refusal of Nutrition and Hydration: Walking the Ever-Finer Line," *The American Journal of Hospice & Palliative Care* 12:2 (March/April 1995): 8-13; James L. Bernat, Bernard Gert, and R. Peter Mogielnicki, "Patient Refusal of Hydration and Nutrition: An Alternative to Physician-Assisted Suicide or Voluntary Active Euthanasia," *Archives of Internal Medicine* 153:24 (December 1993): 2723-2728; Robert J. Sullivan, "Accepting Death Without Artificial Nutrition or Hydration," *Journal of General Internal Medicine* 8:4 (April 1993): 220-224.

49. Phyllis Schmitz and Merry O'Brien, "Observations on Nutrition and Hydration in Dying Cancer Patients," in *By No Extraordinary Means*, 36; Joanne Lynn and James F. Childress, "Must Patients Always Be Given Food and Water?" in *By No Extraordinary Means*, 52-53; Louise A. Printz, "Terminal Dehydration: A Compassionate Treatment," *Archives of Internal Medicine* 154:4 (April 1992): 697-700; J. Andrew Billings, "Comfort Measures for the Terminally Ill: Is Dehydration Painful?," *Journal of the American Geriatrics Society* 33:11 (November 1985): 808-810.

50. Shannon Brownlee and Joannie M. Schrof, "The Quality of Mercy," *U.S. News and World Report*, 17 March 1997, 57.

51. Timothy E. Quill and Robert V. Brody, "'You Promised Me I Wouldn't Die Like This!' A Bad Death as a Medical Emergency," *Archives of Internal Medicine* 155:12 (June 1995): 1251.

52. The double effect principle is discussed in detail by Tom L. Beauchamp and James F. Childress, *Principles of Biomedical Ethics*, 4th ed. (New York: Oxford University Press, 1994), 206-211.

53. Sinclair, *Tradition and the Biological Revolution*, 78.

54. Bleich, *Bioethical Dilemmas*, 75-76; Bleich, *Judaism and Healing*, 137-138; Bleich, "Treatment," 62. See also Rosner, *Modern Medicine*, 209.

55. Bleich, *Bioethical Dilemmas*, 63; Bleich, *Judaism and Healing*, 135-136.

56. Reisner, "A Halakhic Ethic," 66.

57. Dorff, *Matters of Life and Death*, 185-186, 373-374 n. 31; Elliot N. Dorff, "*Teshuvah* on Assisted Suicide," *Conservative Judaism*, 50:4 (1998): 8.

58. CCAR, "Responsum 83. Quality of Life and Euthanasia (1985)," in Walter Jacobs, *Contemporary American Reform Responsa* (New York: CCAR, 1987), 140; CCAR, "Responsum 151. Drugs To Relieve Pain (1991)," *Questions and Reform Jewish Answers*, 239-241. See also CCAR, "Responsum 5754.14. On the Treatment of the Terminally Ill," *Teshuvot for the Nineties*, 343-344; CCAR, "Responsum 76. Relieving Pain of a Dying Patient (1975)," *American Reform Responsa*, 255-257; CCAR, "Responsum 79. Euthanasia (1980),"; ibid., 274.

59. The SUPPORT Principal Investigators, "A Controlled Trial to Improve Care for Seriously Ill Hospitalized Patients: The Study to Understand Prognoses and Preferences for Outcomes and Risks of Treatments (SUPPORT)," *Journal of the American Medical Association* 274:20 (November 1995): 1591-1598.

60. Timothy E. Quill, Bernard Lo, and Dan W. Brock, "Palliative Options of Last Resort: A Comparison of Voluntarily Stopping Eating and Drinking, Terminal Sedation, Physician-Assisted Suicide, and Voluntary Active Euthanasia," *Journal of the American Medical Association* 278:23 (December 1997): 2099-2104.

61. Vittorio Ventafridda et al. "Symptom Prevalence and Control During Cancer Patients' Last Days of Life," *Journal of Palliative Care* 6:3 (1990): 7-11 report that 63 out of 120 advanced cancer patients needed sedation to unconsciousness.

However, in another study only 16 of 100 patients required some type of sedation to achieve pain and symptom relief. Robin Fainsinger et al, "Symptom Contol During the Last Week of Life in a Palliative Care Unit," *Journal of Palliative Care* 7:1 (March 1991): 5-11.

Chapter 6

Facing a Life Threatening or a Chronic Illness: The Jewish Tradition and End of Life Decisions

Facing a life threatening illness, knowing that you are dying or chronically ill, is difficult. It strikes terror in your heart.

There is no medical definition of a "terminal" illness. You probably know someone who outlived a physician's prognosis of the time left. Doctors cannot be certain when our earthly time is "short." Sometimes it is difficult to pinpoint exactly when an illness is terminal and when it is likely to be fatal. With a terminal illness, you go downhill. It is only a matter of time from the diagnosis to death. On the other hand, a chronic condition, whether physical or mental, generally does not progress quickly to death. However, with any illness trajectories can change abruptly; patients can encounter a sudden spiral downward.

With advanced heart disease, the most common cause of death in United States, physicians have difficulty predicting patients' life spans. Sufferers usually face a severely impaired existence for one or two years at the end stage. It is often a roller-coaster existence, with life threatening episodes interspersed between relatively tranquil periods. Some patients live longer than their physicians expect.

With cancer, physicians can tell with more certainty when one becomes terminal and roughly but still not with a high degree of accuracy how long he or she might live. Again, physicians' guesses may be less than accurate.

Chronic, irreversible neurological conditions, such as Lou Gehrig's or Alzheimer's disease, are particularly tragic. It is difficult to determine when the condition becomes terminal. Lou Gehrig's disease, a deadly neurological illness, slowly but inexorably eats away nerves and atrophies muscles. The nerves serving the large muscle groups, arms, legs, and mouth die first. Next are the nerves controlling swallowing and breathing. As each neural pathway shuts down, there is ever increasing anguish. Victims become completely paralyzed, they cannot move, eat, swallow or breathe, but their mind remains completely alert. The disease usually runs its course in three to five years.

Patients in the late stages of Alzheimer's disease, a progressive, presently incurable, neurological disorder, usually of the elderly, lose substantially all memory of their earlier lives. As the condition progresses they generally cannot, except occasionally and in a fragmented way, recognize others. Often they cannot remember the names of family members. They are typically incontinent, unable to walk, incapable of saying more than one or two words. Victims lose the capacity to think about their lives; they cannot plan or have projects. Death occurs in a debilitated, immobile state.

When you are diagnosed with a terminal illness or chronic, degenerative condition disease, as discussed in Chapter 1, most of us become afraid of dying in pain, being left alone, being hooked up to life-support equipment in a hospital, becoming dependent on others, facing hopelessness and a very poor quality of life, and becoming a burden by running up medical bills that may bankrupt our family. We are worried about experiencing anguishing deaths ending up on high tech machines, powerless to determine our own treatment.

Whatever your fears are regarding your impending physical and mental deterioration and the accompanying pain and suffering, you often in fact become increasingly dependent on others for your intimate physical care. The loss of control may become unbearable. Your life may become devoid of meaningful activity. You face the possibility of an intolerable end of life, accompanied by physical, emotional and spiritual suffering. Continued invasive treatments can also be uncomfortable and disheartening, compounding your plight.

When you or a loved one faces a terminal or a degenerative chronic illness, thinking about hastening death often hits home. It becomes an urgent question. You or a beloved may be so despairing that you want to end it all -- now or at least before you or your dear one face one or more protracted periods of hospitalization or a long spell of dependency.

You may think of killing yourself -- suicide -- or having someone else do it, seeking physician-assisted suicide or voluntary active euthanasia. Suicide connotes taking your own life in your own way and at your own time. Uncertainty surrounds a do-it-yourself suicide. There is a fear of a botched, "homemade" attempt. The dosages of drugs can be inexact; they may not stay down. Weakened, terminally ill patients may be unable to end their lives by their own hands.

In a physician-assisted suicide, a doctor writes a prescription for a lethal dose of a drug which you, the patient, must take. Thus, your physician knows you may use the means he or she supplied to kill yourself.

With a physician-assisted suicide, patients may lack courage to do it or the drug may not work. Because self-administration is not always effective, the attempt may fail and leave one worse off then before if, for example, brain damage occurs. The dose of pills may be insufficient. Sufferers may vomit up some or all of the medication. Damaging physical and psychological consequences likely follow from the failure for patients, their families, and their physicians. By the time they are ready to end their lives, some may be physically unable to do so; they may be too feeble to take the pills. In other words, physician-assisted suicide is limited to those physically capable of taking medication themselves. It will not help those who have an illness preventing them from swallowing and keeping down the pills.

Also, death may not come quickly in the case of physician-assisted suicides. There may be longer than acceptable time between taking the lethal drug and death. It is a difficult time for loved ones, even if they are not present. They will have difficulty in going about their normal business, eating or sleeping until they know it is over.

These considerations naturally lead some to request more active physician intervention: voluntary active euthanasia. Voluntary active euthanasia represents the act of killing someone else who wants to die. A physician carries out the final step typically by administering a quick and effective fatal injection. Patients do not need the ability to swallow, manual dexterity, or a functioning gastrointestinal system. Thus, the difference between physician-assisted suicide and voluntary active euthanasia turns on who administers the lethal dose: the sufferer in a physician-assisted suicide, or the physician who intentionally kills a passive patient by giving a lethal injection in the case of voluntary active euthanasia.

When facing a terminal illness or a chronic condition, not everyone thinks of ending it or actually does. Consider the world-renowned cosmologist, Sir Stephen W. Hawking.[1] Although obviously brilliant, he was not a good student. As an undergraduate at Oxford University in England, he nearly failed out because he did not apply himself to his studies. He cultivated the less-than-noble image of being lazy and overly fond of alcohol. Soon after starting in a doctoral program in physics at Cambridge University, he was diagnosed with Lou Gehrig's disease. Hawking's physician gave him a death sentence, telling him he had at the most about two years to live. Although his mind remained intact, during his physical decline, his body deteriorated in fits and starts. His motor coordination worsened. He lost his ability to hold a pen; then he lost the ability to walk; as his speech slurred, he could no longer lecture.

Yet Hawking found meaning in his life, beyond what he had previously regarded as a "pointless existence." He got engaged and seriously plunged into his doctoral program. Now, nearly thirty years later, Hawking, having revolutionized the field of cosmology, is still alive. His condition progressed much more slowly than generally is the case. He has minimal use of his hands, with which he operates a motorized wheelchair and a computer-driven voice synthesizer; the rest of his body is basically immobile.

Maintaining a positive attitude, Hawking did not lose hope. Once while in a hospital, Hawkins saw a boy he vaguely knew die of leukemia in the bed opposite to him. The experience left a lasting impression. There were people worse off than he was. Hawking's condition did not make him feel depressed. "Whenever I feel inclined to be sorry for myself," Hawking recalled, "I remember that boy."

Not everyone is like Stephen Hawking, either in terms of our abilities or our reaction to the diagnosis of a terminal illness or a chronic condition. Not everyone finds meaning in suffering or is able to be a "good sport" about his or her physical or mental plight.

After presenting two examples of physician-assisted suicide, this chapter discusses the American legal background and the Jewish tradition's approach to suicide and physician-aided death. The chapter urges allowing physicians to help patients achieve a peaceful and dignified death. If a sufferer wants to accelerate the dying process at a chosen time and manner, a physician, who aids one to accomplish his or her demise acts compassionately, in accordance with the virtues of Spiritual Judaism. Quality of life considerations do and should enter into end of life decision-making. As discussed at the end of this chapter, from the perspective of Spiritual Judaism, we must frame the issue, particularly, our consideration of the sanctity of biological life principle, in terms of our immortal soul, not our mere physical existence.

Facing a Terminal or Chronic Illness: Examples of Physician-Assisted Suicide

Let's take two examples of physician-assisted suicide, one involving Diane, a terminally ill cancer patient, and another, Janet Atkins, an Alzheimer's sufferer. These two put in perspective the terror facing those who are terminally or chronically ill.

Diane's death was imminent. She chose not to live through two or three more weeks of diminishing consciousness and control. Although not terminally ill, Janet Atkins did not want to be condemned to a life of increasing dementia and loss of personality. Diane made a choice over weeks; Janet over years and years.

In 1991, Timothy E. Quill, M.D., published an account of Diane, a forty-five-year-old artist, who had been a patient of his for eight years, during which time he had seen her through alcohol abuse and recovery as well as watching her return to creative work.[2] Then Diane developed acute leukemia. Without treatment, the disease would kill her within a few months, a classic case of a terminal illness. The recommended therapy consisted of an intensive form of chemotherapy, followed by a bone-marrow transplantation. The probability that she would survive the intervention and recover was no better than 25 percent.

After thinking about these procedures, Diane decided not to go ahead with them. The chances of long-term survival, she concluded, were not worth enduring so severe a course of treatment.

Some days later, Diane told Dr. Quill that she was worried about the prospect of dying slowly. She feared a loss of control and becoming totally dependent. Diane expressed a desire for his assistance with suicide which she made clear after her decision not to have chemotherapy. She asked for enough sleeping pills to kill herself when the time came. Although she discussed the subject openly with Dr. Quill, her specific request was that he prescribe "barbiturates for sleep." Rather than writing the prescription under the cover of responding to her insomnia, he insisted that Diane discuss her plans with him. Dr. Quill probed to make sure she was not irrationally depressed. He concluded that if he did not help her she would become preoccupied with how she might die and would be unable to make the most of the time she had left. He wrote out a prescription for barbiturates. He took pains to inform Diane of the amount needed for sleep and that the dose would be lethal.

Diane, an "incredibly clear, at times brutally honest thinker and communicator," lived another three months with her family around her, a time described by Dr. Quill as "very intense and important for Diane." She spent these months in a hospice program where she received the best that comfort care had to offer. She was wonderfully supported by her husband and her son. Her closest friends regularly saw her. Then, she began to decline rapidly. High fevers persisted despite antibiotics; her weakness progressed despite repeated blood transfusions; the leukemia gradually invaded her skin, which became red and swollen.

Diane saw Dr. Quill one last time. As Quill remembered: "When we met, it was clear that she knew what she was doing, that she was sad and frightened to be leaving, but that she would be even more terrified to stay and suffer."

Two days later, Diane's husband called Dr. Quill to say she said her final good-byes to him and her son that morning. She asked them to leave her alone for an hour. When they returned, she had died. As Quill recalled, "There was no sign of struggle. She seemed to be at peace."

Those encountering nonterminal, chronic situations, involving the gradual deterioration of bodily functions, such as Lou Gehrig's disease, multiple sclerosis, Parkinson's disease, or lupus, not once, but every day must continue to make the choice between hope and despair, between life-and-death. Some of those who suffer from incapacitating neurological diseases, characterized by the deterioration of mental capacities, but who, unlike Diane, are not terminally ill, want to end their anguish rather than having it prolonged.

Janet Adkins, 54 years old, who had taught English at a community college and gave piano lessons at home, faced the early stages of Alzheimer's disease in 1989.[3] She was able to speak quite coherently and play tennis but could not read a book. She could still beat her thirty-two-year-old son at tennis but was unable to keep score. Although she might live another ten years or more, she knew what was coming. In the final phase of Alzheimer's, which can last several years, she would be unable to recognize or communicate with anyone. Her mind would be gone. She would be huddled in bed, debilitated in mind and body.

After trying an experimental, pharmacological treatment which failed, Janet decided she did not want to live a life of progressive mental degeneration. She talked with her minister. Her cognitive ability and independence gave her life its meaning and without which she had no desire to live. As her husband recalled, "Her mind was her life."

Hearing about Dr. Jack Kevorkian's poison-injecting machine, she contacted him and in 1990 became his first assisted suicide. Dr. Kevorkian discussed with Janet her desire to die. He asked Janet to get her doctor in Oregon to send him her medical records. After studying them, Kevorkian, a pathologist, agreed to help Janet.

In June 1990, Janet came to Michigan with her husband, Ron, and her sons. Dr. Kevorkian met them in a motel room and videotaped his conversation with Janet and her husband. On the tape, she smiled and chuckled from time to time. She spoke of things she could no longer do and her desire to "get out with dignity." She satisfied Dr. Kevorkian that she was of sound mind, had reflected on the matter, and wished to die.

The Adkins family spent the night thinking things over once again. Janet had not changed her mind and the family expressed their support for her decision. The next afternoon, Janet met Dr. Kevorkian again and told him she wanted to go ahead.

Dr. Kevorkian had installed a bed in the back of his old Volkswagen van. He drove the van to a public campsite. Inside the van, Janet rested on the bed made with clean sheets and a pillow, hidden behind windows draped with curtains. He put an intravenous line into her arm and explained what she had to do. A harmless mix of water and salt flowed down the line. Janet pushed a button that changed the fluid to a sedative and started a timing device allowing a lethal infusion of potassium chloride to flow into the drip. As a result of the sedative, Janet fell into a deep sleep. After the potassium chloride took effect, her heart stopped.

American Legal Background

As we reflect on suicide, physician-assisted suicide, and voluntary active euthanasia, you should be aware of legal aspects of each of these alternatives in the United States. As we will see, although physician-assisted suicide is legal in Oregon, subject to specific restrictions, physician-assisted suicide and voluntary active euthanasia are otherwise illegal throughout the United States.

Suicide

Suicide or attempted suicide is no longer a criminal offense in any state. Suicide has been decriminalized for a variety of reasons. It is impossible to prosecute or punish a dead person. It is also unfair to deprive an innocent family of their possessions. We want to avoid stigmatizing the person and his or her family. The concept of personal autonomy plays out here. We recognize that people should have the freedom to end their lives. It is a fundamental liberty to decide when and how to exit life.

However, in thirty-five states assisted suicide is expressly illegal by statute and in seven more and the District of Columbia, it is, by judicial decision, a common law crime. The legal status of assisting a suicide remains unclear in the other states.[4] These legal barriers are sufficiently severe to discourage many family members and physicians from assisting those who want to take their lives.

As suicide moved to the province of healthcare professionals, the public stigma of suicide also decreased. Most suicides in the United States result from temporary mental aberrations, from an array of emotional illnesses, especially depression or mood disorders, or from addiction problems.

Despite decriminalization, we remain ambivalent about suicide. Suicide is still deemed inappropriate. Life insurance policies contain a standard clause limiting or nullifying coverage if a policyholder commits suicide. Many states have statutes allowing individuals considered to be a suicide risk to be taken into custody and confined, typically in a mental health facility, until the risk is judged not likely.

Physician-Assisted Suicide and Voluntary Active Euthanasia

In 1997, the United States Supreme Court held that laws in Washington State and New York prohibiting physician-assisted suicide were constitutional.[5] Although unable to identify a constitutional right for individuals to request a physician's help in dying, the High Court gave the green light to public discussion and experimentation at the state level through the legislative and referendum processes. Currently, physician-assisted suicide is illegal in every state except Oregon. Also, the Assisted Suicide Funding Restriction Act of 1997 prohibits the expenditure or use of federal funds in support of any type of physician-assisted death.[6] Unless you are a resident of Oregon, a physician who knowingly prescribes lethal pills for you to take to kill yourself engages in an illegal activity, assisting in your suicide.

Oregon, through its Death with Dignity Act,[7] has taken the lead in legalizing physician-assisted suicide for its residents only, thereby preventing others from traveling to that state to seek physician aid-in-dying. Oregon requires that patients be mentally capable of making the choice and that they make this decision voluntarily without pressure from family or healthcare providers. Specifically, patients must be told by their physician that they have an incurable and irreversible disease that will, within reasonable medical judgment, produce death in six months. Their attending physician must advise them not only of the diagnosis and prognosis but also of feasible treatment alternatives. The medical diagnosis must be confirmed by another physician. Patients must be mentally capable and act voluntarily at the time of their request. There must be no evidence of any emotional disorder, clinical depression causing impaired judgment, or untreated pain or other physical symptoms. They must make two oral requests and a written request, witnessed by two other individuals, for help in dying. A 15-day waiting period between oral requests is designed to ensure that sufferers definitely want to die. The second oral request must be followed by a written directive and a further 48-hour wait before a physician can provide a prescription. Patients must take the physician-prescribed lethal drug without a doctor's help. Finally, the prescribing physician must send certain documents to the Oregon Health Division.

Engaging in voluntary active euthanasia is, at present, illegal in every state, including Oregon. Not only is it a crime, it is also a breach of a physician's professional ethics that may be the basis for disciplinary action, including the loss of a medical license.

A Reality Check

Practice of physician aid-in-dying, although mostly hidden, occurs daily in various forms throughout United States. Physicians write legal prescriptions for sedatives and painkillers, thinking, suspecting, and even knowing, as did Dr. Quill, that a patient may consume them to end his or her life. Doctors quietly help patients die. It is underground; it is "hush-hush."

In a chapter entitled, "How Do You Get the Magic Pills," Derek

Humphry in *The Final Exit*,[8] a how-to-do-it best selling manual, describing various methods of suicide, tells sufferers how to fool physicians into prescribing lethal quantities of prescription drugs by lying about insomnia or finding a cooperative medical practitioner. Humphry suggests the use of Dramamine or alcohol to prevent vomiting the suicide drugs. He also recommends having a plastic bag in abeyance to put over one's head as a fail-safe back up to the pills. In the twenty-first century, access to the Internet furthers the availability of this type of self-help information.

At the risk of violating legal and professional standards, thereby subjecting themselves to criminal and disciplinary sanctions, including the loss of medical licenses and suspension of hospital privileges, clandestine assistance in dying has been and continues to be a common, but hidden, medical practice. Physicians take these risks knowing that coroners rarely perform autopsies, especially on "older" persons. Loved ones refuse to disclose their involvement in physician-aided deaths for legal reasons or to protect others from knowing how the end actually occurred. In short, the assisted nature of many a demise is hidden to protect those involved.

We do not know the exact extent of assisted dying in the United States -- women with metastatic breast cancer, men with advanced prostate cancer, elderly suffering from chronic, degenerative conditions or terminal illnesses. Patients find the means of killing themselves quietly at home. This is typically done without counseling and lacks a full assessment and discussion of the realistic alternatives.

Many studies show the existence of a national pattern of underground physician-assisted suicide and even voluntary active euthanasia. Although the exact number of medical doctors who have in some way assisted their patients die remains shrouded in mystery, as does the number of physician-aided deaths, it is already being done. A significant number of physicians in the United States knowingly and deliberately help their patients die. Anonymous polls show that 13 to 19% of all American doctors participated in a physician-assisted suicide; 2 to 13% provided voluntary active euthanasia on request.[9] This is borne out by national, regional and state specific surveys.

The authors of a national study, based on 1902 completed questionnaires received from physicians in ten specialties in which doctors were likely to receive patients' requests for assistance with suicide or euthanasia, concluded that physician-aided deaths are "not rare."[10] A little more than 3% of respondents indicated they had written prescriptions for lethal drugs mostly for patients who had less than six months to live. Just under 5% said they administered fatal injections to patients on their death beds. Overall, about 6.4% of physicians surveyed reported having complied with at least one request for physician-assisted suicide or voluntary active euthanasia.

A similar pattern surfaces in four regional and state-specific surveys. In a survey of 355 New England oncologists, almost one in seven (13.5%) said they participated in an assisted suicide; 1.8% provided a lethal injection.[11] Nearly one in five (18%) of Michigan oncologists surveyed acceded to a request for a prescription for a lethal dose of medication; 4% provided a fatal injection.[12] A study of physicians caring for patients with AIDS in the San Francisco Bay Area showed 53% of the 117 respondents had granted, at least once, the request of a terminally ill AIDS patient for assistance in ending his or her life.[13] A survey of 1443 Washington State physicians showed that over a one year period they complied with about one quarter (24%, 38 of 156) of all patient requests for physician-assisted suicide. Of 58 patients who asked for euthanasia, 14 received lethal injections from their physicians.[14]

With this legal background in mind and recognizing that physician-assisted suicide and voluntary active euthanasia, together with the assistance provided by family members and friends, occur more frequently than most of us realize, without any guidelines or safeguards, let's examine the overwhelming opposition of modern Jewish commentators to these practices.

The Jewish Tradition and Physician Aid-in-Dying

When discussing physician-assisted suicide and voluntary active euthanasia, contemporary Jewish authorities reach a nearly unanimous conclusion, a resounding "No." Under Jewish religious law and ethics, any form of physician aid-in-dying is prohibited and forbidden as acts of murder, based on one of the Ten Commandments (Exodus 20:13, 21:14; Leviticus 24:17, 24:21; Deuteronomy 5:17). Jewish sages expressed a similar conclusion in the Babylonian Talmud (Sanhedrin 78a).

According to traditionalists, no one has the right to destroy God's property, a biological life. Lord Jakobovits put it rather starkly: "There is no question, therefore, to Judaism, of the absolute and unconditional opposition to any form of direct or active euthanasia, of deliberately hastening the end. . . . Any physician deliberately causing a patient to die, under whatever conditions of debility or suffering, is regarded as committed an act of first degree murder. Nor would any account whatsoever be taken of the wishes of the patient."[15] Physician Fred Rosner and Rabbi Moshe D. Tendler similarly conclude: "Judaism condemns any deliberate induction of death, and considers it an act of murder, even if the patient requests it. Life is not ours to terminate."[16]

Conservative and Reform authorities echo a similar theme. Conservative Rabbi Elliot N. Dorff writes, in a responsum adopted by the Conservative Movement's Committee on Jewish Law and Standards, that aiding a suicide is forbidden, whether the assistance provides the means for the patient to commit suicide thereby making it possible for the patient to do what is forbidden or knowingly administering a lethal drug with the intent of bringing about a person's demise thereby murdering the victim. Dorff concludes: "The tradition bids us . . . to maintain a firm line separating permissible withholding and withdrawal of medical efforts, on the one hand, and illegitimately helping a person actively to take his or her own life, on the other. To fail to do that would be to violate Jewish law and to destroy creatures belonging to God . . . . Judaism . . . requires us to evaluate our lives in light of the ultimate value in us because we were created in God's image. Jewish ideology and law therefore strongly oppose committing suicide or assisting others in doing so, for life is sacred regardless of its quality or usefulness."[17]

Likewise, one Reform responsum states, "To abridge in some positive and direct manner the duration of life by a single second is tantamount to the shedding of blood."[18] In reaching this conclusion, the Reform rabbis rely on the Babylonian Talmud (Shabbat 151b), which provides, "Our Rabbis taught: One who closes [the eyes of a dying person] at the point of death is a murderer. This may be compared to a lamp that is going out: If a man places his finger upon it, it is immediately extinguished." They also cite the Talmudic example of Rabbi Hanina ben Teradyon, previously discussed in Chapter 5, who was condemned by the Romans to be burned at the stake in the second century C.E. His disciples counseled him to let the consuming flames surge into his body and put a speedy end to his suffering. The celebrated martyr is reported to have said: "It is best that the Eternal Who has given the soul should take it away; let no person hasten his or her own death." (Babylonian Talmud Avodah Zarah 18a).

As you will see, analysis of Jewish views on physician-assisted suicide and voluntary active euthanasia, focusing on the mainstream views of the Orthodox, Conservative, and Reform movements, points to a consensus when it comes to mercy killing. All agree that Jewish law prohibits any action designed to actively take a person's life. However, a small number of commentators view physician-assisted suicide and voluntary active euthanasia in a different light.[19] Before discussing physician-aided death, let's first consider the traditional prohibition against suicide set forth in Jewish law as well as the exceptions to the general rule.

The General Prohibition in the Jewish Tradition Against Suicide and Its Exceptions

Overwhelmingly, Jewish commentators firmly state that suicide represents an act of murder under Jewish law. This long-standing prohibition is strongly rooted in Judaism's fundamental value of human life and the Jewish tradition's affirmation of the sanctity of existence considered in Chapter 2, based on the assumption that the biological life of each of us belongs to God Who retains the ultimate say regarding its termination. However, other considerations come into play, including taking one's life in circumstances of martyrdom or while under mental and physical stress, giving rise to exceptions to the anti-suicide rule.

Traditionally, Jewish law has prohibited suicide as a forbidden act of murder -- the murder of oneself. Writers of the Jewish law codes, looked to the Book of Genesis (9:5) where God states: "If anyone takes human life, he or she will be punished."

The traditional and liberal branches of Judaism continue to object strongly to suicide.[20] Suicide is prohibited under Jewish law because it is said to violate our respect for human life and God's ownership of our bodies. The Eternal endowed biological life with inestimable value by creating humans in the Divine image. In return, we must take care of our lives and our health; however, the proprietary interest in our physical bodies remains with God, the Owner. Thus, the argument runs, a person may not intentionally harm or destroy what belongs to the Holy One.

Taking one's life goes against the Eternal's will. As the author of the Book of Deuteronomy tells us in a statement attributed to God: "I [God] will kill and I give life." (Deuteronomy 32:39). Suicide usurps the Eternal's power over life-and-death, representing the Supreme Sovereign's decision, not ours. A person who takes his or her own life is said to renounce a belief in the Divine creation of the world and of humanity and, according to Jewish sages, has no share in the afterlife World to Come, previously considered in Chapter 3.

Some traditional authorities maintain that suicide is in many ways even more tragic than homicide.[21] By killing oneself, the perpetrator dispenses with any future possible earthly repentance for violating God's laws. The perpetrator is dead and unable to atone for his or her actions. Apart from certain exceptions, a person who commits suicide, according to Jewish commentators, must answer to God's judgment in the World to Come as a murderer and as one who denies the Divine ownership of his or her body.

Under Jewish law, however, suicide is permitted in certain instances, namely, to avoid idolatry, sexual transgressions, or murder.[22] Numerous examples exist of suicide as a form of martyrdom where the goal is not simply to end life but to accomplish some greater objective. In these situations, taking one's life testifies to God's sovereignty by preventing the defilement of the Eternal's name. For example, the Babylonian Talmud (Gittin 57b) speaks in praise of four hundred boys and girls who committed mass suicide, by jumping into the sea, when they realized the Romans had captured them for immoral purposes. Their martyrdom represented the sanctification of the Divine name, a symbol of their utmost faith in God; therefore, their action was regarded as praiseworthy.

Furthermore, an exception to the general prohibition against suicide in Jewish law exists for suicides occurring as a result of "overpowering" or "extraordinary" circumstances, including extreme mental or physical stress. One Reform responsum cites authorities who maintained that the act of taking one's own life "to escape extreme pain and degradation" is, in fact, not a suicide. Such a person has been forced to act by "overpowering circumstances."[23]

King Saul's attempt to commit suicide represents a notable historical example. The Hebrew Bible, in I Samuel 31:1-6, tells the story of King Saul's defeat by the Philistines. On seeing his three sons slain and his army defeated, King Saul knew that the end was also near for him. He asked his armorbearer to kill him. When the armorbearer refused, King Saul fell on his own sword. As we'll see later in this chapter, what happened afterwards is not clear and remains subject to various interpretations. However, it is clear, at the very least, that King Saul attempted to commit suicide. The usual explanation permits King Saul's act under the "unusual circumstances" rubric. King Saul neither wanted to be taken prisoner nor did he want to be tortured by the Philistines. His act was viewed as forgivable and pardonable.

Beyond these exceptions to the general prohibition against suicide in Jewish law, authorities have focused on the concept of "intentionality," specifically whether those who commit suicide under extreme physical or mental strain and anguish are "wilful" suicides. The Jerusalem Talmud (Semachot 2:2) defines suicide as the rational, premeditated, intentional taking of one's life. Thus, under Jewish law, suicide occurs when an adult, with a clear mind, who previously announced his or her intention, kills himself or herself by the method he or she declared earlier. A suicide, calmly and with explicit resolve, calls out: "Look, I am going to the top of the roof and will jump off that I may die." When others see him or her go up to the top of the roof, after announcing his or her certain intention, and immediately plunge to his or her death, he or she is considered to have committed suicide. Thus, the concept of a suicide requires an unambiguous, intentional act, by a rational adult, who is neither under the influence of alcohol or drugs nor mentally ill.

Conservative Rabbi Dorff amplifies the concept of intentionality. He notes that modern Jewish authorities assert that the term "suicide" encompasses only those with "competence of mind and freedom of will."[24] Thus, those who suffer from (or who are presumed to suffer from) temporary insanity cannot commit suicide; they lack the requisite intentionality and wilfulness. Although maintaining that Jewish law prohibits suicide, traditionalist Rosner also concludes that people "under extreme physical or mental strain" or "not in full possession of their faculties" are not "wilful" suicides.[25] Because the definition of "wilful" is so detailed and specific, only rare cases come within it.

Traditionally, Jewish law prohibited the performance of mourning rites, such as rending garments, delivering eulogies, and performing other rituals after burial, for one who committed suicide, a determined act of self-destruction. Despite these strictures, an intentional suicide could be buried in a Jewish cemetery but at least six feet from any other graves, often near a cemetery's border.[26]

Over the centuries, Judaism has evidenced a willingness to grant ever greater rights of burial and mourning for those who took their own lives, by excluding from the definition of suicide those suffering from depression or temporary insanity, those under the influence of alcohol or drugs, or those motivated by extreme suffering or terrible anxiety.[27] Although increasingly allowing a Jewish burial and the performance of mourning rituals,[28] including a eulogy, for suicides, Jewish commentators continue to regard the act of suicide as unacceptable.

Thus, while contemporary Jewish authorities conclude that Jewish law, subject to limited exceptions, condemns suicide, a distinct minority notes that suicide is permissible when "continuing to live violates a fundamental principle of what life is all about."[29] These progressive Jewish commentators are concerned about one's anguish. In instances of extreme, unmitigated pain and suffering, suicide, they urge, should exist as an option, at least for the terminally ill.

Reform Rabbi Peter Knobel advocates the decriminalization of suicide in Jewish law.[30] According to Knobel, Jewish law in the twenty-first century should place suicide in the category of acts that are not valid at first, but that are valid after the fact. Knobel does not argue that Judaism should approve of suicide as a mode of ending one's life. Rather, he points out that a difference exists between "may" and "should." He emphasizes that Judaism always will have a preference for life over death. His point, however, is that in order to allow one to die speedily so as to lessen his or her suffering and humiliation, Jewish law, in evidencing more compassion in dealing with those who are terminally ill, should acquiesce in one's suicide under these circumstances.

In case of a terminal illness, accompanied by incessant pain and suffering, a patient, according to Knobel, should have the option of ending his or her life. This action should not only be permissible but may in fact be praiseworthy.[31] Under this analysis, ending one's life is viewed as making a statement about one's dignity and one's beliefs. Humans may choose not to continue to suffer from debilitating and extremely painful conditions or diseases diminishing their understanding of what it means to be created in God's image.

Knobel analogizes the biblical and rabbinic examples of martyrdom to the present-day anguish faced by some terminally ill patients. He maintains that sometimes these sufferers are subject to endless numbers of ineffective, but invasive, interventions. When syringes and tubes become too much for a patient, these modern day, aggressive medical treatments become implements of torture. Knobel compares the condition of some today to the plight of King Saul, who, as we have just seen, was mortally wounded in battle. Looking around and seeing that his army had been defeated, Saul realized that the Philistines were about to capture him. He attempted to commit suicide in order to escape torture and the indignities the Philistines planned for him. King Saul thought that living was not in his best interests. He chose death to suffering.

From the example of the children in the Babylonian Talmud, anticipatory suffering may present a justifiable reason for preemptive suicide. At the time the four hundred children committed suicide, they did not presently suffer. They foresaw indignities and a "life of shame," but had experienced neither. From this tragic story, progressive Jewish commentators conclude that anticipated suffering certain to result in death may present a sufficient justification for taking one's life. Thus, one may choose to commit suicide in a preemptive manner prior to the foreseeable end of one's life.

Physician-Assisted Suicide and Voluntary Active Euthanasia in the Jewish Tradition

As discussed in Chapter 1, new medical realities bring into focus society's ethical and religious beliefs concerning dying and death. Some argue that authorities from the past could not have foreseen today's medical developments. Ancient thinkers about life-and-death had no idea that second half of the twentieth century would, among other examples, bring mechanical means to replace bodily functions. Others argue that prolonging patients' lives with technology and drugs is cruel and inhumane. Hence, proponents for physician-assisted suicide and voluntary active euthanasia have coined the term "mercy killing."

Although Jewish authorities, across the spectrum of the Jewish tradition, appreciate the difficult dilemmas patients face, they all come to the same conclusion -- opposition to any form of mercy killing or physician aid-in-dying. For example, in reaffirming the sanctity of biological life and the supreme value of each human being, a report to the Central Conference of American Rabbis, the international rabbinic association of Reform Judaism, stated that euthanasia is "contrary to. . . moral law."[32] Expounding the traditional Jewish teachings regarding the incalculable value of earthly life, one recent Reform responsum reasons in some detail as follows:[33]

> . . . If the doctrine of life's essential holiness means anything at all, it means that we must stand in reverence before the very fact of life, the gift of God that renders us human. And this reverence does not diminish as human strength declines, for the dying person still possesses life, a life stamped

> indelibly with the image of God until the moment of death. It is an awesome and awful responsibility we take upon ourselves when we determine to kill a human being, even when our intentions are good and beautiful. Such an action is the ultimate arrogance, for it declares that we are masters over the one thing - life itself - that our faith has always taught must be protected against our all-too-human tendency to manipulate, to mutilate, and to destroy.
>
> . . . [W]e do not believe that the existence of pain and suffering constitutes a sufficient Jewish justification for killing a human being in the name of compassion. It is true that none of us wants to endure a state of physical or psychological agony, and none of us wants this for our loved ones. We have every right to administer treatment to relieve pain. . . . It remains a fact, however, that pain and suffering are part and parcel of the human condition. We do not cease to be human, that is, when we experience suffering, even that of a terminal illness. The choice we face when we are ill is essentially the same choice we confront at every other moment of our lives: to determine what we, human beings in covenant with God, propose to do with the time and the strength available to us on this earth. All of life, its end no less than its beginning and its middle, is the arena in which we act out our humanity. Judaism, for its part, bids us to respond to the challenges of life by *choosing* life, to praise God whether that life brings us joy or sorrow. Even in debilitating illness, when our freedom of action is severely limited, we yet sanctify the divine name by *living* our relationship with God, by striving toward nobility of conduct and of purpose, by confronting our suffering with courage. To say this is not to ignore the agony of the dying but to recognize a fundamental truth: that even when we are dying we have the power to choose how we shall live. We can kill ourselves, thereby accepting the counsel of despair, or we can choose life, declaring through our actions that despite everything life -- all of it -- is blessed with the promise of ultimate meaning and fulfillment.

Traditionalist and other more liberal authorities echo a similar conclusion. Orthodox Rabbi J. David Bleich points out: "Any positive act designed to hasten the death of the patient is equated with murder in Jewish law, even if death is hastened only by a matter of moments. No matter how laudable the intentions of the person performing the act of mercy-killing may be, his deed constitutes an act of homicide. . . ."[34] Also, Conservative Rabbi Dorff writes, ". . . Jewish sources view all forms of active euthanasia and assisted suicide as forbidden acts of murder."[35] Although Dorff confidently asserts his conclusion, backed by the nearly unanimous view of modern Jewish commentators, a small minority exists within Judaism, advocating looking anew at these acts in a more positive manner.

Despite their grudging acceptance of some, if not most, forms of passive euthanasia, as developed in Chapter 5, Jewish authorities overwhelmingly evidence particularly strong feelings in opposition to any form of physician-assisted suicide or voluntary active euthanasia. In addition to the sanctity of biological life principle and our being enjoined to "Choose life" (Deuteronomy 30:19), contemporary Jewish authorities rest their opposition on two basic points: first, the duty of a physician to cure, not kill, human beings, and second, dismissal of any quality of life considerations. They also look negatively on the Dutch experience with voluntary active euthanasia. Let's begin, however, by looking at two historical examples.

Looking at Two Historical Examples

As we will see, modern Jewish commentators interpret two historical examples, first, the death of King Saul in a battle against the Philistines, and second, the death of Rabbi Judah Ha'Nasi, to suit their positions, pro or con, on the topic of physician-aided dying.

Earlier in this chapter, we considered King Saul's death. II Samuel 1:1-10 tells us that after King Saul's attempt to commit suicide failed, he then saw an Amalekite. King Saul asked the young man to kill him. The Amalekite agreed to kill him because he thought King Saul would not have survived his wounds.

According to one Reform responsum, King Saul's death at the hand of the Amalekite represented an act of martyrdom, because he chose not to be abused by the Philistines; it was not an ancient example of voluntary active euthanasia.[36] If the Philistines had captured King Saul, the Israelites would have been compelled to rescue him. More people would have been killed in any attempt to save King Saul. Thus, his death represented an act of martyrdom to save others' lives. The responsum further notes that Saul was correct in committing suicide because he feared being tortured into violating the Jewish laws against idolatry.

In contrast, Reform Rabbi Knobel argues that King Saul's death provides a basis in the Jewish textual tradition for permission today to engage in voluntary active euthanasia.[37] The young Amalekite ended the plight of King Saul, who told him: ". . . [F]or I [King Saul] am in agony and am barely alive." (II Samuel 1:7). King Saul chose to accelerate his death rather than prolong his suffering. He did not choose death to escape abuse by his enemies. He sought to preserve his dignity. Furthermore, in II Samuel 1:13-16, we are told that King David had the Amalekite put to death for killing King Saul. Rabbi Knobel believes that David did not punish the Amalekite for *halakhic* reasons. Rather, political expediency forced King David to sanction the young man who killed King Saul. If David had not punished the Amalekite, others would have questioned his allegiance to Saul by allowing his killer to go untouched.

The passing of Rabbi Judah HaNasi, the redactor of the Mishnah, raises questions about the Jewish view of physician-assisted suicide and voluntary active euthanasia for those who are terminally ill as well as for other sufferers. In the Babylonian Talmud (Ketubot 104a), we know that Rabbi HaNasi suffered greatly from a debilitating intestinal disorder. The rabbi's maidservant, a woman of the highest piety and moral character, realized that her master was in pain and beyond the point of any cure. However, the rabbi's followers ceaselessly prayed that he might be kept alive a little longer. The maidservant went up the roof of the house and prayed for the rabbi's passing. When she heard his followers' continuous prayers, she threw a vase from the roof. Her act interrupted the followers' prayers and allowed the rabbi to pass away. The Talmud tells us,"[For a moment] they ceased praying and the soul of rabbi departed to its eternal rest."

One recent Reform responsum[38] asserts that the maidservant did not directly kill the rabbi. Rather, she merely removed an impediment to his death; in modern terms, she facilitated a form of passive euthanasia. In this responsum, the Reform rabbis maintain that taking positive steps to kill someone is qualitatively different from removing impediments to one's natural passing. Although recognizing that rabbinic stories may be viewed as supporting assisted suicide or voluntary active euthanasia, the Reform rabbis conclude that they have never been understood in that way. In the long history of Jewish study of the Hebrew Bible and the Talmud, the texts in question have never been interpreted to support acts of murder, they conclude, even if consented to by a victim. For more than fifteen centuries, they assert that Jewish learning has "consistently and unequivocally" stood against any form of mercy killing.

In contrast, Reform Rabbi Knobel asserts that Rabbi HaNasi's death illustrates a favorable opinion of Jewish sages regarding voluntary active euthanasia.[39] The prayers of the rabbi's followers were similar to a powerful, artificial life-support system. However, the maidservant realized that these prayers impeded the rabbi's dying process. In so doing, the prayers became a form of "abuse and torture," keeping the rabbi alive when it was unreasonable to do so. The maidservant understood that the rabbi's followers, consumed with their own needs, had replaced their master's interests with their own desires. Thus, she threw a vase from the roof. The disciples paused in their prayers when they heard the crash. During the pause, the rabbi passed away.

Knobel presents Rabbi HaNasi's death as analogous to modern medical situations. The rabbi's students represent, in today's terms, a patient's family or physician who often forget the sufferer's best interests. The disciples were determined to keep Rabbi HaNasi alive, similar to some contemporary family members (or physicians) who strive to keep loved ones (or patients) alive at all costs. As his followers prayed, the rabbi's condition remained stable, but he continued to suffer. When the maidservant distracted the disciples from their prayers that had lost their therapeutic value, she precipitated the rabbi's death. Knobel notes that she did not merely remove an impediment to dying. The maidservant not only prayed, but she also performed a positive physical act, throwing a pot down from the roof. The Talmud indicates no disapproval of her action. Thus, Knobel maintains that Judaism does not prohibit physician-assisted suicide and voluntary active euthanasia, at least for those who are terminally ill.

Reconsidering the Role of Physicians

Assisted suicide or voluntary active euthanasia typically involves a physician. In many cases, the assistant to the act, for instance, a physician, such as Dr. Quill, may provide an overdose of pills. Or, a physician, such as Dr. Kevorkian, may set up a machine for the patient or provide a lethal injection. The cases of assisted suicide and voluntary active euthanasia bring into question a physician's duty.

In his classic article, "Neither For Love Nor Money: Why Doctors Must Not Kill," the philosopher Leon R. Kass concludes that killing patients who ask for death violates meaning of the healing vocation of medicine.[40] Physicians must always strive, according to Kass, to prolong life and not cause death. However, from the perspective of Spiritual Judaism, even if a physician has an obligation to cure, in some situations he or she has a conflicting duty, perhaps an even higher duty, to engage in "mercy killing."

Jewish authorities assert that physicians must cure (or at least care) for patients and prolong their lives, not serve as dispensers of death.[41] They see this mandate based on the literal biblical phrase, "And heal they shall heal" (Exodus 21:19). The Babylonian Talmud (Bava Kamma 85a) views the duplicative use of the word "heal" to mean that God authorizes physicians to heal. Arguably, when physicians participate in an assisted suicide or perform active euthanasia, they negate the Biblical obligation to save an endangered life. They also act in violation of the negative commandment, "Do not stand idly by the blood of your neighbor," (Leviticus 19:16) as well as the positive commandment, "You shall love your neighbor as yourself." (Leviticus 19:18). Furthermore, the Babylonian Talmud tells us: "He or she who saves one life is as if he or she saved the whole world." (Sanhedrin 37a).

However, healing is only one of several appropriate medical objectives. Physicians, even with the best of knowledge and equipment, in some situations cannot cure a patient. Viewing disease as the enemy, they strive to defeat and banish illness from a sufferer's body by any and all technological and pharmacological means. But the ravages of an illness or condition may thwart medical efforts to restore useful and dignified bodily function. Some patients simply cannot be restored to health characterized by living well without the presence of intractable pain, severe disability, a deteriorating mental or neurological condition, or a terminal illness.

For some, experiencing chronic, debilitating conditions become a permanent feature of living. Because medical doctors cannot restore their physical well-being, those who are chronically ill need to learn to live in the continued presence of their illness.

Not all pain and other physical symptoms, such as nausea, fever, diarrhea, can be controlled for those who are terminally ill. Some die in unspeakable agony. Some types of pain and other physical symptoms are difficult to relieve without producing someother discomfort or other harmful side effects.

Many with a chronic, degenerative condition or those encountering a terminal illness face intractable suffering on one of several levels: physical, emotional, or spiritual. At some point, compassion and mercy by providing relief from severe anguish in its various forms, engendered by a pitiable or degrading physical and/or mental condition, if requested by the patient (or his or her surrogate), supercede a physician’s duty to cure. More harm may be done by allowing a patient to undergo a slow, agonizing death rather than a quick, gentle physician-assisted demise.

Physician aid-in-dying thus represents, in my opinion, a natural extension of Spiritual Judaism's virtue of compassion into the ambit of medical care. By helping one who is in an extreme state of suffering, whether physical, emotional, or spiritual, to die peacefully, a physician acts compassionately and mercifully. Medicine should not be a callous discipline guided by a blind obeisance to the sanctity of biological life principle or by the technological imperative. Rather, compassionately and mercifully responding to a patient's pain and suffering, striving to optimize a sufferer's control and autonomy, and minimizing harm to a patent and his or her loved ones by avoiding inhumane interventions should serve as the beacons for modern medical care. Physicians should be able to: consider their patients' pleas for help, listen deeply to their innermost thoughts, ask searching questions, have them ponder their reasons for wanting to die, show heartfelt concern, and respond compassionately and mercifully by providing safety at the end of life, preserving a person's dignity which it took a lifetime to acquire and preventing unnecessary suffering.

The relationship of trust existing between patients and their physicians also enters into the equation. Some may lose their trust in physicians if doctors may legally assist in deaths. Others will find increased confidence if they know that physicians will follow their wishes and provide aid-in-dying on request when they can no longer endure their anguish. For the latter group, into whose camp I fall, continued medical interventions evidencing a lack of compassion and mercy only exacerbate the public's lack of trust in the healthcare professionals to their relieve pain and suffering. Thus, by making assistance in dying legally available, under strict guidelines, fear of the dying process may diminish, thereby increasing public trust in physicians.

Let's also return to our image of God, the loving and benevolent Deity, portrayed in Chapter 3. The Eternal does not want any of us to experience anguish. In the Jewish tradition, suffering is not a virtue; it lacks any redemptive value. The Holy One provides us with modern medical knowledge, technology and drugs to offer ways, such as physician aid-in-dying, to end our pain and suffering as gently and mercifully as possible. When a terminally or chronically ill person's disease or condition contradicts his or her image of God, Judaism should not bar the acceleration of the end of life.

The Dutch Experience: Are We on the Slippery Slope?

Contemporary Jewish sources comment negatively on the Dutch experience with physician aid-in-dying. In the Netherlands, physician-assisted suicide and voluntary active euthanasia are publically condoned and practiced under highly regulated conditions (and may in the near future be legalized).[42]

In 1973, a Dutch court excluded physicians who aided a patient in dying from criminal sanctions if a number of requirements were met. Although physician aid-in-dying should remain illegal, the court stated that when a conflict of duties confronts physicians they may argue that necessity obliged them to act as they did. The conflict arises when a physician's ethical obligations to honor a patient's request to die with dignity forces a doctor to act inconsistently with provisions of the Dutch Penal Code that forbid killing. The validity of the necessity defense rests on an investigation into whether the physician made a responsible medical judgment, linking the provisions and concepts of Dutch criminal law to the criteria derived from medical ethics.

In 1984, the Royal Dutch Medical Association sought to clarify the criteria accepted within the medical profession in favor of physician aid-in-dying under specific conditions, including voluntariness on a patient's part, a well-considered request, and stability of desire. These guidelines do not require that the patient be in a terminal condition, only that his or her suffering is intolerable and without hope of improvement. The guidelines, as further revised in 1995, have come to favor physician-assisted suicide over voluntary active euthanasia. Patients are urged to take the fatal drugs themselves, whenever possible, rather than having a doctor give a lethal injection, thereby reducing the emotional stress on physicians but raising problems with completion of the process, including technical and other impediments to assisted suicide.

In 1993, the Dutch Parliament, although not repealing the law making mercy killing a criminal offense, gave formal legal status to a notification procedure, taking effect in 1994, for physicians to report medical decisions resulting in aid-in-dying to a local medical examiner and a regional review committee. The conclusion of the review committee is then submitted to the Dutch Public Prosecutions Service that decides, on a case-by-case basis, whether or not criminal prosecution should follow. Great weight is given to the opinion of the review committee with respect to the criminal prosecution question. However, as a general rule, a physician offering assistance in dying in accordance with the guidelines of the Royal Dutch Medical Association and the case law criteria will not be prosecuted.

To make a long story short, at present, the Dutch Ministry of Justice will not criminally prosecute physicians for assisting in a suicide or carrying out euthanasia, provided certain due care requirements are met. First, physician must be convinced that the patient's request is voluntary, well-considered and lasting; second, the patient must face unremitting and unbearable suffering, either physical or mental, but the patient need not be terminally ill; third, the patient must be informed concerning his or her situation and prospects; fourth, the physician must have reached a firm conclusion, together with the patient, that there is no reasonable, alternative treatment to the patient's situation; fifth, the attending physician must have consulted at least one other independent physician (having no professional or family relationship with either the patient or the doctor), who examines the patient and forms a judgement concerning the requirements of due care in items 1-4; sixth, the attending physician must carry out the termination of life in a medically appropriate fashion. In addition to conforming to these due care guidelines, physicians must also report the circumstances of any assisted death.

With this background in mind, let's consider several research studies dealing with the Dutch experience. In 1990, three studies of the practice of euthanasia in the Netherlands were undertaken.[43] The first study involved detailed personal interviews with 405 Dutch physicians regarding patients who died in their care. In the second study, a questionnaire was mailed to physicians of 7,000 persons who died from August 1 to December 1, 1990, resulting in nearly 5,200 completed questionnaires. In the third study, 322 physicians in the Netherlands documented their medical decisions in 2,257 patient deaths.

Two follow-up studies were conducted in 1995. The first involved interviews with 405 physicians and the second involved questionnaires mailed to physicians attending some 6,000 deaths from August 1 to December 1, 1995.[44] None of these studies reflected the experience under the revised 1995 guidelines for physician aid-in-dying.

About one in 50 deaths in the Netherlands, some 2,300 per year, results from voluntary active euthanasia. Also, there are 400 cases per year in which physicians help their patients commit suicide. In almost all of these 2,700 deaths, the patients were terminally ill, usually with some form of cancer, and had only a short time to live. In three-fourths of these 2,700 deaths, it was estimated that the physician-assisted suicide or voluntary active euthanasia shortened life by less then four weeks.

The studies indicated that about 1.8% of all deaths in the Netherlands in 1990 occurred through voluntary active euthanasia with some form of physician involvement; by 1995 the figure exceeded 2.3%. About .3% were the result of physician-assisted suicide in both years. A further .8% of the deaths in 1990 (and .7% in 1995) were characterized as life terminating acts without the patient's explicit request.

Euthanasia in the Netherlands is, in theory, voluntary. Jewish critics of the Dutch experience stress on the seemingly involuntary nature of a number of cases of active euthanasia. For example, one recent Reform responsum notes that Dutch government records show that involuntary active euthanasia took place in at least 1,000 cases (and perhaps in excess of 6,000 cases, counting about 5,000 intentional morphine overdoses given with primary purpose of ending life) constituting a "'deliberate action to terminate life without the patient's consent.'"[45] According to this responsum, these cases involved physicians supplying, prescribing or administering a lethal drug with the purpose of hastening the end of life, but without an explicit request from a patient, thereby reflecting a move from voluntary to involuntary euthanasia.

In going behind the numbers, we see a quite different picture. The overwhelming percentage, 86 percent to be specific, of the involuntary cases in 1990 involved patients considered to be within a few days or hours of death. The others, although suffering greatly, had a longer life expectancy, perhaps upwards of one month, but verbal contact with them was no longer possible.

In more than half of the involuntary deaths in 1990 and 1995, physicians had information about their patient's wishes, but not an explicit request. There was some previous patient involvement with their medical doctors as to what they would want if their suffering became unbearable. Others had discussed the possibility of euthanasia at earlier points in their illness, but were not fully capable of requesting euthanasia when physicians actually administered the drugs.

In nearly all of the other cases, discussion with a patient was impossible and the patient had not previously expressed a wish regarding euthanasia. In these situations, because the patients were unconscious or in a reduced state of consciousness, they lacked the ability to assess their condition as well as to formulate and verbally express their choices in a clear manner. Nearly all of these decisions to hasten death were taken in consultation with other healthcare professionals and/or the patient's family.

Assistance in dying in the Netherlands thus represents a carefully considered option for a small number of people at the end of life. In nearly all the cases of life terminating acts without a patient's explicit request, the patients were suffering unbearably, no chance of improvement existed, and comfort care possibilities were exhausted.

From my perspective, the Dutch experience with euthanasia does not point to the slippery slope, a plunge into depravity, more specifically, to physicians performing involuntary active euthanasia on the very old, the physically or mentally disabled, or those financially, emotionally, or otherwise burdensome, as opposed to voluntary euthanasia. As the authors of the 1995 study conclude, the "data do not support the idea that physicians in the Netherlands are moving down a slippery slope."[46]

Carefully constructed safeguards can be devised in the United States to restrict, but perhaps not completely eliminate, potential abuses by family members, physicians, or healthcare cost managers. As with nearly everything, perfection may be impossible. Obviously, we need to prevent involuntary active euthanasia of three groups: first, those who do not want to die; second, those lacking medical care decision-making capacity, such as the comatose, senile, demented, depressed, or psychotic; third, those facing the financial or other pressures from healthcare professionals and insurers who consider a patient too costly to maintain or from family members who may want to speed up an inheritance or have malevolent intentions.

From a public policy perspective, we must insist on clear-cut evidence of a patient's informed, uncoerced choice. Various safeguards to achieve this objective may include requiring: first, a psychological evaluation of the patient designed to identify temporary, reversible depression or other disturbances of reasoning; second, some sort of waiting period between the initial request for physician aid-in-dying and the provision of these services, making the choice stable and enduring (or the existence of a previously executed written advance care directive); third, assurance that a patient has received high quality care to relieve pain and other physical symptoms; fourth, the documentation of any procedure involving physician aid-in-dying, including a clear expression that patient's request is his or her idea, freely made, independent of financial, family, or other sources of coercion, a record of treatment alternatives discussed with the patient, forms of pain relief offered including comfort care options; fifth, the reporting of the physician's aid-in-dying to a local, state, or federal public agency.[47] Although the likely subject of much controversy, I would permit, under the above conditions, preemptive physician aid-in-dying for those who are terminally ill or facing an incurable and debilitating physical or mental condition, even if not yet experiencing unrelievable suffering.

Naturally, overtime these guidelines may require revision. I have considerable faith in state legislatures and the American legal system to design and enforce guidelines to prevent abuses.

For me, there is an even greater risk of abuse, if physicians, as some do now, help sufferers die, secretly, and without accountability or scrutiny from their peers, the judicial system, or anyone else. Failure to regulate physician-assisted dying may create an even greater potential for the very abuses critics fear. Thus, these guidelines, designed to legalize physician-assisted suicide and voluntary active euthanasia, would reduce the problems of inappropriate physician assistance in dying.

Quality of Life Considerations

In contrast to advocates of physician aid-in-dying who maintain that quality of life considerations currently and repeatedly enter into end of life decisions, contemporary Jewish authorities of nearly every stripe reject any notion of incorporating subjective, individualized judgments about a patient's condition into the decision-making process. Quality of life considerations are said to have no theological basis in Judaism. Each moment of physical life is intrinsically valuable independent of its quality.

The mainstream of Jewish commentators -- traditional and more liberal -- assert that the value of biological life must always be measured from God's perspective.[48] In the Holy One's eyes, all humans possess infinite worth regardless of whether or not they are healthy. Thus, the quality or usefulness of one's present and future earthly life is irrelevant. We should recognize the Divine nature of those who are terminally or chronically ill, regardless of what we or they perceive as the quality of their lives. As Rosner writes, "Evil has small beginnings. When the quality of life replaces the sanctity of life, society has done itself irreparable harm."[49]

The rejection of any quality of life considerations spans the Jewish spectrum. One recent Reform responsum unconditionally rejects any and all arguments for mercy killing based on the "quality of life."[50] The Reform rabbis argue that a quality of life standard is inherently subjective and "is virtually impossible to determine." Furthermore, "it cannot be quantified, verified, or tested against any principle other than the conviction that one's suffering is no longer tolerable." If a patient in a coma or in a persistent vegetative state lacks an acceptable quality of life, then, the responsum asks, using a slippery slope argument, who is to say that a paralyzed patient, or one who is aged and infirm, does not have the "right to die?" The responsum asserts, "Once we have adopted 'quality of life' as our standard, we have no principled reason to oppose the suicide of *any* person (with the possible exception of children and the insane, who by definition cannot make a "responsible" choice), no matter how flimsy the justification, whether undertaken in response to terminal illness, or to chronic illness, or to psychological or emotional distress."

It is also useful to mention an earlier Reform responsum dealing, in part, with a completely paralyzed person unable to communicate because a segment of her brain providing intelligence seemed to be damaged beyond repair. With respect to the quality of life issue, the Reform rabbis noted, "Judaism does not define human life only in terms of mental activity. Every person has been created in the image of God . . . and so even those individuals who may be defective . . . have always been considered as equally created in the image of God; their life is as precious as any other. . . . [W]e can . . . not utilize a 'low quality' of life as an excuse for hastening death."[51] In short, for these Reform authorities, their underlying concern seems to turn on their interpretation of the term "quality of life."[52]

Like the Reform rabbis, other Jewish commentators overwhelmingly reject any subjective judgments about a person's condition. For instance, traditionalist Fred Rosner, a medical doctor, unconditionally turns aside any consideration of "quality of life" or "quality of existence factors" as embodying "within them a concept of worthiness with connotations of personal character and social status."[53] Orthodox Rabbi Bleich states that when humans were created, we were, according to tradition, commanded by God to nurture and sustain life. Even if we do not find meaning or value in our lives, we must obey this commandment and preserve physical life. Although the trials of our existence represent a Divine mystery to us, Bleich asserts that our obligation to sustain biological life remains. He concludes, "The quality of life that is preserved is thus never a factor to be taken into consideration."[54]

Likewise, Conservative Rabbi Avram Israel Reisner opposes the balancing of the benefits and burdens of anyone's life.[55] Rejecting quality of life calculations, he encourages patients to assert their personal autonomy by adhering to God's mandate to choose life. Conservative Rabbi Dorff also concludes that Judaism "strongly affirms the value of human life regardless of its usefulness or quality."[56]

Another Reality Check

Despite the overwhelming weight of modern Jewish authority, both traditional and more liberal, a certain amount of realism and common sense are in order. Many of us fear the over treatment with life prolonging medical technology and pharmacology long after any return to meaningful function is possible. Also, some interventions may be only partially successful, leaving a sufferer lacking important elements of function and dignity. Also, comfort care techniques are not effective one hundred percent of the time.

Even if medical interventions address one's physical distress, emotional and spiritual suffering also exist. In other words, unacceptable anguish, on a number of levels, can still occur in the midst of excellent care, whether taking an aggressive form or even of a palliative nature. In short, it is simply impossible to achieve an idealized, pain and suffering-free death for everyone.

As indicated in Chapter 2, the infinite value of each moment of life -- the sanctity of biological life principle -- cannot be and, except for the most strictest of traditionalists, is not an absolute standard. Patients (or their surrogates) and their physicians do take into account other factors. The implicit balancing of the benefits and burdens of treatments as well as quality of life judgments are unavoidable, unless one adopts the view that earthly life has an absolute value in and of itself and each patient must be treated with every available mode of technology and medication until death is absolutely certain.

To be consistent, someone who takes the view that human life as such, regardless of its condition, always has the same value and all biological life must be prolonged, no distinction exists between passive and active euthanasia. Those supporting this position should oppose both.

Yet, we do not see unqualified support for the preservation of life at all costs and under all conditions. With most Jewish commentators acquiescing in some forms of passive euthanasia, as discussed in Chapter 5, the prevailing intransigence with regard to physician-assisted suicide and voluntary active euthanasia may, in coming decades, abate. Judaism recognizes that "there is a time to die." (Ecclesiastes 3:2). Except for the most devoted followers of the sanctity of biological life doctrine, efforts to hold the line may prove futile. A greater degree of reality may lead to a reinterpretation. A new standard will, in my opinion, be drawn in the twenty-first century. Otherwise, it seems to me, we engage in a cruel exercise of the powers of modern medical science to extend the dying process far beyond what previous generations could ever have imagined.

Let us grant that it is not easy to consider the various consequences of life threatening disease or a chronic, degenerative condition, to weigh the benefits and burdens of any treatment or procedure, and the quality of life offered. Each of us has a different tolerance for risk as well as various thresholds of and susceptibilities to pain and suffering. Thus, the quality of life considerations remain inherently subjective for each sufferer. None of us can define the quality of life for anyone else. It is a lot easier to cite the sanctity of biological life principle, thereby finding a sense of security, order, and continuity, based on a belief that the physical life of every human being, as a reflection of the Divine, must be preserved as long as possible. Perhaps the sanctity of biological life principle reflects human reluctance to come to terms with our mortality. However, text-oriented Jewish commentators, whether traditionalists or more liberal interpretators, must face the realities of the twenty-first century.

In our everyday lives we, even traditionalists, engage in a multitude of behaviors inconsistent with and detrimental to the single value of maximizing longevity. Facing a life threatening illness or a chronic, debilitating condition, most of us, from my experience, do not want our care shaped solely by the value of prolonging our physical existence regardless of its quality. Most of us, from my experience, express strong negative feelings toward existing in a state of extreme pain and suffering, extreme physical disability, or extreme mental incapacity. We commonly share concerns about these elements of an undignified dying process; when each of us reaches a level of degradation we subjectively deem intolerable and undignified, we want to avoid any form of life sustaining intervention, if not end it all.

Jewish commentators may continue to look away from the way we are actually living. However, quality of life judgments are inevitably made, nearly all of the time. Let's make them openly, not covertly, thereby reducing arbitrary or unjustified assessments.

It is easier to accept, both as the American legal system and the Jewish tradition currently do, indirect, rather than direct, action. Allowing one to die has more appeal than killing. As we saw in Chapter 5, the withholding or withdrawal of medical intervention, viewed as passive euthanasia, receives approval by the American legal system and many Jewish commentators. In these situations, death occurs either as a result of allowing a fatal, underlying pathological condition to take its natural course, or because of the need to stop doing something useless.

In the twenty-first century, as technology gives us more and more control over the physical dimensions of our lives, we will need to rethink the distinction between passive and active euthanasia. Whether it is passive or active euthanasia, someone, typically a physician, plays a part in enabling death. Whether someone supplies a lethal means which the patient then uses, or someone withdraws the feeding tubes, the means of continued biological life, in accordance with a sufferer's request, that someone and the patient act together to bring one's physical life to a close. The fact that a terminally ill patient is on a life-support system in the second situation should not make a difference.

The line between allowing one to die by removing a feeding tube and actively killing by lethal injection remains elusive. In both cases, biological processes take place in the patient's body culminating in death. The difference is not in what happens to the patient, but in what the helper intends, does, and is responsible for. Withdrawing treatment, removing a respirator or taking out a feeding tube, involves an act. Someone, a physician or another under his or her authority and acting on his or her direction, does something resulting in a patient’s death. There is nothing passive about taking a sufferer, who is incapable of breathing on his or her own, off a ventilator. It is not something refrained from. It is a positive act.

The withholding or withdrawal of treatment represents a form of physician-assisted suicide, a form of physician assistance in a process leading to death. A doctor remains as responsible for an act of omission as for an act of commission. We, as well as physicians, may be helped, perhaps emotionally, if we think that we are only allowing "nature to take its course"; however, passive and active euthanasia are on a par as far as "nature" is concerned. It will take its course from whatever circumstances we present: not-doing, stopping-doing, or doing. Because of our ability to intervene, we cannot avoid our participation in the process, claiming that "nature" alone is responsible. In my mind, there is not a sufficient distinction between the withdrawal of life sustaining treatment and actively bringing on death. In fact, the latter may be more compassionate.

Although we may assume that a passive omission will allow a patient to die, a physician actually has no control over when he or she dies. Letting a disease kill someone presents the potential for considerable pain and suffering. The result may be a prolonged, painful, agonizing process, taking several days, requiring, as we have seen, terminal sedation to unconsciousness. It is the functional equivalent of causing death, a painful demise, rather than an easy one. Loved ones also suffer witnessing a withering away over days.

In contrast, with physician-assisted suicide or voluntary active euthanasia, one can choose the time and manner of death. Particularly with voluntary active euthanasia, it is quick and painless. Once someone desires and accepts death, it is more humane to end life quickly. For me, it shows more respect for life's sanctity.

Spiritual Judaism and the Acceleration of Death

From the perspective of Spiritual Judaism, a sufferer may want to accelerate the release of his or her immortal soul from a degenerative physical body. The earthly body fails, but as we have seen in Chapter 3, our soul lives on in the afterlife World to Come. Each of us should be able to liberate our soul earlier, if one so desires, on the body's or the mind's downhill course, particularly, but not exclusively, when one is terminally ill, facing an approaching death.

Viewing souls as coming into biological life and again departing from it, enables us to put a different perspective on physician aid-in-dying and formulate a new Judaic approach to life-and-death. The cessation of biological functions does not constitute the end of life, but a transition to another phase of existence. We must focus on our immortal soul, not our mere physical being.

Let's next consider how patients might go about rational, end of life decision-making. As we will see, it is not a clear-cut, black or white issue: hold on to the bitter end or have someone help you die -- today.

Notes

1. John Noble Wilford, "Scientist At Work: Sailing A Wheelchair To the End of Time," *New York Times*, 24 March 1998, sec. C1; Sonja Carberry, "Physicist Stephen Hawking," *Investor's Business Daily*, 30 September 1998, sec. A6.

2. Timothy E. Quill, "Death and Dignity -- A Case of Individualized Decisions-Making," *New England Journal of Medicine* 324:10 (March 1991): 691-694. See generally, Timothy E. Quill, M.D., *Death and Dignity: Making Choices and Taking Charge* (New York: Norton, 1993).

3. Timothy Egan, "As Memory and Music Faced, Oregon Woman Chose Death," *New York Times*, 7 June 1990, sec. Al; Melinda Beck, "The Doctor's Suicide Van," *Newsweek*, 18 June 1990, 46-47, 49.

4. Alan Meisel, *The Right to Die*, vol. 2, 2nd ed. (New York: Wiley Law, 1995), 478, table 18-1.

5. *Washington* v. *Glucksberg*, 521 U.S. 702 (1997); *Vacco* v. *Quill*, 521 U.S. 793 (1997).

6. 42 U.S.C. §14401 et seq.

7. Oregon Revised Statutes §§127.800 -- 127.880.

8. Derek D. Humphry, *The Final Exit: The Practicalities of Self-Deliverance and Assisted Suicide for the Dying* (Eugene, Oreg.: The Hemlock Society, 1991).

9. Charles F. McKhann, "Is There a Role for Physician-Assisted Suicide in Cancer? Yes" in *Important Advances in Oncology 1996*, ed. Vincent T. DeVita, Samual Hellman, and Steven A. Rosenberg (Philadelphia: Lippincott-Raven, 1996), 272.

10. Diane E. Meier et al, "A National Survey of Physician-Assisted Suicide and Euthanasia in the United States," *New England Journal of Medicine* 338:17 (April 1998): 1193-1201.

11. Ezekiel J. Emanuel et al, "Euthanasia and Physician-Assisted Suicide: Attitudes and Experiences of Oncology Patients, Oncologists and the Public," *Lancet* 347:9018 (June 1996): 1805-1810.

12. David J. Doukas et al, "Attitudes and Behaviors on Physician-Assisted Death: A Study of Michigan Oncologists," *Journal of Clinical Oncology*, 13:5 (May 1995): 1055-1061.

13. Lee R. Slome et al, "Physician-Assisted Suicide and Patients with Human Immunodeficiency Virus Disease," *New England Journal of Medicine* 336:6 (February 1997): 417-421.

14. Anthony L. Back et al, "Physician-Assisted Suicide and Euthanasia in Washington State: Patient Requests and Physician Responses," *Journal of the American Medical Association* 275:12 (March 1996): 919-925. The experience with physician-assisted suicide under the Oregon statute shows that only one in six requests is being granted. Linda Ganzini et al, "Physicians' Experiences with Oregon Death with Dignity Act," *New England Journal of Medicine* 342:8 (February 2000): 557-563.

15. Sir Immanuel Jakobovits, "Ethical Problems Regarding the Termination of Life," in *Jewish Values in Bioethics*, ed. Rabbi Levi Meier (New York: Human Sciences Press 1986), 90. See also Dr. Immanuel Jakobovits, *Jewish Medical Ethics: A Comparative and Historical Study of the Jewish Religious Attitude to Medicine and Its Practice* (New York: Bloch, 1975), 123-124, 276.

16. Fred Rosner and Moshe D. Tendler, *Practical Medical Halachah* (Northvale, NJ: Jason Aronson, 1997), 54.

17. Elliot N. Dorff, "*Teshuvah* on Assisted Suicide," *Conservative Judaism* 50:4 (Summer 1998): 8-9. See also Elliot N. Dorff, *Matters of Life and Death: A Jewish Approach to Modern Medical Ethics* (Jewish Publication Society, 1998), 183-188.

18. Central Conference of American Rabbis (CCAR) "Responsum 78. Euthanasia (1950)," in *American Reform Responsa: Collected Responsa of the Central Conference of American Rabbis*, ed. Walter Jacob (New York: CCAR, 1983), 263. CCAR, "Responsum 79. Euthanasia (1980)," ibid., 271-274, concludes, "We would not endorse any positive steps leading toward death. . . . We would reject any general endorsement of euthanasia. . . ."

19. Peter Knobel, "Suicide, Assisted Suicide, Active Euthanasia: A *Halakhic* Inquiry" in *Death and Euthanasia in Jewish Law*, ed. Walter Jacob and Moshe Zemer (Pittsburgh: Rodef Shalom Press, 1995); Byron L. Sherwin, *In Partnership with God: Contemporary Jewish Law and Ethics* (Syracuse: Syracuse University Press, 1990), 85-101; Byron L. Sherwin, "Euthanasia as a Halakhic Option" in

Jewish Approaches to Suicide, Martyrdom, and Euthanasia, ed. Kalman I. Kaplan and Matthew B. Schwartz (Northvale, N.J.: Jason Aronson, 1998); Byron Sherwin, "A View of Euthanasia" in *Contemporary Jewish Ethics and Morality: A Reader*, ed. Elliot N. Dorff and Louis E. Newman (New York: Oxford University Press, 1995); Rabbi Byron L. Sherwin, "Euthanasia: A Jewish View," *The Journal of Aging and Judaism* 2:1 (Fall 1987): 35-57.

20. J. David Bleich, *Judaism and Healing: Halakhic Perspectives* (New York: KTAV, 1981), 158-161; Fred Rosner, "Suicide in Jewish Law" in *Jewish Approaches to Suicide, Martyrdom and Euthanasia*, 61-77; Fred Rosner, "Suicide in Jewish Law," in *Jewish Bioethics*, ed. J. David Bleich and Fred Rosner (New York: Hebrew Publishing, 1979), 317-328; Fred Rosner, "Suicide in Biblical, Talmudic and Rabbinic Writings," *Tradition* 11:3 (Summer 1970): 25-40; Sidney Goldstein, *Suicide in Rabbinic Literature* (Hoboken, NJ: KTAV, 1989); Dorff, *Matters of Life and Death*, 18, 182-183; Virginia L. Trimble, "Masada, Suicides, and Halakhah," *Conservative Judaism* 31:2 (Winter 1977): 45-55; Seymour Siegel, "Suicide in the Jewish View," *Conservative Judaism* 32:2 (Winter 1979): 67-74; CCAR, "Responsum 5754.14. On the Treatment of the Terminally Ill," in *Teshuvot for the Nineties: Reform Judaism's Answer to Today's Dilemmas*, ed. W. Gunther Plaut and Mark Washofsky (New York: CCAR, 1997), 337-363; CCAR, "Responsum 76. Relieving Pain of a Dying Patient (1975)," *American Reform Responsa*, 254; CCAR, "Responsum 81. Huntington's Disease and Suicide (1983)," in Walter Jacob, *Contemporary American Reform Responsa* (New York: CCAR, 1987), 135-136. See also Baruch A. Brody, "A Historical Introduction to Jewish Casuistry on Suicide and Euthanasia" in *Suicide and Euthanasia: Historical and Contemporary Themes*, ed. Baruch A. Brody (Boston: Kluwer Academic, 1989), 40-62.

21. Dorff, *Matters of Life and Death*, 179-180, 370-371 n. 7; Dorff, "Assisted Suicide," 9-10. See also Bleich, *Judaism and Healing*, 158-159; Fred Rosner, M.D., *Modern Medicine and Jewish Ethics*, 2nd ed. (Hoboken, NJ: KTAV, 1991), 257; Fred Rosner, "Suicide in Jewish Law," in *Jewish Bioethics*, 326-327.

22. Rosner, *Modern Medicine and Jewish Ethics*, 257-259; Dorff, *Matters of Life and Death*, 181-183. CCAR, "Responsum 5754:14. On the Treatment of the Terminally Ill," *Teshuvot for the Nineties*, 339.

23. CCAR, "Responsum 5754.14. On the Treatment of the Terminally Ill," *Teshuvot for the Nineties*, 339. See also CCAR, "Responsum 76. Relieving Pain of a Dying Patient (1975)," *American Reform Responsa*, 254; CCAR "Responsum 89. Funeral Service For a Suicide (1959)," ibid., 303-304.

24. Dorff, *Matters of Life and Death*, 181; Dorff, "Assisted Suicide," 5. See also Joseph H. Prouser, "Being of Sound Mind and Judgment: Rethinking Sanctions in the Case of Assisted Suicide," *Conservative Judaism* 49:4 (Summer 1997): 3-16.

25. Rosner, *Modern Medicine and Jewish Ethics*, 259; Rosner, "Suicide in Jewish Law," in *Jewish Bioethics*, 328. See also, Bleich, *Judaism and Healing*, 160.

26. Maurice Lamm, *The Jewish Way in Death and Mourning* (New York: Jonathan David, 1969), 218-220; Rabbi Tzvi Rabinowicz, *A Guide to Life: Jewish Laws and Customs of Mourning* (Northvale, NJ: Jason Aronson, 1989), 67-68.

27. Dorff, *Matters of Life and Death*, 181; Dorff, "Assisted Suicide," 5.

28. CCAR, "Responsum 89. Funeral Service for a Suicide (1959)," *American Reform Responsa*, pp. 302-306, CCAR, "Responsa 90. A Eulogy for a Suicide (1980)," ibid., 306-307.

29. Knobel, "Suicide, Assisted Suicide, Active Euthanasia," in *Death and Euthanasia in Jewish Law*, 41.

30. Ibid., 46.

31. Ibid., 41-42.

32. CCAR, "Responsum 78. Euthanasia (1950)," *American Reform Responsa*, 263. See also CCAR, "Responsa 83. Quality of Life and Euthanasia (1985)," *Contemporary American Reform Responsa*, 138-140; CCAR, "Responsum 79. Euthanasia (1980)," ibid., 274; CCAR, "Responsum 76. Relieving Pain of a Dying Patient (1975)," ibid., 255; CCAR, "Responsum 77. Allowing a Terminal Patient to Die (1969)," ibid., 259-260.

33. CCAR, "Responsum 5754.14. On the Treatment of the Terminally Ill," *Teshuvot for the Nineties*, 340-341.

34. J. David Bleich, *Bioethical Dilemmas: A Jewish Perspective* (Hoboken, NJ: KTAV, 1998) 63; Bleich, *Judaism and Healing*, 136.

35. Dorff, *Matters of Life and Death*, 177. See also Elliot N. Dorff, "Assisted Death: A Jewish Perspective" in *Must We Suffer Our Way to Death? Cultural and Theological Perspectives on Death By Choice*, ed. Ronald P. Hamel and Edwin

R. DuBose (Dallas: Southern Methodist University Press, 1996), 141-173.

36. CCAR, "Responsum 5754.14. "On the Treatment of the Terminally Ill," *Teshuvot for the Nineties*, 356.

37. Knobel, "Suicide, Assisted Suicide, Active Euthanasia," in *Death and Euthanasia in Jewish Law*, 40-41; Fred Rosner, *Modern Medicine and Jewish Ethics*, 249, mentions other Jewish commentators who consider King Saul's death a case of euthanasia. See also Fred Rosner, "Suicide in Jewish Law" in *Jewish Bioethics*, 319 and Byron Sherwin, "A View of Euthanasia," in *Contemporary Jewish Ethics and Morality*, 379 n. 33.

38. CCAR, "Responsum 5754.14. On the Treatment of the Terminally Ill," *Teshuvot for the Nineties*, 357-358.

39. Knobel, "Suicide, Assisted Suicide, Active Euthanasia," in *Death and Euthanasia in Jewish Law*, 44. See also Leonard Kravitz, "Euthanasia," in ibid., 15-16.

40. Leon R. Kass, "Neither For Love Nor Money: Why Doctors Must Not Kill," *The Public Interest* 94 (Winter 1989): 25-46.

41. Bleich, *Bioethical Dilemmas*, 62; Bleich, *Judaism and Healing*, 1-10; J. David Bleich, "The Obligation to Heal in the Judaic Tradition: A Comparative Analysis" in *Jewish Bioethics*, 23-28; Rosner, *Modern Medicine and Jewish Ethics*, 5-11; Fred Rosner, "The Physician and the Patient in Jewish Law," in *Jewish Bioethics*, 47-51; Dorff, *Matters of Life and Death*, 27-28; CCAR, "Responsum 5714.14. On the Treatment of the Terminally Ill," *Teshuvot for the Nineties*, 346-348. See also Sherwin, *In Partnership With God*, 68-77.

42. I have drawn on Robert L. Schwartz, "Euthanasia and Assisted Suicide in The Netherlands," *Cambridge Quarterly of Healthcare Ethics* 4:1(Winter 1995): 111-121 and Marlise Simons, "Dutch Doctors Tighten Rules on Mercy Killings," *New York Times*, 11 September 1995, sec. A3. See also Suzanne Daley, "The Dutch Seek to Legalize Long-Tolerated Euthanasia," *New York Times*, 20 June 2000, sec. A1.

43. Paul J. van der Maas et al, "Euthanasia and Other Medical Decisions Concerning the End of Life," *The Lancet* 338:8786 (September 1991): 669-674; Loes Pijnenborg et al. "Life-Terminating Acts Without the Explicit Request of Patient," *The Lancet* 341:8854 (May 1993): 1196-1199.

44. Paul J. van der Maas et al, "Euthanasia, Physician-Assisted Suicide, and Other Medical Practices Involving the End of Life in the Netherlands, 1990-1995," *New England Journal of Medicine* 335:22 (November 1996): 1699-1705. Johanna Groenewoud et al, "Clinical Problems with the Performance of Euthanasia and Physician-Assisted in the Netherlands, *New England Journal of Medicine* 342:8 (February 2000): 551-556 report the technical problems, complications, and a longer than acceptable time between the taking of a lethal drug and death, especially with physician-assisted suicide.

45. CCAR, "Responsum 5754.14. On the Treatment of the Terminally Ill," *Teshuvot for the Nineties*, 342.

46. van der Maas, "Euthanasia, Physician-Assisted Suicide," 1705. See also Johannes J.W. Van Delden, Loes Pijnenborg, and Paul van der Maas, "Dances With Data," *Bioethics* 7:4 (July 1993): 323-329.

47. I have drawn on Margaret Battin, "Voluntary Euthanasia and the Risks of Abuse: Can We Learn Anything from the Netherlands?," *Law, Medicine, & Health Care* 20:1-2 (Spring/Summer 1992), reprinted in Margaret Pabst Battin,*The Least Worst Death: Essays in Bioethics on the End of Life* (New York: Oxford University Press, 1994), 163-181; Quill, *Death and Dignity*, 161-164; Franklin G. Miller et al, "Regulating Physician-Assisted Death," *New England Journal of Medicine* 331:2 (July 1994): 119-123.

48. Dorff, *Matters of Life and Death*, 187-188; Elliot N. Dorff, "Assisted Suicide," 10.

49. Rosner, *Modern Medicine*, 228.

50. CCAR, "Responsum 5754.14. On the Treatment of the Terminally Ill," *Teshuvot for the Nineties*, 342. See also CCAR, "Responsum 160. CPR and The Frail Elderly (1989)," in Walter Jacob, *Questions and Reform Jewish Answers: New American Reform Responsa* (New York 1992), 265-266.

51. CCAR, "Responsum 83. Quality of Life and Euthanasia (1985)," *Contemporary American Reform Responsa*, 139-140. See also CCAR, "Responsum 156. Living Will (1989)," *Questions and Reform Jewish Answers*, 256.

52. CCAR, "Responsum 5750.5. Hospital Patient Beyond Recovery," *Teshuvot for the Nineties*, 368.

53. Rosner, *Modern Medicine*, 227.

54. Bleich, *Bioethical Dilemmas*, 69, 116. See also Bleich, *Judaism and Healing*, 136, 139.

55. Avram Israel Reisner, "A Halakhic Ethic of Care for the Terminally Ill," *Conservative Judaism* 43:3 (Spring 1991): 54-55, 68-69.

56. Dorff, *Matters of Life and Death*, 188. See also Dorff, "Assisted Suicide," 9-11.

Chapter 7

Ten Suggestions for Patients Facing a Terminal Illness or a Chronic, Debilitating Condition

When you learn that you suffer from an illness that is expected to take your life, your days change. You face new challenges and worries. You experience feelings of loss on a number of levels: pain; physical, emotional, and spiritual suffering; denial; anger; guilt; frustration and fear.

Knowing that a disease or condition threatens your life raises a number of concerns. How long will I live? (More appropriately, what is the shortest and longest that I am likely to live?) What is likely to happen to me before the end? What types of pain and suffering will I experience? What are the available medical options and what will they likely do for and to me? How will I pay for my treatments? Who will care for me? Will I be a burden to my loved ones? What will happen to: my spouse, my children, my partner, my friends?

It is only natural to feel worried and afraid. Your stress will likely affect your condition.

In the twenty-first century, the process of dying can take many forms and may be quite prolonged and deformed. What do you want and why? Does when and how you die matter to you -- a lot, somewhat, or not at all? How do you want to be remembered? Do you care about your image? How others see you in a gravely debilitated and deteriorated condition, facing a protracted demise?

Take Emily, an incapacitated eight-seven year old stroke victim, partly paralyzed, needing a wheelchair to get around, able to speak only with difficulty, who lives at home, with round-the-clock nurses and companions, at a cost of tens of thousands of dollars a year. What should she do? How should she go about making a decision regarding the end of her life?

As Emily tosses and turns at night, she grapples with a number of dilemmas. Does she want to: complete tasks, retain control, resolve family and emotional issues, and accept her pain and suffering? Or, does she want to: drop unfinished tasks, yield control, leave family and other matters unresolved, and avoid further pain and suffering? Does she see her life as hopeless, lacking any realistic options? What does it really mean for her to have a dignified end to her life? In contemplating and planning for a peaceful death, will she act out of: fear, resignation, despair, or a desire to escape?

Leaving aside the legalities, both American and Jewish, discussed in Chapter 6, does Emily want to determine the time and manner of her demise? Does she wish to choose to die at her own time and in her own way? Does she desire to decide when "enough is enough?" Does she wish to reject medical interventions lengthening the process of dying more than she wants it extended? Does she desire to die passively or to try to assert more active control, to a greater or lesser degree, over the process of her dying? In other words, does she want to play some sort of role in bringing about her own death or does she want to allow herself to succumb, more "naturally?" Does she want a planned death where her family and friends gather in an atmosphere of a good-bye party?

It boils down to how does Emily (or you) balance: extending one's life versus avoiding great pain and suffering; maintaining the quality of one's life in all its various aspects as well as one's dignity; ensuring that others remember you as you wish them to. In other words, is one's continued life a benefit or a burden?

This chapter and the next one focus on your decision-making as a patient diagnosed with a terminal illness or an incurable, debilitating chronic condition, in answering one question: do you want to go sooner or later? Do you want the end to be protracted, to live for as long as you possibly can, despite a gradually deteriorating condition, or do you want to avoid the worst (or perhaps any significant) degradation your illness or condition can deliver, at the expense of weeks or months (or even years) of life?

It is not an easy choice. You will struggle with the complexity of what you are doing. Although most modern Jewish commentators will disagree, I do not see your quest as a black or white issue. It is quite complex, with many nuances and shades of gray. In Chapter 6, I suggested, after reviewing the spectrum of opinions, that it is a very personal question, not solved by simply looking at the rules provided by Jewish law or even the underlying sanctity of biological life principle.

This chapter offers ten suggestions designed to assist you as you face a life threatening or even a chronic illness. First, don't blame yourself. Also, second, despite your anguish, try to continue to develop your faith and trust in God. Third, turn to prayer and meditation. Fourth, take on more responsibility for your situation. Fifth, cultivate a lighthearted, positive outlook. Sixth, reframe your pain and suffering. Seventh, participate in social support networks. Eighth, find meaning and purpose in your life, despite your plight. Ninth, engage in selfless service to others. Tenth, achieve emotional and spiritual closure with your loved ones. Before considering each of these in more detail, remember: whether through your spiritual practices, your assertiveness, or your social support network, you need to cultivate the desire to be helped. Cherish hope and gratefully receive encouragement.

Don't Blame Yourself

Guilt often enters into the equation when you are ill. Don't blame yourself for getting so sick. Don't ask: Why me? Rather, thank your limbs, organs, and cells for faithfully sustaining you for as long as they have. Adopt a forgiving, rather compassionate and supportive attitude to your body, your mind and your soul.

Even if you have done the "right" preventive things and you encounter terminal illness or a chronic condition, you are not a spiritual failure. A multitude of causal factors, such as genetic, family, and personal history, environmental, lifestyle, nutritional, general health habits, and accidents, all enter into the picture. Modern Western medical science, as well as alternative healthcare approaches, simply do not know what causes some diseases or their cure.

Do not worry that you brought your condition, physical or mental, on yourself as a result of some type of behavior or personality characteristic. God is not punishing you. Illness is not sent to purify your character. Your misery is not deserved.

Develop Your Faith and Trust in God

Spiritual practices for healing -- achieving a wholeness of your body-mind-spirit -- depend on a clear realization of the Divine Presence, an unfaltering faith in God's infinite goodness, and an unbounded trust in the Eternal's love. As the Psalmist tells us: "How happy are those who trust in You [God]." (Psalm 84:12).

The future remains open, no matter how bleak the present may be and seem. You are not alone. You can draw on the Holy One's Presence as a source of guidance and support in your plight. God is with you in your time of need. Strive to develop a personal relationship with the Eternal.

You can turn to God, the Ultimate Comforter. The Supreme Sovereign nurtures each of us on an ongoing basis. Again, remember the words of the Psalmist: Though I go through deepest darkness, I fear no evil, for You are with me; Your rod and Your staff, they protect me. You have prepared a banquet before me in the presence of my enemies; You welcome me as an honored guest and fill my cup to the brim. Surely Your goodness and mercy will be with me all my life; and I shall dwell in Your house forever. (Psalm 23:4-6).

Somehow the Eternal suffers when you do. Human anguish represents a source of Divine agony. The Hebrew prophet, the Second Isaiah, writes, "In all their troubles God was troubled." (Isaiah 63:9). In the Babylonian Talmud, Rabbi Meir recounts, "When a person is in pain what does the Divine Presence say? My head aches. My arm aches." (Sanhedrin 46a). As we have seen in Chapter 3, although Divine suffering is beyond human conception, an awareness of God's agony and sorrow may help to ameliorate your anguish.

Keep firmly in mind that you are a Divine being and an integral part of God's plan for the cosmos. Reaffirm daily that you are a child of the Holy One, Who will not desert you. Thus, a positive belief in your spiritual practices, a realization that, for instance, your prayers are acceptable and that God constantly sends each of us beneficent influences, are of vital importance in helping you remain alive, no matter how difficult your physical or mental condition.

Develop and deepen you faith and trust that everything is in God's hands and everything the Eternal does is for the best: your joy and sadness, your health and sickness, your hope and loss. Perceive your life as ultimately being one with God, your Creator and Sustainer. See the Holy One as a partner working with you even in your time of trouble and tragedy.

Turn to Prayer and Meditation

We pray and meditate when we are stricken with illness, physical or mental, and experience the accompanying pain and suffering, especially when we are convinced that human assistance has exhausted its possibility of helping us. When hope in a human agency of curing is dimmed, we turn to God.

Prayer represents a universal way to connect and communicate with God, the Master Healer. By keeping our attention anchored in the present moment, meditation enables us to go deeply within our own experience, our own uniqueness. Prayer and meditation represent powerful healing techniques. Through prayer and meditation we attain wholeness, integration, and harmony. Prayer and meditation can even facilitate physical and mental recovery.

Prayers

You can offer various types of prayers -- petitionary, affirmative, or surrender -- for your own healing and the restoration of health. Experiment with different forms of prayer, including crying out to God.[1] There are many ways of praying: verbally, silently, or with music. Realizing that words are not the only acceptable form of prayer, you need to discover what is appropriate for you. Prayer need not be a conscious, waking activity. You can pray in your dreams, unconsciously. A deep, driving desire is a prayer that is always going on.

To engage in prayer for your own healing or recovery, select a quiet location. Get away from or turn off your answering machine, your beeper, your computer, and your fax. Close your eyes to eliminate distractions. Relax and calm your body and mind with deep breathing. Sit or recline comfortably, but keep your back, neck, and head straight. Do not slouch. Repeat whatever prayer you select once or twice a day, for ten to fifteen minutes, for several weeks. Be patient and positive.

Petitionary Prayers

You can offer one of these petitionary prayers to invoke God's aid:

Bring healing (or a cure) to my suffering, [specify the problem] O God, the most powerful and compassionate Healer.
Blessed are You, O God, Who brings healing (or curing). Please heal me. (Please cure my ---.)
God, please increase in me Your life giving and healing (or curing) power.

Affirmative Prayers

You can offer affirmative prayers for either your general health or a specific malady. For your general health:

God fills me with perfect health and strength, strengthening the parts in me that can do the regeneration.
God expresses the Divine Presence in me through my perfect health and well-being.
God, Who gave me life, repairs me, restores my strength in accordance with the Divine goodness and lovingkindness.
God, the Source of all health, works wonders.

For a specific physical malady or an organ or limb:

The stream of Divine health and goodness flows into my --- [specify organ or limb], filling it with abundant wellness, restoring me to perfect health and strength.
Health and wellness saturates my --- [specify organ or limb], obliterating all my pain and suffering.
God removes the pain from my ---; the Eternal is restoring me to perfect health.

For mental or emotional illness, especially depression:

God, fill me with joy, peace, and confidence.

Prayers of Surrender

You can give the situation over to God, either after or in conjunction with healthcare professionals and alternative practitioners doing or having done the best they can for you. In praying for what is best for you, because you do not know what that is, offer one of the following prayers of surrender. Remember that God has many ways of helping you.

Thy will be done.
Whatever You think is good for me, what You think I should go through, please do it.
I trust in You, O Loving God, Who created and sustains me. I realize I am in Your control, an infinitely loving Presence. I am loved by the Eternal One.
Into God's hands I entrust my spirit, when I sleep and when I wake, and with my spirit and my body also, God is with me, I will not fear. (The last line of the *Adon Olom* (God Eternal) prayer, probably composed by Solomon ibn Gabriel (1021-1058 C.E.), Spanish-Jewish poet, hymn writer, and philosopher.)

If you are in such pain and suffering that you are unable to concentrate on any type of prayer, whether petitionary, affirmative, or surrender, ask for a candle to be lit to represent your prayer and placed where you can see it. Then try to pray whenever you are as calm as you can be. With your eyes closed, repeat very slowly for as long as you can (or up to fifteen minutes): God removes (try to exhale a sigh) all pain from my --- [part of body or mind] and restores (try to inhale) me to perfect health.

Cry Out to God

You may want to cry out to God, the Source of Strength, as do the Hasidic followers of Rabbi Nachman of Breslov, who lived from 1772 to 1810, who roused his followers to heights of attachment to God together with sublime joy. Even today, they engage in secluded prayer.[2]

Daily, they talk to God in private prayer, in their own language and from their own hearts. They speak about whatever is on their minds, about everything and anything.

If possible, find a place where no one else is present, where you can be alone with yourself and God. Set aside a specific time each day for this aloneness. Cry out to the Eternal: "Open my heart. Please help me." Talk to God. Express your concerns, your problems and your needs. Be truthful. Do not hide anything.

In entering into a personal conversation with God, get comfortable and speak as you would to your best friend or closest relative. Do not be concerned about using formal prayer language. Use the language you are comfortable with. Talk in a tone that is best for you. Speak of everything, wherever the spirit leads you. Do not hold anything back. Be confident of being heard with compassion and understanding.

Trust God to have your best interest at heart. Pour out your heart to the Eternal God -- your fears, your worries, your sorrows, your anger -- and ask for the Holy One's help.

After pouring out your heart and entering into an intimate dialogue with God, turn things over to the Supreme Sovereign, making space for the Eternal. By emptying yourself of your mental and emotional clutter, you will become more open and receptive to God. Surrendering yourself to God's care and delivering yourself to the Divine protection, you will be given help in a manner you can accept and understand. Persist in crying out and turning to God.

Meditations

Meditation helps you clear your mind and identify and connect with God. By calming and focusing your mind, freeing it from negative thoughts and helping you relax, meditation enables you to enter into a state of awareness and stillness for a period of time. You begin to experience an inner peace and a transcendent vision. As you forget yourself, you feel the presence of God. You reconnect to the Eternal, the Source of comfort and healing.

In his best-selling book *The Relaxation Response*,[3] Dr. Herbert Benson presents the Relaxation Response, a demystified form of meditation, a turning inward, designed to induce short-term calming and long-term benefits. Researchers have concluded that the Relaxation Response, helps with chronic pain (including headaches and back pain), hypertension, heart disease, diabetes, ulcers, asthma, arthritis, and cancer. Specifically, cancer patients experienced decreased symptoms and better control of nausea and vomiting associated with chemotherapy. Individuals who had undergone open-heart surgery encountered less anxiety and few postoperative heart difficulties. Patients with cardiac irregularities experienced fewer of them. There was less anxiety and less need for medication for those undergoing painful X-ray procedures.[4]

What is going on? The Relaxation Response breaks the pattern of our everyday thoughts. Giving the brain and the body a respite results in a physiological relaxation. A significant drop in the body's oxygen consumption accompanies a downshifting in metabolism. Blood pressure drops, heart rate decreases, breathing slows and becomes deeper, and muscles relax and require less blood. According to Dr. Benson, the point is ". . . when the mind quiets down, the body follows suit."[5]

Six basic steps must be followed:[6] (1) Sit in a comfortable position, with your eyes closed. (2) Let your muscles relax, starting with your face and working down to your feet. (3) Become aware of your breath as you breathe in and out through your nose. Each time you exhale, repeat a word, a prayer, or a phrase, for example, *Shalom*, *Sh'ma Yisroel* or "The Eternal is My Shepherd." (4) Disregard everyday thoughts that come to mind. Do not fight these distracting thoughts. Return to your repetition and your breathing. (5) Continue the repetition for ten to fifteen minutes. Once you finish, do not stand immediately but continue to sit quietly, allowing your thoughts to return. Then open your eyes and sit another minute or so before standing up. (6) Practice this technique once or twice daily; morning and evening are best. The more dramatic effects of using the Relaxation Response are cumulative overtime.

According to Dr. Benson, religious conviction, such as Spiritual Judaism, enhances the beneficial effects of the Relaxation Response. Using a focus that is drawn from a religious tradition reinforces the Relaxation Response. You are more apt to adhere to the routine, to look forward to and enjoy it. Dr. Benson concludes: "When present, faith in an eternal or life transcending force seemed to make the fullest use of remembered wellness because it is a supremely soothing belief, disconnecting unhealthy logic and worries. . . . It appeared that beliefs added to the response transported the mind/body even more dramatically, quieting worries and fears significantly better than the relaxation response alone."[7]

Whatever your spiritual practices they must be sincere; they must come from your own heart. God wants your wholeheartedness, your genuine devotion. Reach out to and connect with the Supreme Sovereign. Pray and meditate with concentration and a total effort of your entire being. Sincerely yearn for healing, a wholeness of your body, mind, and spirit, if not a physical or mental cure.

Take on More Responsibility

Learn to meet your physician as an equal. Each of us has a responsibility to pull our self along. Play an active role now when you face a life threatening illness or a chronic condition.

Take responsibility for all aspects of your medical situation. You are the central factor. Bernie Siegel, the noted oncologist and the best-selling author of *Love, Medicine and Miracles*,[8] concludes that an unshakable relationship with their own internal will and its encounter with God characterizes "exceptional cancer patients," not their faith in a physician's medical skills and powers.

These exceptional patients feel more in control of their fate. They have a strong sense of self-efficacy. They perceive that they are the masters of their destiny. They believe that they can make things happen. They maintain close vigilance over their medical treatments. They are willing to participate in and take responsibility for decisions related to their health. They want to enter into more equal relationships with their healthcare professionals.

They are not submissive, passive sufferers. Rather they are responsible, assertive participants, who express their personal rights and communicate their feelings. Taking charge of their medical care, they argue with their healthcare professionals. Seeking solutions, they remain open to exploring new treatment avenues. If you choose to become one of these exceptional patients, you may find a procedure or treatment that increases the acceptable physical or mental quality of your life for a longer period.

These exceptional patients manifest a fighting spirit, an attribute of optimism, an intense desire to live and experience joy, a willingness to fight for as full a life as possible, hoping for the best and believing in their ability to survive and affirming their belief that their illness will not kill them, although they have a realistic appraisal of their situation and can be prepared for the worst. They communicate clearly and openly with their healthcare professionals and express appropriate emotions. They are also willing to look at their lives beyond their illness or condition, to what they have contributed in the past and to what they hope to accomplish with the time they have left.

As part of this new healing paradigm, healthcare professionals and alternative practitioners will serve as valuable resources for these confident, resilient, more self-reliant, high self-esteem, empowered individuals, who will define their own personal visions of health and learn from and respond to life's adversities. Armed with new skills, resources and capacities, a more expansive understanding of health and disease, their faith and trust in God Who is able to contribute to human emotional and spiritual empowerment, they will assert a primary role in healthcare decision-making. They will make more conscious and self-directed choices. Increasingly, they will not look to medical professionals as the final authority on issues of health and healing.

Cultivate a Positive, Lighthearted Outlook

Hope and optimism help in healing, leading to a wholeness of mind-body-spirit and to better medical outcomes. Drugs and procedures are more effective when you are in a hopeful state of mind. Our thoughts have a magical power. Our mental attitude does impact on disease progression. You have probably heard stories of critically ill people whose cheerful attitudes help them recover.

When you are ailing, try not to be fearful or to worry. Do not sink into a morass of negativity, hopelessness and depression. Of course, this is not easy; however, strive to face life with optimism and courage. Sometimes illness may appear to crush us, mentally and emotionally. Do not brood over your ailment; otherwise, you will encourage it. Try to minimize your physical or mental problems, make light of the dangers, and strive for cheerful thoughts and talk. Ask family members and friends to take a positive attitude toward your condition and to continue to relate to your life as they have done in the past.

In *Anatomy of an Illness*,[9] Norman Cousins champions the ideal that humor can help restore one's health. Cousins provides anecdotal evidence of the benefits derived from his own use of old episodes of the television show "Candid Camera," Marx Brothers movies, and humor books to overcome a rare and painful illness. As the saying goes, "laughter is good medicine."

Cousins notes that laughter has rejuvenating effects on the body and the mind. It relaxes muscles and reduces blood pressure and heart rate. Laughter, what Cousins term "internal jugging," gets your attention off of you and your plight. It provides the distance needed for a new and better perspective on your situation.

Reframe Your Pain and Suffering

Strive to reframe your situation, searching out positive ways of viewing your difficulties. Focus on the meaning and value to you of your continued suffering. Do you see your illness or condition as a challenge, a creative opportunity, an invitation to "come up higher" and to contribute more profoundly to the creation perfection of the world? Remember: God believes in you.

Ask yourself: What is it you need to learn from my illness or condition? Ask God: "Teach me." If you have only a little time left, your spiritual learning - healing - creating curve may accelerate enormously.

Begin by trying to reframe your situation.[10] Recognize how your negative, automatic thoughts cause you to feel anxious, depressed, angry, guilty, or helpless. Realize that some of these thoughts are distorted, illogical, or exaggerated. Challenge your negative thoughts. Is it correct? Am I jumping to conclusions? What is the evidence? Am I exaggerating the bleak aspects of my situation? How do I know what will happen? Is it as bad as it seems? Is there another way to look at it? Replace your negative thoughts with more positive statements and affirmations. Use journal writing to help you identify vulnerable areas, where your buttons are pushed as well as patterns of distorted thoughts.

Also, regularly reevaluate whether you think you are contributing or learning anything valuable by delaying your death. Does your pain and suffering serve a constructive purpose? Can the positive energies you are generating spread to others? Try to reassess the significance of your illness or condition in terms of the possibilities it offers for your spiritual growth and development and in helping you face and attempt to resolve difficult emotional and relational issues. Those who need to meet you part-way to reach such resolution may attain a significant opening and reconstruction of their views and feelings by responding to your personal stance in these testing circumstances. They may be blessed with repentance and atonement. You were stricken; they may be healed. Delaying your demise may enable you to grow personally and contribute to the growth of others.

Specifically, do you need to cultivate patience, courage, or faith? Do you need to learn to receive care, particularly through your dependency on others, as part of the dying process? Are you willing to accept dependency for the benefit of those who love you? For example, you raised your children and did so much for them, now they want to reciprocate and care for you. Are you able to let them provide care as a means of completing the relationship? Or, does the shift from caretaker to care recipient, accompanied by a parallel loss of control and status, represent a devastating blow to your self-esteem and you ability to cope?

Elisabeth Kübler-Ross, the death-and-dying pioneer, tells the poignant, personal story of her seventy-nine year old mother who throughout her life gave and gave, but could not receive. "One day," she writes, "we got a phone call saying that Mama had been found in the bathroom with a massive stroke. She was paralyzed, unable to speak, unable to move anything, unable to do anything." After her mother suffered another massive stroke, "she just had to let people wash her, feed her, take care of everything for her." Kübler-Ross and her sisters found an excellent nursing home for their mother, who remained there four years before dying; learning the lessons she needed to learn. Kübler-Ross recalled:[11]

> I was furious with God. I cannot tell you, I could have shred Him to pieces if I'd had the chance. I used every language, Swiss, French, Italian, English, everything. He didn't budge. He gave no response. No *nothing*.
>
> And I said to Him, "You S.O.B." . . . in *our* language. And got absolutely no reaction from Him. That made me even more furious.
>
> You know, you can call Him every name, and He just sits there and loves you. . . . You know, it is like when you are really mad and somebody says "Sweetie Pie" to you. . . . And you could kill Him. . . . And I went through all the rage, the bargaining, the depression and the guilt trip and the whole works.
>
> This rage of mine lasted not only for the four years that she continued *existing* in that body, but weeks and months after she died I still tried to review my opinion of God. I really needed to come to grips with this. I thought, "He can't be such an S.O.B. But how can a loving, compassionate, understanding God let this woman suffer who has been seventy-nine years loving and giving and caring and sharing?" I mean, that is not God. . . .
>
> And then, months after she died -- needless to say we were very relieved and glad when she finally died. . . . I don't know how to say it, but one day I reviewed my opinion of God. And the moment I realized what this was all about I almost jumped out of my skin. And I said, "Thank you, thank you,

thank you, thank you, you are the most generous man that ever existed.". .

You know, what suddenly came to me on that day is that you get your lessons one way or another, you understand, and *you* yourself are responsible for what lessons you *get* -- and, since I at least *knew* this, I shouldn't have had such a tough one -- and at last I realized what He did for her, and that you are only able to see that from a distance. . . .

And with my distance from my horribly suffering mother who laid guilt trips on me with her looks, I finally saw that this is the most generous God because he allowed her to give and give and give and love for seventy-nine years and she only had to learn to receive for four years.

You understand that? Generous -

Nowadays if I see somebody who just has to learn it the hard way because he didn't learn it the easy way, I know for sure it's His doing. . . .

To help you see your situation in a new light, set aside sometime each day to offer, for ten to fifteen minutes, the following focused, personal prayer.[12]

Learning Life's Lessons Prayer

O dear God, help me understand
that life's difficulties are
life's opportunities,
that life's bitter disappointments are
life's finest teachers.

Even if you make previously impossible leaps of spiritual development, how long are you willing to endure the continued physical, emotional, and spiritual anguish? At what point does your unremitting pain and suffering, reaching excruciating, uncontrollable levels, serve no purpose? When do you reach the point of no further opportunity for spiritual growth and development and begin to turn toward the next phase of your larger life? When is "enough, enough?" Not because you have no more resources or capacity but because your earthly work is truly finished, it is enough. Only you can answer these questions. Listen to your inner voice.

Participate in Social Support Networks

Participate in social support networks. Social support helps us. We realize that we are not alone in facing life's challenges and hardships. Friends and family can offer practical help and information, emotional support, and spiritual encouragement. All this is beneficial.

In addition, you may need to find a support group where you can experience understanding from strangers with whom you can share your losses, fears and thoughts. You will be able to hear how others find strength in their plight, learn new ways to deal with life's spiritual, physical, mental, emotional, and social challenges, listen to what others say about what is helpful to them, and share stories and laughs. When you encourage others and they encourage you, the emotional - spiritual power is increased.

Empirical studies show that social contact helps extend the length and quality of life. In a widely cited study, researchers found that women suffering from advanced breast cancer who participated in support groups lived an average of eighteen months longer than those patients who did not -- a significant difference.[13] This study demonstrates the power of an interpersonal connectedness to improve life extension.

Groups composed of people linked only by a common illness or a chronic condition offer particularly effective emotional support. Sufferers experience the benefits of being linked to and participating in a growing relationship, even with strangers. They learn new and more effective coping skills and new levels of connectedness. They let down their defenses, begin to communicate openly, and get in touch with and honestly share their feelings through close, self-revealing discussions with others. They talk about who and what they really are, without judgment, criticism, or rejection. Support groups provide safe spaces where people are able to talk about what is going on in their lives and enable them to create a sense of intimacy they may not have experienced for a longtime, if at all. Members offer nurturance, reassurance of each person's worth, and a general sense that they can always turn to other participants. Hearing others' stories, one's own story falls into perspective.

The breast cancer support group participants, for instance, discussed how to cope with cancer. They expressed their feelings about their illness, their grief, their anger, and its impact on their lives, thereby enabling them to better carry on with their daily existence. The support group also helped them overcome the alienation that often divides cancer patients from well-meaning but anxious family members and friends. It helped them improve their communication with relatives and physicians, better control their pain and suffering, and face and master their fears about death and dying.

Find Meaning and Purpose in Your Life

We all need to find a sense of meaning and purpose in our lives, especially in the last stage of our existence. Within the limitations imposed by our physical and mental capabilities, we want to do something meaningful and significant, thereby overcoming our spiritual distress, our inner emptiness.

Have you ever asked yourself: "What's my life all about?" Or, "What is the meaning of my life?" Now may be the time to reflect and find a purpose for your continued earthly existence, despite your present physical or mental condition. Searching for sources of strength may enable you to reframe your current situation and help you through your moments of despair.

The courage to continue to exist despite pain and suffering becomes a matter of choice linked to your belief that you have unfinished business in life, even in the most traumatic and tragic moments. Out of his Nazi concentration camp experiences, the late Viktor E. Frankl, the renowned existential psychiatrist, found meaning in suffering. He was impressed by the courage of those who survived their ordeal by focusing on the opportunities, presented in their situation, to respond well. They adapted to where they were in life; they turned suffering into human triumph. Individuals are free to choose the ways they confront life; they may find a "why" for life, enduring the most unbearable "how." For Frankl, the search for meaning represents a primary force in one's life. As he wrote regarding his concentration camp experiences:

> A man who let himself decline because he could not see any future goal found himself occupied with retrospective thoughts. In a different connection, we have already spoken of the tendency there was to look into the past, to help make the present, with all its horrors, less real. But in robbing the present of its reality there lay a certain danger. It became easy to overlook the opportunities to make something positive of camp life, opportunities which really did exist. Regarding our "provisional existence" as unreal was in itself an important factor in causing prisoners to lose their

> hold on life; everything in a way became pointless. Such people forgot that often it is just such an exceptionally difficult external situation which gives man an opportunity to grow spiritually beyond himself. Instead of taking the camp's difficulties as a test of their inner strength, they did not take their life seriously and despised it as something of no consequence. They preferred to close their eyes and live in the past. Life for such people became meaningless.[14]

Strive to elicit meaning and purpose for your life, even in a seemingly hopeless situation -- your terminal illness or chronic, debilitating condition -- through reframing your circumstances. Try to make the most of your predicament.

A life threatening illness often opens the pathways to self-examination. What is your purpose in life? What are your values, interests, and priorities? What are your short-term and long-term goals? What are your strategies for attaining your goals? Where do you want to put your remaining time and energy?

Through your illness or condition, you may come to see what you truly believe in life. Your continued search for meaning and purpose in life may give you the strength to endure. There is always one more challenge, one more mountain to climb, one more opportunity to actualize your values. For instance, you may need to learn to open your heart in love and compassion to others, your family and friends -- even to God -- and to forgive. Ask yourself what is preventing you from living your days with as much lovingkindness and forgiveness as you possibly can?

Fever, exhaustion, and pain, of course, may make sustained introspection difficult, if not impossible. Yet your suffering may be conducive to deeper insight and self-understanding, resulting in your emotional and spiritual evolution.

Even if you are exhausted from the self-defeating cycle of being unable to do things or go out and the sameness of every day, having a compass, a sense of positive direction regarding the end of your life, will help reawaken your spirit for living. Try, if possible, to widen the spectrum of meaning and purpose beyond a focus on yourself. Reorder your life to reflect this awareness. Ask yourself: What it is that I am here for? From the perspective of Spiritual Judaism, to it is contribute love and compassion to the world as well as to express and experience unconditional love. Find your fulfillment in these spiritual virtues and in your interactions with others.

In committing yourself to a new set of priorities, you may find a connection to something far greater than yourself. As many have found, the transcendent realm, God, your immortal soul, and the afterlife World to Come, assume a greater prominence. Your illness may facilitate a profound spiritual change and deepening. Projecting yourself, that is to say, your immortal soul, into the future may help restore a sense of hope and meaning in the present.

Embark on a spiritual journey at the end of life as a chance to learn and grow. Rethink what really matters. Strive to find your own meaning and purpose. Focus on your goals and priorities. There are only so many hours in a day, only so many days left, so fill your time with your priorities.

Let me suggest several ways, namely, listen to your inner voice, engage in a life review by means of the Life Roadmap Exercise, use the Meaning of Life Meditation to pursue your search for meaning and purpose, thereby transcending your current physical or mental limits.

Listen to Your Inner Voice

Ask yourself: Would prolonging your life over several months serve any purpose? Do you want to complete certain life tasks? Is there something you want to do? Read a book? Learn? Complete an unfinished project? How important is your continued ability to do something with your life?

You may want to set aside some time each day to offer, for ten to fifteen minutes, the following focused, personal prayer:[15]

Life's Priorities Prayer

O Eternal One
help me find the enduring truths of life.
Let my every word and action be directed
toward life's ultimate goals.
How eager I am to face You,
my Creator,
help me devote my days
to preparation for the moment

when I will meet You.
How I long to come into
Your Presence!
Liberate me from my
fantasies and illusions,
Set me free to be You.
From the unreal,
lead me to the Real,
From darkness lead me to Light,
From death lead me to
Immortality.

Daily, be quiet and listen to your inner voice, hear God's call to you -- the Eternal's still, small voice (1 Kings 19:12). Offer a prayer that God direct your mind and all your conscious processes and that the Holy One will indicate to you what to do. Sit and wait. Does the voice repeat itself, nudging you toward something? As directions come to you, write them down. If they seem reasonable, carry them out. If not, if you feel uneasy and doubtful, wait for further direction. The right direction will feel correct from the beginning, and you will be drawn to it. There will be no doubt.

The Supreme Sovereign will reveal your unique function. The more you are able to pursue a task you understand to be uniquely yours, the more your life will have meaning and purpose. You will come to know what to do with your life and you will feel fulfilled in doing it, whether it "succeeds" in worldly terms or not, because it is yours -- your creative contribution to God's artwork, this world. It will give you deep satisfaction.

You may also want to seek out others, your spouse, family members, or friends, whether older or younger, who may be on a spiritual journey. Discuss with them your quest for meaning and purpose. Perhaps they will share theirs. You can learn from one another and draw closer together.

Engage in a Life Review

A life review may help you find meaning and purpose in your remaining days, weeks, and months. A life review will let you see your life as a whole. Take stock and reflect on your life and its events and relationships, good times and bad times. Ask yourself: What events, experiences, and interactions with people and places have had a major impact on my life? What were my emotions and feelings then? What are my emotions and feelings now? What insights did I gain? What do I now understand?

A life review will enable you to see what your life has added up to overall as well as your specific accomplishments and disappointments. It will let you forgive yourself for your shortcomings and regrets. It will enable you to achieve an inner peace within yourself, reconciling yourself to not having done all the things you wanted do or thought you wanted to do. Come to terms with who you are, what the world is about, your place in it. Perhaps you will discover a wider view of your life.

Also, contemplate what your earthly presence has meant to others. Ask yourself: How has my life affected others? What does my presence mean to them now and in the future?

Create a Life Roadmap

To find meaning in your life and gain a new set of goals and priorities for the time remaining to you, many have found it helpful to create a Life Roadmap.[16] Use this exercise as a means of short-term and long-term goal setting.

Get a big, make that a really big, sheet of paper. Use flip chart paper or the back of a sheet of giftwrap. Begin with a story of your life -- your first significant event, situation, or person. Put some representation of that event on the paper. Then, go forward from that event to the present, using freehand drawings or taping pictures from magazines or old photographs to the paper. Show your life's positive and negative events; the people who influenced you, your mentors, teachers, role models; the road blocks and hurdles you encountered. Don't worry about how it looks. Focus on what has been meaningful for you in the past and present.

Then, where do you want to go in the future? What would you like for yourself in terms of your career, relationships, creativity, material objects, play, spirituality, health? Again, represent your goals in some way on the paper.

Each day try to do something meaningful to achieve your goals, even if only you have a short time to live. Strive to do something new and good for yourself and for others, each and every day.

Use the Meaning of Life Meditation

Many have found that meditation helps facilitate the search for meaning and purpose in life. Meditation aids our inner journey, enabling us to realize our true and authentic being. Meditation in the Jewish path provides intimacy with God in every aspect of our lives. We become aware of the Divine Presence and directly encounter God.

Use the following meditation for ten or fifteen minutes once or twice daily, for several weeks, if possible. Be patient. Open yourself to God and invite the Holy One into your heart and your being.

Meaning of Life Meditation

Introductory Instructions. Create a warm, welcoming atmosphere, and environment of serenity and spaciousness for the journey within. Lower the lights in your room.

Close your eyes, sit quietly, calm and relax your body by sitting, reclining or lying down, breathing in and out normally, feeling where your breath flows into and out of your body. Adjust your breaths so that the in and out breaths are the same length thereby bringing about both a relaxation of your body and an alertness of your mind. (Obviously, vary these instructions depending on your situation).

Contemplate what are the three most important things for you to do with your remaining time: Consider areas such as work, creativity, inner life, and relationships. From these choose three for priority concentration.

For each close relationship, ask what would be left undone if you were to die before important things were said?

Reflect on what is your significance in the great scheme of things. Breathe in the power of purpose; exhale your confusion.

Reflect on: what is hope and where do you find it? Consider: your family, nature, God. How do you know when you have hope?

Concluding Instructions. Now come back to the here and now. Take time to ease yourself back. Slowly bring your awareness back into your being. Feel yourself back in your room and open your eyes.

You may find it helpful to write down: the three most important things for you to do with your remaining time; your significance in the great scheme of things; what is hope and where you find it? Each day repeat these to yourself as affirmations.

Some Concluding Thoughts on Finding Meaning and Purpose in Your Life

Try to live life fully and make the most of each day you have left. Focusing on meaningful activities and commitments raises your self-esteem, engendering hope and joyfulness. It also helps to shift your viewpoint from being a patient twenty-four hours a day to being someone with important things to do and to look forward to. It will help you look at and reframe your illness or condition as a challenge, a learning experience, however difficult.

Set daily, realistic goals. Strive to complete significant, unfinished projects. Focus on and finish one thing at a time.

Strive to improve the quality of your life in small increments within your capacity to manage. Make your life more meaningful, for example, by increasing your mobility for a brief time period by moving from your bed to a chair; entering into conversations about life and family situations thereby increasing the scope of your involvement and interests which you have not engaged in for a while; or taking control of your pain medication.

Even if your physical or mental abilities and energies are at a low ebb, accomplishing a goal, such as making even one telephone call, sending one email, or performing a specific task, will help your self-esteem and continue to provide meaning to your existence. However, remain flexible. Your energy level may not be up to the task you set for yourself. In that case, you can at least say a prayer for someone else in need.

If you have the strength and the time, you may want to embark on a new endeavor. For instance, you may want to take up a hobby you put aside long ago or learn a new skill.

Benefits of Selfless Service to Others

Love, compassion, and selfless service may enter into healing and even into curing physical or mental symptoms. Love and compassion influence the effectiveness of our spiritual practices. Conversely, if love and compassion are not present, prayers, meditations, and visualizations are less effective.

To facilitate your healing -- achieving a wholeness of body - mind - spirit, -- develop a sense of altruism, a fuller life shared with the rest of humanity, through your unconditional love, your selfless service, and your participation in the life of the community. There is a healing power in "doing good."

Begin by performing small acts of kindness toward others in daily life, out of your unconditional love for them. Look at each person you meet during the day and love him or her without expecting anything in return. You will soon experience the fact that you are not alone. By extending your love, your very essence, you will gradually forget about your pain and suffering, whether physical or mental. You will gradually detach yourself from your mental image of weakness, isolation, or hopelessness.

Within the limitations of your physical or mental abilities, strive to help repair the world through selfless service. Do what you can for others. This will bring new meaning to your existence. Experiencing the joyfulness of living through a useful, other-directed activity, will help you begin to transcend your pain and suffering.

In his book *The Healing Power of Doing Good*,[17] Allan Luks summarizes surveys he conducted involving the relationship between altruism and well-being. Luks concludes that people who regularly engaged in helping activities involving personal contact, particularly with strangers who needed assistance, without regard to the outcome, experienced "feel-good" sensations directly associated with better self-perceived physical health. Luks calls this phenomenon the "helper's high." Volunteers surveyed indicated they experienced relief from pain and other physical symptoms, including chronic headache, back pain, and stomachache. Biochemical changes, particularly increased production of endorphins, muffle the pain message and distract the sufferer from his or her discomfort. Also reported were relief from symptoms of chronic diseases, including arthritis, lupus, and asthma, as well as a hastening of recovery from surgery. Volunteers also claimed emotional benefits, both short-term -- a sense of euphoria, a greater sense of calmness and relaxation, increased energy, and a general sense of emotional well-being -- and long-term -- a feeling of tranquility, improved self-esteem, increased optimism, and decreased depression.[18]

The benefits of helping strongly correlated to the consistency of the helping behavior. For instance, the long-term emotional benefits occurred only when people engaged in a regular regime of helping activities over sustained time periods. The frequency of helping is also critical: weekly (about two hours a week of one-to-one helping) is much better than monthly or one-time volunteer endeavors. It is also important to let go of the results, Luks maintains, and just feel close to and empathize with the person you are trying to help. Exert yourself to reach out; extend yourself, physically or emotionally.

The act of helping others may be an especially effective means of developing a network for healing social support. Volunteering enables helpers to develop close relationships and provides purpose and meaning to their lives. A sense of social connection paves the way for the sensation of the "helper's high." By enriching the lives of others you enrich and heal yourself.

Achieve Emotional and Spiritual Closure with Your Loved Ones

The dying process can be a profound time for personal transformation. It offers important opportunities for spiritual growth and enlightenment.[19] As relationships are repaired or strengthened, some of the most valued of all human experiences can occur between diagnosis and death. You probably need time to resolve interpersonal issues, attain relational closure, and say your good-byes. You may have one last chance to be the person you have always wanted to be.

It is a period for love and emotional sharing with your dear ones. Express your unconditional love to others. Spend time at the end of life with those who are most important to you. Ask yourself: Are there people -- family and friends -- you want to see before I die? Each of us looks forward to meaningful hours with our loved ones. Enjoy the time you have with them, sharing memories and your love. In the words of one breast cancer sufferer's son, in the visits of those last days of life, "There was a great energy and love in that room, and it was emanating from her, and flowing through us, and gave us the strength to overcome our fears, our own weaknesses, and stay, and be with her." Of what was shared during those final days, when the battle was acknowledged to be over and the family had become reconciled with reality, her ex-husband stated, "It was the richest of times."[20]

Give away treasured items, things special to you or of significance to family members and friends.

Gather photos of yourself and family members, especially if others will not recognize people from the past. Organize a scrap book for those you will leave behind, creating and perpetuating memories of shared times.

The writing of an "ethical will" offers tremendous opportunities for closure. Create a legacy for those who love you by writing a letter, or making a tape or video recording. Impart to your survivors your values, hopes, insights, beliefs, and perhaps some stories and advice. Share with your dear ones the lessons in life you have learned.

Is there anything previously hidden that you now want to reveal? Ask yourself: What parts of my life, thoughts, and feelings, my best kept secrets, do I want to share with others? This previously private knowledge about you and your passions, motivations, desires, and longings as well as your beliefs often provides something of value to others and helps them with their lives.

In addition to sharing your memories, values, and feelings, try to make up with family members and friends, by addressing failed relationships, old grievances, and hurts inflicted on or by others. You may be ready to apologize, to ask for forgiveness from others, and to send forgiveness to others as well as to yourself.

Engage in an end of life conversation with your beloved. Discuss with your loved ones any unresolved issues, apologize for your shortcomings and failures, address old hurts and grievances, extend or receive forgiveness for earthly wrongdoings, and achieve a sense of closure. How much unfinished emotional business do you have with your dear ones? Do you have relational debris you have never fully faced that you need to work out with others? Do you wish to try to resolve and complete this interpersonal business before you die?

Forgiveness is often quite difficult. Each of us continues to fear being hurt or rejected again. We may be unable to let go of our past perceptions. What has been done to us in the past, especially if we have been victims of physical or verbal abuse or violence, may approach being an unforgivable transgression. Forgiveness is not condoning an act; it is getting past continuing to feel hurt, maligned, abused, or injured. This is a shift in your own feelings, to your own comfort and freedom. It is not a shift in your judgment of the rightness or wrongness of what occurred. It is finding that you no longer hate the person who hurt you. However, forgiveness does not necessarily mean that you once again enter into an active relationship of friendship, trust, and intimacy with that individual. That would be reconciliation, which is something else. You may choose to that as well, or you may not. You can forgive, this breaking the bond of hatred that tie you to the other, without instituting a renewed relationship. You need not feel that you ought to be willing to reconcile; it may not be emotionally possible, or it might not be wise or prudent. What you can do toward the other is offer unconditional well-wishing: that the other should find, in the Universal Love that is God, healing, growth, joy, and goodness.

An admission of past mistakes and asking for forgiveness is often quite powerful. It offers opportunity for healing old wounds and tapping the power of love. By facilitating possible reconciliation between estranged children, parents, siblings, and others, the quest for forgiveness often enables the achieving of closure with and the opening into unconditional love for your closest relatives and friends.

I have observed individuals before their death reconnect and heal relationships torn apart with estranged parents, children or siblings. Some of these difficult family situations go back decades; for instance, stubborn siblings who long ago had a quarrel and had not spoken until one of them was dying. Seemingly intractable interpersonal conflicts may be amenable to compromise. On one's deathbed what once triggered anger often dissolves in the light of one's life meaning and the bigger picture of our transcendent existence.

In contrast to a sudden, unexpected death -- a heart attack, a car accident, or a plane crash, a slowly developing illness with a fatal outcome, such as cancer, gives a dying person, as well as his or her beloved, time to express regrets, ask for forgiveness, and the chance to resolve old, unfinished emotional business. In addition to affording the opportunity to heal previously strained relationships, the dying period also gives time to express affection and to accept gratitude and appreciation.

Bringing closure to life takes time. It requires a conscious effort to open hearts, share final words, express last wishes. It is a difficult period, if you are in pain or experience physical symptoms. Try to start it early.

Open lines of communication to express and seek forgiveness. Reflect on your unresolved emotional dilemmas, your psychological baggage, things left undone or unsaid. If possible, make time to deal with these issues. Try to know close family members and friends as individuals. Move toward forgiveness and unconditional love. Let go; see things differently; don't hold on to the past. Right old wrongs. Make an intimate, heart-to-heart connection with others. Do what your inner voice tells you; what feels right in your heart. Don't die with unresolved emotional issues or something you are ashamed of. Until these matters are resolved, your immortal soul may not be able to rest or progress emotionally and spiritually.

If you have time, open a safe avenue of communication through a letter or a note to a relative or friend, expressing love and forgiveness. Writing it out may help you see past irrationalities and restore relationships. Use others as intermediaries. Or, arrange a tentative meeting. Explore alternatives if your efforts to express forgiveness fail to achieve positive results. Remember: even as you offer your forgiveness, closure may be one sided. The other is not yet dying, so does not have the insight and motivation you now have.

Depending on the circumstances of your dying process, there may not be sufficient time or energy for you to heal personally old resentments and fears, either face-to-face or over the telephone. In such a situation, perhaps you can give yourself inner peace by leaving a message with your caregiver that you wish to exchange forgiveness with this one and that one. Then you can use prayer and meditation to open the heart and enable you to let go of the resentments that block your openheartedness. Remember that there are different paths in Spiritual Judaism, depending on your personality. Some will experience God's Presence in prayer, others in meditation. As developed in Chapter 9, your loved ones also can help you.

Set aside some time each day to offer, for ten to fifteen minutes, one or more of the following focused, personal prayers:[21]

Finding the Good Prayer

O God, please let me see the
good and Godliness that lies hidden within
everyone shine forth
and emerge as a grand reflection
of beauty and light.
Show me the goodness, the beauty,

the kindness in everyone.

The Power of Love Prayer

O God, help me search for the fine
qualities in others and to recognize
their immeasurable worth.
Help me cultivate a love for all Your
children for no one is without redeeming value.
Help me to be loving and kind just
as you are loving and kind to all Your Creations.

Prayer for Forgiving

O merciful and forgiving God,
You alone know how urgently I need
to learn to forgive.
Help me extinguish the anger
that burns within my heart.
Help free me of resentment
against those who have wronged me.
Help me abandon all the
animosity clogging my heart.
Help me turn my anger into
love and my hostility
into compassion.

You may also want to meditate. You do this by going within, quieting your mind, calming and centering your being, and bringing yourself to a still place. In this quiet place in which you can reveal yourself, you can make contact with and listen to God, aligning yourself with the Higher Energy. You attain a space to receive; a place to commune with your Creator, Sustainer and Deliverer. You connect with your Godlike nature, often receiving a new openheartedness, facilitating the process of forgiveness.

In asking for or communicating forgiveness, as appropriate, use the

Forgiveness and Lovingkindness Meditation daily, for ten to fifteen minutes, to facilitate the process of forgiveness and reconciliation with others as well as self-forgiveness. You can choose to forgive at any time, whenever you are ready to forgive or to ask for forgiveness. Many have found this meditation very powerful; however, be patient. Remember that the desire to forgive is part of your standing in the Presence of God. That desire is the act of your will, which is free and able to do whatever it chooses. Your emotions are not quite so free, though they also can change. The essential thing is that you will forgiveness, whether or not you can bring your emotions into line right away. Your righteousness, your share in the World to Come, depends on your will. You can will the good, even with your emotions pulling in the opposite direction.

Forgiveness and Lovingkindness Meditation

Introductory Instructions. Create a warm, welcoming atmosphere, an environment of serenity and spaciousness of the journey within. Lower the lights in your room. Close your eyes, sit quietly, calm and relax your body, breathe in and out normally feeling where your breath flows into and out of your body. Adjust your breaths so that the in and out breaths are of the same length. (Obviously, vary these instructions depending on your situation).

Feel yourself surrounded by warmth and love. Allow any anger, envy, or other emotions you feel to dissolve into the warmth. Feel the warmth nourishing you. Breathe in love and feel the openness that love creates in you. Allow the warmth and love to give rise to forgiveness. The power of forgiveness is so very great. It is coming out of a narrow, constricted place.

Visualize another person. Within a new state of openness, invite him or her into your heart. Try to let him or her through to your heart. Notice what blocks his or her approach to your heart -- the problem, the hurt, the fear, the anger, the envy, the guilt, or whatever it is. Enter into and continue a dialogue until there is nothing more to say. Then try again to let him or her through to your heart. Let go of the pride that holds onto resentment. Allow the pain of old hurts to dissolve.

In your heart say, "I forgive you for whatever you did in the past, whether intentionally or unintentionally, through you deeds, words, or thoughts, that caused me pain or hurt." Repeat the words "I forgive you." Allowing the forgiveness to grow, let go of your resentments, your anger, and your hurt and open unconditionally into love and compassion.

Continue to visualize this other person. Does he or she resent you? Did you cause him or her pain? Did he or she put you out of his or her heart? With a new state of openness invite him or her into your heart. Notice whatever blocks his or her approach to your heart. Try to let him or her through to your heart.

From the bottom of your heart ask for forgiveness. Say: "I ask for your forgiveness for what I did in the past, whether intentionally or unintentionally, through my deeds, words, or thoughts, that caused you pain or hurt." Repeat the words "Please forgive me." Again, let yourself be touched by the possibility of forgiveness. Ask him or her to let go of his or her anger and hurt and let you back into his or her heart. Feel his or her forgiveness.

Repeat for as many of your significant others as is necessary.

Let your heart fill with forgiveness and lovingkindness for yourself. Say to yourself: "May I be happy and at peace, free from anger, pain, fear, and doubt. May I be filled with love."

Concluding Instructions. Come back to the here and now. Take time to ease yourself back. Slowly bring your awareness back to your being. Feel yourself back in the room and open your eyes.

Strive for emotional and spiritual closure, filled with love, compassion, and forgiveness for your loved ones.

Let's turn and consider a number of questions that go into your end of life decision-making. The next chapter organizes these issues around three general topics: first, spiritual and religious issues; second, the physical and mental quality of your life; and third, emotional, social and economic concerns. These questions will stimulate your thinking, helping you make end of life choices grounded in and consistent with your values.

Notes

1. Adapted from Lewis D. Solomon, *Jewish Spirituality: Revitalizing Judaism for the Twenty-First Century* (Northvale, NJ: Jason Aronson, 2000), 47-55, 208-210.

2. Rabbi Nathan of Breslov, *Rabbi Nachman: Advice*, trans. Abraham Greenbaum (Brooklyn: The Breslov Research Institute, 1983), 80-87; Chaim Kramer, *Crossing the Narrow Bridge: A Practical Guide to Rebbe Nackman's Teachings*, ed. Moshe Mykoff (New York: Breslov Research Institute, 1989), 137-165.

3. Herbert Benson, M.D., *The Relaxation Response* (New York: William Morrow, 1975).

4. Herbert Benson, M.D. with Marg Stark, *Timeless Healing: The Power and Biology of Belief* (New York: Scribner, 1996), 146-147.

5. Ibid., 127.

6. Ibid., 134-137.

7. Ibid., 155.

8. Bernie S. Siegel, M.D., *Love, Medicine & Miracles: Lessons Learned About Self-Healing from a Surgeon's Experiences with Exceptional Patients* (New York: Harper & Row, 1986), 161-204; Jeanne Achterberg, Stephanie-Matthews Simonton, and O. Carl Simonton, "Psychology of the Exceptional Cancer Patient: A Description of Patients Who Outlived Their Predicted Life Expectancies," *Psychotherapy: Theory, Research, and Practice* 14:4 (Winter 1977): 416-422; Paul Charles Roud, "Psychosocial Variables Associated with the Exceptional Survival of Patients with Advanced Malignant Disease," *Journal of the National Medical Association* 79.1 (January 1987): 97-102. Catherine Classen et al, "Coping Styles Associated with Psychological Adjustment to Advanced Breast Cancer," *Health Psychology* 15:6 (November 1996): 434-437 concluded in a study of 101 women that a fighting spirit and emotional expressiveness were associated with better adjustment to metastatic breast cancer.

One recent study of 578 women with early stage breast cancer over a five-year period found that although optimism and a fighting attitude may help breast cancer patients cope with their illness, positive thinking is unlikely to increase their chances of survival. Persistent hopelessness, however, may raise a woman's risk of suffering a relapse or succumbing to breast cancer. M. Watson et al,

"Influence of Psychological Response on Survival in Breast Cancer: A Population-Based Cohort Study," *The Lancet* 354:9187 (October 1999): 1331-1336; Erica Goode, "'Fighting' Spirit Little Help in Cancer Fight," *New York Times*, 19 October 1999, sec. D10. In an earlier study of 69 breast cancer patients, researchers found that patients who had a fighting spirit or who had initially reacted to the diagnosis by denial had a higher survival rate than those who responded with stoic acceptance or feelings of helplessness and hopelessness. S. Greer, T. Morris, and K.W. Pettingale, "Psychological Response to Breast Cancer: Effect on Outcome," *The Lancet* 2:8146 (October 1979): 785-787.

9. Norman Cousins, *Anatomy of an Illness as Perceived by the Patient: Reflections on Healing and Regeneration* (New York: Norton, 1979).

10. Solomon, *Jewish Spirituality*, 146-148. See also Herbert Benson, M.D. and Eileen M. Stuart, "How Thoughts Affect Health," chap. 11 in *The Wellness Book: The Comprehensive Guide to Maintaining Health and Treating Stess-Related Illness* (New York: Birch Lane, 1992), 189-202.

11. Elisabeth Kübler-Ross, M.D., *Death Is Of Vital Importance: On Life, Death and Life After Death* (Barrytown, NY: Station Hill Press, 1995), 145- 146, 148-149.

12. Adapted from *The Gentle Weapon: Prayers for Everyday and Not-So-Everyday Moments: Timeless Wisdom from the Teachings of the Hasidic Master Rebbe Nachman of Breslov*, adapted by Moshe Mycoff & S.C. Mizrahi with the Breslov Research Institute (Woodstock, VT: Jewish Lights Publishing, 1999), 72.

13. David Spiegel et al, "Effect of Psychosocial Treatment on Survival of Patients with Metastatic Breast Cancer," *The Lancet* 2:8668 (October 1989): 888-891; Fawzy I. Fawzy et al, "Malignant Melanoma: Effects of an Early Structured Psychiatric Intervention, Coping, and Affective State on Recurrence and Survival 6 Years Later," *Archives of General Psychiatry* 50:9 (September 1993): 681-689. Manuela M. Kogon et al, "Effects of Medical and Psychotherapeutic Treatment on the Survival of Women with Metastatic Breast Carcinoma," Cancer 80:2 (July 1997): 225-230 conclude that support group participation was the determining factor in the survival of participants.

14. Viktor E. Frankl, *Man's Search For Meaning* (New York: Washington Square Press, 1984), 92-93. See also Ira R. Byock, "Consciously Walking the Fine Line: Thoughts on a Hospice Response to Assisted Suicide and Euthanasia," *Journal of Palliative Care* 9:3 (Autumn 1993): 25-28.

15. Adapted from *The Gentle Weapon*, 18.

16. Adapted from Ann Webster, Ph.D., *Creating Your Life's Road Map*, Mind/Body Medical Institute, n.d..

17. Allan Luks with Peggy Payne, *The Healing Power Doing Good: The Health and Spiritual Benefits of Helping Others* (New York: Fawcett Columbine, 1991).

18. Ibid., 60-61, 67-68, 82, 88-91.

19. See generally Ira Byock, M.D., *Dying Well: The Prospect for Growth at the End of Life* (New York: Riverhead, 1997) and Ira R. Byock, "The Nature of Suffering and The Nature of Opportunity at the End of Life," *Clinics in Geriatric Medicine* 12:2 (May 1996): 237-252.

20. Robert Lipsyte, *In the Country of Illness: Comfort and Advice for the Journey* (New York: Knopf, 1998), 219, 230.

21. Adapted from *The Gentle Weapon*, 42, 46, 47, 54, 84.

Chapter 8

Questions for Patients Facing a Terminal Illness or a Chronic, Debilitating Condition

As you go about your end of life decision-making, having considered the suggestions in Chapter 7, I am assuming you care about how your existence terminates and that you want it to end appropriately for you. You want your death and your dying process to keep faith with how you have lived. You want to die the way you have lived. In other words, you want your values and interests to guide the last phase of your earthly adventure.

This chapter will help you sort out your values, goals, and priorities in life and in death. You will be guided in answering the following questions: How do you see the value of your life? What is a meaningful life for you? What is special to you about your life? What makes your life worth living? What are your significant needs and interests? What is a loss of self -- yourself? Given your illness or condition, will you be able to continue to pursue a life consistent with your basic values, goals and aspirations?

You want to come up with an informed choice, a course of action based on a sound decision-making process. From my experience, most individuals, suffering from a life threatening illness, can make rational decisions regarding the time and manner of their death, based on realistic assessment of their situation. You will want to reflect on and examine your life-and-death in the context of your values, interests, needs, and goals. I want to trace the possibilities for such an examination as amplified by the principles of Spiritual Judaism, beyond our obvious preference for pleasure and the avoidance of pain. In that context, how could one choose wisely, not out of ignorance, fear, or confusion? This chapter offers to aid you in making prudent choices: what you really want for yourself.

As part of the decision-making process, many have found it useful not only to write out their answers to the questions posed in this chapter but also to keep a daily journal. In your journal, write about your crisis, record your physical, mental, and emotional symptoms, your adherence to your prescribed treatment regime, your ability to engage in daily activities, any changes in sleep patterns, variations in your appetite. Try to keep track of: what is bothering you; your powerful emotions; your attitude to living and dying; your gratitude and joyfulness. Journaling will help you explore your feelings and accept your emotions. It will prevent you from getting stuck in a particular mood. It will also aid in recognizing the family, religious, and cultural influences on your emotional expression. Or, if journaling does not come naturally to you, try drawing, or any other way to track and interact with your deep processing.

As a patient, you face a whole cluster of issues in your decision-making at the end of life. To begin, let's consider three basic categories: first, spiritual and religious issues; second, the physical and mental quality of your life; and third, emotional, social and economic concerns.[1] Then, we will discuss the need to be sensitive to the impact of your death, its timing and manner, on your loved ones. Your release from pain and suffering may harm others. Or, perhaps family members experience more misery from your living in distress than from your accelerated dying.

Spiritual and Religious Issues

As part of your decision-making process, focus on what is of importance, spiritually and religiously, for you. As you consider how you want to deal with the process of your dying, reflect on the following:

1. What do you believe about God? Do you believe that there is God? If so, does the Eternal care about you and your pain and suffering? Do you believe that only the Holy One can take life or that you can be a partner with God in controlling your dying process and your death?

2. What is your attitude toward the sanctity of biologcal life principle? Is every moment of physical life, your life, precious? Is your physical body solely your own, does it belong to God, or to you and the Eternal as copartners? Do you feel an "unnatural" ending of earthly life represents

an insult to God and the Eternal's gift of life? Do you believe that one can accelerate the end of one's life (alone or with assistance) yet respect the sacredness of human existence? What is the basis for your beliefs? Are your beliefs based on the Jewish tradition, your rabbi, someone else, or your own experience, study, and reflection?

3. Do you want to remain alive as long as you possibly can and at all costs, emotional and financial, to you and your loved ones, no matter what your physical or mental condition, regardless of your pain and suffering, even if you lose your enjoyment of living? In other words, is mere biological life so inherently precious to you that nothing can justify ending it, short of your imminent demise from an absolutely hopeless condition? Do you want to endure prolonged physical or mental deterioration, no matter how severe? Do you want to continue to spend your declining years, demented or incontinent, if modern medicine has helped you overcome a lethal disease, such as cancer? Do you think it is important to be defiant even in the face of your inevitable demise? If so, as we will discuss in Chapter 10, instruct your physician not to disconnect life-support systems and to continue artificial feeding and hydration.

4. Do you want a "dignified" closure to your life? Do you dread being kept alive, permanently vegetative or sedated to unconsciousness, intubated, treated as a vegetable? Does any of these conditions degrade what is valuable in your life? Do you want to die with your mental capabilities intact? Do you view life as worth living only if you retain some minimal, meaningful quality of life?

5. Do you see some sort of spiritual benefit from suffering until the very "end"? Or, do you perceive your suffering as unconstructive in any meaningful way? If so, at what point?

6. Do you want to hold out for the possibility, however slim, of a miracle[2] or a cure? Longshot cures are rare, but they do occur. There are always new studies, new machines, new organs, new drugs upon drugs. There are also, very rarely, medically unexpected and unexplainable spontaneous recoveries. Are you prepared to face (and die in) miserable conditions if a miracle does not materialize? If physicians can predict the course of your disease with great accuracy, of course, there is less room for unfounded hope.

7. Do you view suicide as wrong or acceptable?

8. Is it right or wrong for a person to have another end his or her life if he or she is suffering from a terminal illness or a chronic, incurable, progressively debilitating condition that ultimately will prove fatal? In

taking such action, do you believe one is denying or rejecting or not properly trusting God?

9. What do you believe about the afterlife? Do you believe that there is life after your present earthly existence? Is each of us an immortal being that survives our physical death? Are you comfortable with the notion that we are far more than our earthly bodies?

How will the manner of your death impact on your soul? How will your suicide or an assisted death impact on the departure of your soul from your body? In a violent or quick death by suicide or physician-aid-in-dying, do you believe your soul will experience difficulty in overcoming the Pangs of the Grave, discussed in Chapter 3? How will a drug-induced coma, as a means of pain control, affect not only your death moment visions but also your soul?

10. How do you feel about death: scared, excited, hopeful? Does the prospect of death cause you to feel despair or hopelessness? Are you able to come to terms with your death and dying? Do you look forward to it with happy expectation?

11. What do you see as the meaning and purpose of your life, now? Do you find meaning and purpose in your present existence? Does your personal life have meaning because of what you can do, think, and feel, or because of its intrinsic value? Do you believe that a person's worth is judged by one's productivity, one's capacity to produce, to be useful or do something? Do you see your life as rooted in its physical or mental dimension? Do you seek spiritual meaning in your life? Have you found it? Do you want to continue your search?

Some, however, bear tragedy less ably than others. They may not be able to continue to say "yes" to life. Some who are physically imprisoned by pain and other physical symptoms may be able to better contemplate their situation and reflect on their lives, leading to even more profound suffering.

Only you can answer the following questions: What if you cannot find meaning in your suffering? What if you cannot make any sort of success out of your misery? What if you do not have the strength or courage to continue to face the future? What if your circumstances or abilities do not enable you to triumph over your adversity? What if you are unable to see yourself as part of a transcendent existence?

12. Have you sought counseling regarding your religious and spiritual issues?

The Physical and Mental Quality of Your Life

Questions about the physical and mental quality of your life will enter into your decision-making process. Consider the following:

1. Do you have: a terminal, irreversible sickness; a progressive, incurable chronic illness; a physically or mentally debilitating or deteriorating condition; or chronic, intractable pain or physical, emotional or spiritual suffering leading to a quality of life that is unacceptable to you?

Do you face severe, but nonterminal incapacitation, unlikely to be relieved soon by death? Are you chronically disabled? Is your chronic condition irreversible?

2. What do you value about your physical and mental existence? At what point does the loss of your physical or mental capabilities become unacceptable?

3. Do you have a realistic assessment of your situation? Specifically, do you understand: your condition; the range of treatment options and their consequences; your prognosis; your illness trajectory -- the probable course of your disease -- as inexact as it may be?

Discuss these questions with a physician having first-hand knowledge of your situation, who can provide predictive information, either statistical data or generalizations from familiar cases, on the medical events a person with your illness or condition will likely encounter along the way. Obviously, your own situation and particular susceptibilities must be considered. Also, remember that doctors may feel uncomfortable when pressed to predict your survival time and its experiences. They tend to err on the side of optimism,[3] often widely overestimating how long their patients will live.

For lucid descriptions, from a mechanistic perspective, of how the common causes of death, including heart disease, stroke, Alzheimer's, and cancer, progress and how affected organs cease to function effectively, you may want to read the bestseller, *How We Die* by Sherwin B. Nuland, M.D.[4]

4. Is there any possibility of error in your diagnosis and prognosis? Get a second opinion and, if necessary, a third opinion, from a specialist in your illness or condition.

5. What is your current physical condition? Do you suffer from any of the following symptoms: fatigue, severe weakness, fever, insomnia, dizziness, shortness of breath, nausea, vomiting, inability to eat or

swallow, constipation, or diarrhea? Are you presently exhausted from a prolonged process of physical deterioration? Are you suffering from the treatments themselves?

6. Are your current physical symptoms treatable? Are you receiving effective, aggressive symptom control and management? Can some of your symptoms be treated with little effort and minimally invasive procedures? Have you considered a range of treatment options?

Carefully consider and weigh the benefits as well as the burdens and risks of any intervention alternatives. What are the likely side effects of any procedure or medication? What is the goal of any option: to improve your health, alleviate discomfort, postpone death? Will a procedure or treatment entail loss of physical function, distress disproportionate to benefit, or bodily mutilation? Will a procedure or treatment have only a small (how small?) chance of achieving any benefit? What happens if nothing is done?

Remember: a trial intervention may be an attractive option because it permits the testing of a potentially beneficial therapy without your committing to a course of treatment not leading to a cure. You may be more comfortable with an intervention if it is understood that it will not be continued should it prove of little or no benefit to you. In other words, your physician will end the trial intervention if continuing it would unlikely provide further benefit and would likely cause harm.

Do you regard with horror certain hospital paraphernalia, such as feeding tubes or dialysis machines, and want to avoid them? What about constant sedation? How do you feel about being hooked up to a respirator or other life-supporting machines? Are you apprehensive about receiving the wrong level of medical care -- too little or too much?

Do you understand what medical treatments can and cannot accomplish for you? Have your physician explain your choices in ordinary language, describing the likely consequences of each option in sufficient, realistic detail. Indicate to your doctor what terms or phrases make no sense to you. Urge your physician to translate medical jargon into everyday language. It is helpful to prepare a written list of questions before you talk with your physician. The bottom line: ask your doctor would he or she recommend this treatment if the patient were his or her parent, child, or best friend?

Ask your physician about the signs and symptoms to be encountered during the terminal phase of your illness, such as respiratory distress, bleeding, agitation, seizures, generalized weakness, an inability to eat or speak. Do you suffer from an illness or condition with an end stage likely involving severe physical, emotional, and spiritual suffering that cannot effectively be treated? Will these symptoms and your suffering be unrelenting? Do you know how your physician plans to deal with and control your symptoms and anguish? How do you feel about anticipating such a future?

Do you face terminal decline which, depending on your illness or condition, may be marked by a range of predictable medical events, with a known probability of specific outcomes and possible events? Or, are the early stages of your mortal disease comparatively benign with a sudden, rapid downhill course at the very end? Does your future promise weeks (or months) of continued pain and fatigue?

7. What kinds of deteriorating physical conditions do you consider intolerable? What types of physical debilitation can't you live with? What are your fears regarding the symptoms of your future physical condition? Consider the following: loss of one or more bodily functions, immobility, other motor skill impairments, alteration in body image, decreased physical attractiveness, fatigue or exhaustion, weakness, sleeplessness, dizziness, nausea, uncontrollable diarrhea (or the opposite), shortness of breath, inability to eat or swallow? Do you fear concurrent medical problems? How bad will it be if things turn out as you fear?

8. What is your current level of pain and suffering? Are you experiencing intractable pain accompanied by suffering from physical symptoms or loss of function? What is your likely future level of pain and suffering? In the future will your pain lessen or is it irreversible, or becoming only more severe? Do you fear excruciating, unrelenting pain during an extended dying process? Does your pain (or will it) interfere with your mental functioning? Can your pain be controlled?

What is your tolerance for and willingness to accept pain? Do you want to "tough it out" -- to be a hero, stoically accepting your fate? Will you surrender yourself to God in trust, no matter what happens?

Do you fear addiction to pain control medication, even if you face a life threatening condition or are terminally ill? Do not worry addiction. It is truly ridiculous to think that an incurably ill patient will end up "hooked" on painkillers. You will not become an addict by taking your pain medication. Tell your physician to treat your pain. Take your pain medication. Do not say "no" to good palliative (comfort) care.

Learn about the causes of your pain. Ask your physician about how he or she will treat your discomfort. Explore your palliative care options.

Discuss with your physician alternative nonpharmacological techniques, such as acupuncture, massage, or meditation (breathing) exercises, to control your pain. Find out how successful both the standard and the alternative methods are. Do this early, while you still have the energy. Ask friends and other patients for their help and guidance.

Modern techniques can alleviate physical pain in nearly all cases. It can nearly always be managed well enough so a terminally ill patient's life can be comfortable. However, not all pain from a mortal illness or a chronic condition can be controlled. Also, the best medical treatment for pain can cause horrible side effects, including nausea, vomiting, sleeplessness, constipation, and dizziness.

Many physicians are inadequately trained to provide the highest quality palliative care. Does your physician (or your team of physicians) have experience in caring for the terminally ill, especially with respect to pain control and comfort care? Is your physician underprescribing (or overprescribing) pain medication? Seek a second opinion from a pain control specialist.

Do you want to make peace with death and accept the reality that is a part of our existence? If so, and if your condition is terminal and you have less than six months to live, consider hospice care because hospice healthcare professionals are often better trained to manage pain. A hospice provides comfort and supportive care for the dying and their families. Palliative medicine offers an interdisciplinary team approach focusing on a patient's physical, psychological, social and spiritual concerns as well as those of his or her loved ones. It is designed to care for someone who is fatally ill as a person. It has the goal of alleviating one's pain, other physical symptoms, and suffering, but not curing the underlying disease. Seeking to make the process of dying as natural and humane as possible, it recognizes the many levels of suffering, physical, emotional, and spiritual, accompanying the dying process. It strives to make the end of life more comfortable and death less difficult for patients and their families based on a philosophy of comfort care, not aggressive treatment. Comfort care provides human contact, emphasizing the patient as a person, not a medical problem, offering care either in your own home (or that of a loved one) or in a residential facility devoted to caring for the dying. Because hospice care views the patient and his or her family as one unit of care, it attends to both the patient's and his or her family's emotional and spiritual needs.

The heart of palliative medicine focuses on pain relief and symptom control. New pharmaceutical and other physical treatment methods are used to control pain, and other physical symptoms otherwise depriving the mortally ill of their strength, their will to live, and their dignity. Because patients are expected to die, life-support machines are not used.

Hospice care seeks to provide a supportive and pain-free environment. Enabling the terminally ill to live their remaining days as fully, as comfortably and as alert as possible, it aims to keep one alert, able to enjoy his or her family, visitors, and surroundings, not desensitized by pain, suffering, and anxiety. However, hospice care is sometimes marked by extensive sedation to control pain and suffering, especially at the end, in which case a dying person experiences heavy drowsiness and loss of cognitive skills.

The principles of palliative medicine are most often put into practice in home hospice care for the dying. Hospice services include physician and nursing care, inpatient medical care (if necessary), medication, supplies and equipment, and counseling and respite help. A team of visiting nurses, home health aides and volunteers provides this array of care and services.

With Medicare's hospice benefits (and most private insurers, if they cover hospices at all) limited to those with a prognosis of six months or less to live, the brief final course of cancer, with a generally predictable trajectory toward death, fits the service-rich hospice care model. Patients with chronic conditions, such as dementia, stroke, or heart disease, generally do not have access to hospice care because their illnesses follow a much longer, far more uncertain trajectory. These patients may be referred too late or not at all for hospice care; thus, they may not derive solace from living their last days at home. Often they are just too sick by the time they are referred to hospice programs offering them merely brink-of-death care. Also, the undue optimism physicians may continue to evince when death is near, often delays referrals to hospices.

9. Can you describe a stage in the future, when, in the course of your dying process, life will become too painful or undignified? What for you is an unacceptable level of physical dysfunctionality, a degree of physical pain, a physical quality of life that is no longer tolerable? When would you want aggressive treatment to stop and just go with comfort care?

10. Have you witnessed the intolerable deaths of others -- family members or friends? Did they experience a variety of invasive medical procedures with little curative value? Did they receive inadequate pain relief, experience a lack of concern from physicians, or suffer from

harmful side effects of medications and interventions?

11. How important is your capacity to think clearly and make your own decisions? Does your fundamental interest in this life involve a logical, clear view of the world? How would you react to the onset of dementia and the beginning of your inability to mentally process experiences and activities?

If you suffer (or were to suffer) from Alzheimer's disease or some other form of dementia, are you repelled by the thought of someday living in a severe, permanently demented state, incapable of understanding the world beyond you, a contravention of reason and sense? Do you regard a passive life, for instance, just watching daytime television, as worse than no life at all? Or is a demented existence, filled with childlike pleasure, better than no physical life at all? Would you accept being "pleasantly" senile, being aware of your environment and capable of extracting some pleasure from interacting with others, but with a limited ability to initiate activities and communicate? What for you is a personally unacceptable level of mental disfunctionality, a mentally debilitating or deteriorating condition, a mental quality of life that is no longer tolerable?

12. How do you want to spend your last days? Good, but not perfect, control of physical pain can be provided most of the time, but there may be a period before your death when your pain is out of control. In some cases, no amount of medication, short of terminal sedation, can control the pain. To deal with otherwise unbearable pain, for instance, if you have cancer, do you want to be sedated to the point of unconsciousness before you die?

In addition to considering these questions, it is important to begin a dialogue with your primary care physician about your pain and suffering as well as the physical, mental and emotional quality of your life, now and in the future. Talk openly about all your concerns or find a new primary care physician who listens and responds with information and recommendations enabling you to make your best medical care decisions. Find a doctor with whom you discuss your healthcare questions, get answers (or at least information and recommendations), allaying your concerns and uncertainties about your diagnosis, treatment alternatives, and prognosis. This is perhaps easier said than done.

Your physician needs all necessary information from you to provide you with meaningful answers. Open a dialogue and discuss as soon as possible all your concerns as well as your interest (if you are interested) in an assisted death. To ensure you have adequate time for this type of discussion, if possible, set up an extended appointment.

Look to various web sites on the Internet to increase your knowledge base, including the National Institutes of Health databases (www.nih.gov/health), as well as those assembled by university medical centers and the Mayo Clinic (www.mayohealth.org). The technical information provided by MEDLINEplus, (www.ncbi.nlm.nih.gov/PubMed/), the medical database managed by the National Institutes of Health's National Library of Medicine, may also be helpful. Other websites include original peer-reviewed reports and journal articles organized by medical specialty (www.medscape.com) and links to government agency health sites, online publications, and medical dictionaries (www.healthfinder.com). Use your Internet research to open a dialogue with your physician. If you find a specialist, who is doing groundbreaking work, ask your primary care physician for an opinion or even a referral.

Emotional, Social, and Financial Concerns

Beyond physical and mental quality of life issues, a life threatening illness or a chronic condition presents a number of emotional, social, and financial concerns.

Emotional Issues

Sickness, the dying process and ultimately death bring with them a multitude of emotional transformations, including the loss of independence, a sense of isolation and loneliness, feelings of depression, sadness, anger, helplessness, the loss of future goals, regrets over lost opportunities or the inability to live your life as fully as you wished, fears of becoming a physical, economic or emotional burden to others, and guilt in leaving loved ones.

To help you reflect on your negative (and positive) feelings and emotions, consider the following:

1. What are the negative feelings and emotions you most often experience, when do they occur, how are you feeling physically, and

whom are you with? Do you find yourself thinking, "I have no joy in life" or "I feel hopeless with what I see in front of me?" Note your sleeping and eating patterns. Are you having difficulty in sleeping? If so, what's keeping you awake? What physical conditions or social factors trigger particular feelings or emotions on your part?

The presence of persistent diarrhea, having to labor with each breath, being unable to speak or recognize family members, for instance, may produce emotional suffering as excruciating and as unbearable as pain and other physical symptoms. Are you frustrated or humiliated from living in a body that does not work?

2. Do you experience more positive feelings and emotions? If so, when, what are you doing, and whom are you with? Do you find small pleasures in life, such as engaging in any of your favorite activities?

3. Is there any logical pattern to your negative or positive feelings and emotions? Do these occur at particular times of day, before or after meals or taking medication, while you are engaged in certain activities, or with certain people? Consider your family patterns of expressing feeling and emotions and how these impact you now.

Try to change the circumstances that trigger negative feelings and emotions. Avoid activities and personal contacts resulting in or exacerbating negative feelings and emotions. Conversely, increase activities and personal contacts generating more positive feelings and emotions. Talk with your physician and/or pharmacist about the possible mind-altering impact of any medication you are taking. Be aware of the interactions: drug-drug, drug-food, drug-vitamins, drug-herbs, drug-natural remedies. You cannot rely entirely on professionals. Professionals make mistakes. Try to learn about your condition and your medicines yourself. Arrange to have those close to you continue to do this when you become incapable.

4. Are you more than sad? Are you depressed? Is your depression narrowing your view of the possibilities still open, restricting your view of alternatives, screening off human relationships and experiences in the time left to you?

It is natural to feel sad as you contemplate the end of your life -- what you have already lost as a result of your illness or condition -- health, job, independence -- and what you will lose when you die -- personal relationships and your physical existence. Sadness differs from depression. The desire for physician-aid-in-dying is a symptom of depression.[5]

Sadness is not, however, depression, which rules out hope and renders a person helpless, energyless, and withdrawn. A number of symptoms, with varying degrees of intensity, characterize clinical (major) depression. These include feelings of powerlessness, irritability, a sense of guilt, discouragement, lowered energy and diminished participation in and enthusiasm for enjoyable activities, changes in appetite or weight, sleep disturbances, decreased sexual drive, preoccupation with thoughts of death or suicide, difficulty in making decisions, decreased levels of concentration, and inability to cope with small demands. Someone who is depressed sees only the bleak side of things, evidences an absence of interest in what is going on, displays a lack of emotion no longer taking pleasure in things he or she usually enjoyed, and lacks any positive or hopeful feelings. The future seems one of unending bleakness. A depressed person's perspective is not at all what it should be.

The diagnosis and evaluation of depression in mortally ill patients remains challenging because the typical emotional symptoms of a life threatening condition overlap those same symptoms of depression, such as a preoccupation with death, loss of interest in daily life, poor concentration, fatigue, and sleep disturbances.

Some symptoms are perfectly normal in the face of terminal illness. Thoughts of death are natural as is sadness and a loss of ambition, as long as you do not become preoccupied with them. However, you can go from being sad to being depressed. Also, you can go to transcendence and freedom instead of a sense of "loss."

If you suffer (or think you suffer) from presence of clinical depression, obtain treatment or counseling referrals to deal with it. In most cases, you can be helped. If you take medication for your depression, be sure it is compatible with the drugs you are taking for your primary condition.

Consider antidepressant medication to help in bringing your biochemistry back to normal. However, these drugs have their own side effects.

Also, actively attempt to resolve your emotional concerns through nonpharmacological means. Walking (if you can), laughing, listening to music can help as do hugs. Understanding one's larger spiritual life, your immortal soul, aids in undercutting sadness or depression. Counseling for unresolved emotional issues provides a means to vent your feelings and offers learning strategies to help you better cope with your condition. Look into joining a support group to receive mutual encouragement and nonjudgmental openness. There, you can share your feelings about death and the dying process and issues pertaining to the physical, mental, emotional and social qualities of your life. A support group lets you consider the emotional issues and consequences regarding your decision-making, especially assisted dying.

Getting help for your depression will give you the chance to think more clearly about your life and your death, unimpaired by psychological problems or severe emotional distress. Remember: your biological future may in fact be limited and bleak. Your depression may merely confirm and correspond to what a realistic view of your situation shows. However, does your depression impair your judgment and preclude rational decision-making?

5. Even if you are not clinically depressed, do you have concerns about your loss of control and independence? Can you adapt?

Have you always valued a high degree of personal control in your life? Are you a "control freak?" Finding meaning in your suffering and for your remaining days may alleviate, at least to some extent, the need for a sense of control in your life.

How important are independence and self-sufficiency for you? How do you define your personal independence: your career, job, volunteer activities, club memberships, engaging in your favorite pursuits, living alone in your own residence, taking care of your home, driving, shopping, walking, cooking, bathing, thinking clearly to make household and personal financial decisions? Is the maintenance of an independent lifestyle an absolute necessity for you? Do you want not to need anyone, answer to anyone, burden anyone?

Are you able, and will you in the future be able, to deal with the difficulty, if not the impossibility, of fulfilling your old roles at work and at home, including handling finances, maintenance, errands, shopping, and meal preparation? Now, or in the future, physical problems, such as vision, dexterity, or mobility, or mental challenges may interfere with your in-home activities, such as reading, using a computer, cooking, doing the laundry, listening to TV or radio, watching videos. Out-of-home activities also may become too difficult.

Are you experiencing or will you face: anger and grief over loss of meaningful tasks that provided you with identity and self-esteem; an inability to be a contributing member of society; guilt from seeing a loved one, as caregiver, work harder, while you feel useless and an increasing burden; frustrations in watching a loved one perform tasks "incorrectly" you once did effortlessly?

You probably face the likelihood of increased dependency. Is it degrading for you to be dependent? Are you ashamed to ask for help? Do you regard dependence, a progressive loss of activity, mobility, and freedom, as a bad thing, a horrific weakness? Is it an affront to your concept of dignity to be incontinent, unable to feed or dress yourself, to get in and out of a bath or shower independently, to speak, move, or think, to cut your toenails, or to change your position in bed by yourself? Do you feel humiliated in needing help with using the toilet or in dressing? How do you regard being dependent to the point of having to ask for everything? Do you see your loss of autonomy and your dependence on others as lowering your self-esteem?

Or, is dependency something you must learn in order to give meaning to your life? Are you able to deal with the loss of control, to welcome others' care, to be dependent, to accept passivity?

Are there other ways to maintain a sense of independence over your life, for example, keeping control over your healthcare decisions? Can you see how your personal reality, your central selfhood, is not dependent on all these physical "independencies"? As these are removed, your realization of your essence comes out, large and bright, its value and dignity in itself.

Is your physician addressing your needs for control and independence?

Is your consideration of suicide or aid-in-dying a way of seeking control in a situation over which you feel little or no mastery? Does access to one of the means for accelerating your demise, for example, a supply of lethal pills, serve as a sort of safety net you could, if necessary, access, thereby providing comfort and giving you not only the freedom of choice but also sense of control, a guarantee of your autonomy, a weapon against powerlessness?

6. Do you fear becoming a burden to others? Do you worry that their care for you will physically and emotionally exhaust them? How realistic are your concerns?

If you feel like a burden on others, whether you remain in your own home or another's, or are a burden, what are the options? Can you and your family members and friends, who serve as your caregivers, adjust their expectations and better mesh their lifestyles and behaviors with your needs? If everyone knows what is expected, it will help your caregivers maintain their schedules and their specific roles, thereby reducing your caregivers' stress, minimizing the disruption of their daily lives, making more enjoyable your time together, less like a death watch. Discuss your concerns with your caregivers.

7. Where do you want to die -- at home, in a hospital, in a nursing home, or in an inpatient hospice?

Do you fear living in a nursing home, especially if you suffer from a degenerative condition that may continue for years, warehoused with strangers, losing your independence and control, becoming dependent on others to bathe you, change your diapers, walk you like a puppy and not come when you call or take seriously your account of your problem?

Assess your alternatives. Will you be able to live at home (or with a loved one) until your death? Look into home nursing care and in-home hospice care combining skilled nursing assistance with daily nursing visits. Get information on the alternatives and share your concerns with loved ones and discuss the various care options with them.

If realistic alternatives exist, do you want to die in a hospital room, an often impersonal setting where you are isolated from your family and friends and sustained in life by artificial means for as long as possible, or the warmth of a family home? Or, will your hospital room be quite nice? Will the hospital let your family stay, even providing beds? There may be care advantages in a hospital over a family home. Hospice care, which encourages an environment in which healthy persons are present, generally represents home care. A hospice will provide adequate pain relief, while a hospital may not.

Remember: too often patients are referred to a hospice to treat distress, not disease, and provide emotional succor only in the final days of their lives. It is often much too late for anything beyond crisis management. Many patients, their family members and physicians do not want to give up. If you want to go the hospice route, identify the right time to use this alternative.

8. What do you really fear: dependency, helplessness, hopelessness, frustration, decreased income or an inability to work, being depressed, loss of control, being a burden to others, loss of meaningful tasks providing identity and self-esteem, unfulfilled aspirations, isolation, meaninglessness, being identified mainly in terms of your medical problem, the emotional toll imposed on loved ones resulting from a prolonged deathwatch if you become extremely debilitated, physically or mentally, being undignified in how you look, being abandoned? Do you fear the dying process, dying an "undignified" or physically or mentally disturbed death? Do you want an assisted death as an escape from your fears or as a release from your actual distress?

9. Is there some special event, a particular milestone that would add a good deal of meaning to your life? Do you want the opportunity to hang on and experience (or at least live for) a significant life cycle event, for instance, the birth of a grandchild, a college graduation, a wedding, or a special birthday? Do you want to give a family member one last gift, by letting another say "I'm sorry," thereby lightening his or her grief later on and setting him or her free from needless guilt? Do you want to tie up some loose ends or make amends with family members? Do you want to hear, in person, one last "I love you" from someone special? Do you need some time to say "good-bye," "I'm sorry" or "I forgive you?"

10. Have you sought counseling for your emotional issues?

The Social Quality of Your Life

Your illness will likely constrain your ability to participate in the social world and engage in pleasurable activities outside your (or another's) home or a healthcare facility. Consider the following:

1. What are all the social elements and pleasurable activities of your life that have made your existence worthwhile?

2. As a result of your physical or mental condition, what aspects of these previous elements, activities, or abilities are presently lost to you? What elements, activities or abilities will likely be lost in the future? Are, and will, these missing features be temporarily or permanently lost? After medical intervention, will any of these again be available to you? Are these present and future missing features vital to your enjoyment of life? Through what alternatives can you find enjoyment, now and in the future? To help you accept the permanent loss of these elements, activities, or abilities, you may need to find a support group where you can grieve their loss.

3. What other elements, activities, or abilities, unaffected by your present (or foreseeable future) physical and mental condition have given (or will give) your life value?

Try to use these unaffected abilities. Adapt your abilities or alter your activities to meet your physical or mental constraints. For example, you are a perfectionist pianist but arthritis of the hands sets in and you find it difficult to play well. Are you able to redirect your interests to teaching or writing? Are you (and will you be) able to relate to others in a way that is of value and is meaningful to you?

4. Are you currently lonely? Is there someone you can turn to for practical help, financial support, or caregiving as your illness or condition requires?

Do you fear future isolation, increased loneliness, a lack of outside experiences and a variety of social contacts? Do you fear being abandoned and left alone because there is no one who really cares for you and on whom you can depend?

It is often difficult to reach for other topics of conversation when physical needs, symptoms, and concerns loom so large. The dullness of everyday life often narrows scope of one's attention. There may be far too little to stimulate you. The absence of challenge results in sufferers paying less attention to what happens around them. The number of people who populate one's life often plummets dramatically; one's world shrinks. If one is homebound, there are not even contacts with store clerks. One becomes even more dependent on relatives' and friends' visits, phone calls, and e-mails for social needs. One seeks to prolong visits and calls beyond others' endurance. The ever increasing, vacuous chatter may prevent you from speaking intimately with others.

5. In light of your present and likely future physical, mental, and emotional situation, who or what is your social support system? Has your life been rooted in your family and friends, holidays, and celebrations? How does (and will) your condition impact on these activities? Can you call on others, for instance, a relative, a friend, or someone from a Jewish organization, for help? Do you have someone to confide in and talk to about yourself or your problems? Whom can you count on? Is there someone you can have a good time with?

Many have found it helpful to engage in the Social Contacts Exercise.

Social Contacts Exercise

Place a small photo of yourself in the center of a large piece of paper. Draw the faces of those who provide you with support. Who is missing from your life? Draw the faces of those whom you want to get closer to. Are there people in your life who are causing you stress? If so, move them to the edge of the paper.

6. Have you taken (or are you taking) the initiative in searching for help and overcoming your isolation, for example, by contacting a Jewish

organization or joining a patient support group?

Financial Considerations

Financial considerations, focusing on whether you are or will be an economic drain on loved ones, include the following:

1. Do you see your own value, primarily or solely, in terms of monetary resources?

2. Does the process of your dying pose the fear or the prospect of actual financial difficulties because of a lack of adequate medical care insurance, financial reserves, or Medicare or Medicaid benefits? What is (and will be) the economic impact of your medical care expenses on your loved ones, going from a diminished inheritance for them to a dependence on the resources of others? Does your family face financial ruin from your catastrophic illness?

Do you want to preserve the funds you have saved? Are your savings better spent for your survivors, for instance, a grandchild's college education, rather than giving you a few more weeks or months of life? Are a few more weeks or months of severely compromised life worth the loss of the economic security for your survivors you have worked so hard to achieve?

3. Do you feel an obligation to die so as to end the financial burden you are imposing on your family? Do you want to die sooner rather then later to conserve your resources for others? Are you being pressured, directly or subtly, by your relatives or friends to accelerate your death thereby maximizing the wealth they will inherit?

4. Are your concerns realistic? What is your financial status and what are the current and likely future costs of your medical care?

5. What are your medical insurance benefits, your long term care insurance benefits (including in home healthcare coverage), your Medicare or Medicaid coverage?

If you are terminally ill, investigate whether your life insurance company allows you to cash in your policy, more technically known as viatical settlement, for a part of its face value generating assets and thereby lessening your feelings of being a financial burden on others.

6. In comparison to the physical, mental, and social quality of your life factors, how strongly are realistic financial factors influencing your decision-making?

7. Do you have any unfinished financial and legal matters, specifically, debts, wills, trusts, other financial or business arrangements, you need time to complete?

Putting It All Together

Strive to pull together your answers to the questions in these three key areas: first, spiritual and religious issues; second, the physical and mental quality of your life; and third, emotional, social and economic concerns. Assess and discuss the alternatives, reflect on your feelings and motives, consider fully the consequences, be concerned for your loved ones, and strive to minimize the harm to them as well as to yourself.

Do not act in haste or out of unsound reasoning. Take time to reflect, unless your condition or your quality of life deteriorates markedly. If you are still well enough to do the research, explore your options. You likely will vacillate between wanting to live and considering it might be better to die. Does your decision tend to settle one way or the other so as to be consistent, unwavering, certain, over a reasonable period of time -- several days or one week? Listen to your inner voice.

Before you make a final decision, reflect on the following more holistic concerns:[6]

1. Are your reasons sound and is your timing right? Have you gotten the most out of life, as you see it, for as long as possible? Has the quality of your life in all its dimensions and your baseline conditions for living become intolerable (or at what point will they become intolerable)?

Rarely is uncontrolled physical pain the exclusive reason for requesting physician assistance in dying. As shown by studies of those who availed themselves of physician-assisted suicide in Oregon,[7] the dimensions of suffering are far deeper than pain or physical symptoms. The choice of physician-assisted suicide in Oregon is most strongly associated with concerns about a loss of autonomy, loss of control of bodily functions, a poor quality of life, an inability to participate in activities making life enjoyable, a desire to control the circumstance of death, and a fear of future suffering.

Similarly, in the Netherlands, unrelieved pain was the sole reason for life termination requests in about 5% of the cases, part of the problem (a contributing factor) in 46% (with the 5% of the cases included in the 46%), and not reported in the remaining 54%. The most common reasons for accelerating one's demise were: intolerance of physical disintegration, dependence and being a burden on others, and a life lacking meaning.[8] In short, most requests were motivated by a mix of personal and existential issues, together with physical suffering.

2. Do you have a realistic assessment of your present situation and what your future may hold? Have you exhausted every reasonable effort to stay alive? Have you explored all reasonable alternatives to improve the quality of your life and relieve your pain and suffering? Have you consulted with objective professionals, your rabbi or your physician?

3. Are you mentally up to this type of decision-making? Can you make an informed choice regarding your medical care? Are you mentally "clear"? Is your decision-making free from distorted judgment? Are your mental processes unimpaired by psychological illness, for example, depression or severe emotional distress? Can you appreciate the major characteristics of your illness or condition? Do you understand the impact of the main treatment options? Can you judge the relationship of these alternatives to your beliefs and values? Are you able to deliberate about your choices? Can you communicate your decision in a meaningful manner?

Are you at peace or are you physically exhausted, emotionally numbed from being a patient and the constant battle you have waged against your illness or condition? Have you had it with your illness or condition -- the treatments, office visits for examinations and tests, dealing with new drugs and their side effects, endless discussions about your diagnosis, prognosis, and medical options?

Have you consulted with a mental health professional who has made an assessment of your decision-making capacity, particularly, the absence of treatable major depression?

4. Is your decision enduring? Is your mind made up? Does your choice remain firm?

One study of 168 mostly elderly, terminally ill cancer patients, admitted to a hospital for end of life care in the weeks before death, showed significant fluctuations in their will to live.[9] The participants rated themselves twice a day on 100- point scales measuring pain, nausea, appetite, activity, drowsiness, sense of well-being, and the strength of their will to live. Over a twelve-hour period, a patient's will to live could fluctuate by as much as 30% or more; over a thirty day period, the shifts were even greater, on an average of more than 50% to over 70%. Thus, the researchers concluded that the will to live is "highly unstable" among the terminally ill cancer patients they studied.

In this study, researchers found that in the period just after hospital admission, increased anxiety, perhaps resulting from the psychological shift in moving to hospital care, resulted in a decrease in the patients' will to live. After one or two weeks, spiraling depression was most closely associated with a reduced will to go on. In the final days of the life, the study showed a correlation between physical symptoms and the loss of will to live. At the end, physical distress, particularly pain and shortness of breath, lessened the will to live more strongly than the previous psychological suffering.

Do you think you will want to alter your decision to end your life? In the past, have you changed your mind about an important decision? For example, have you broken an engagement or backed out of a decision to buy a house?

In thinking about what to do, you may discover that the time is not right, for any number of possible reasons. Are you absolutely certain about your decision, your reasons and the timing?

5. As you reach a final decision, ask yourself: is this your own choice? Is it voluntary and made of your own free will? Have you been influenced by anyone? Have you been coerced by others, perhaps quite subtly if they are exhausted from caregiving and are beginning to withdraw from you or evidence signs of irritability? Are you under pressure to act by those you love or whose opinion you respect? Are family and friends exerting pressure to spare them emotional pain and financial expense?

Remember: let it be your own decision. However, in making your choice, consider its impact on your loved ones and involve them in your decision-making.

Consider and Involve Your Loved Ones in Your Decision-Making

Try to discuss your concerns, the quality of your life, treatment approaches, and alternatives with your beloved. Involve your loved ones in your decision-making process so as to avoid prolonged negative consequences, such as a legacy of guilt, on their part.

Ask your immediate family members and your close friends: How my death, its timing and manner might affect them? Talk with the people you love. Opening a dialogue enables you to share your innermost feelings and fears, move beyond your isolation, reinforce intimacy in personal relationships, obtain feedback, and achieve emotional closure for yourself and others.

If you do not want to open this discussion, do you have valid reasons for your reserve? Will everyone be honest, frank and guilt free? Will such conversation strain everybody? Do you feel that others will not say what they really feel?

Entering into a dialogue with your beloved is not a one time conversation but an ongoing interaction. You want your decision to be based on the facts of your physical and mental condition, your emotional, spiritual and social needs and values (not your fears), and the concerns of your loved ones. Receive constructive feedback from family members, close friends, healthcare professionals, your rabbi. Discuss practical problems, consider various options, exchange information.

In particular, express your financial fears to those you think you are burdening. Listen to and consider how they assess the economic impact of your medical care on them. Force them to deny that your continued life is financially burdensome to them.

Also, consider the following:

1. As you reach out to others, ponder what you want from them: compassion, a sympathetic ear, approval, or help in dying?

2. Do your loved ones, who will be impacted by your protracted or accelerated death, support your decision, your reasoning, and your timing? Do they fully and completely accept and support your choice, the reasons, and the timing, or only show hesitant or lukewarm support, or outright opposition? Do they want you to go ahead or wait? Do you understand their perspective? Are they willing to let go? Is their viewpoint based on a commitment to principle, a sense of duty to you ("I will always support your decisions"), or their exhaustion as caregivers? What is the basis of their opposition? What are the religious, spiritual, and ethical beliefs of your loved ones regarding suicide or aid-in-dying? What emotions do they express to you now? Are they in denial about your condition and your likely prognosis?

3. What will be the likely impact of your suicide or your taking a lethal pill or injection on your loved ones? Will they face prolonged psychological turmoil? Assess whether your action would lead to feelings of guilt, anger, or intensified grief on the part of your survivors, for instance, their feeling responsible for not relieving your emotional pain. What are other potential after effects on your loved ones? Will there be

a stigma? How will they manage it? What about the impact on those initially unaware of your decision but who learn about it later? Do you intend to leave an explanatory statement?

4. What weight do you want to give to the interests of your beloved? If you favor great weight to the interests of others, rather than your own interests, you may want to review a tentative choice you have made and amend it.

Opening a dialogue with others and letting them share their concerns, also gives your loved ones time to adjust and adapt to the idea and to say their good-byes. Let others talk about what your death will mean to them.

Creating an avenue of communication may delay or reverse your decision to accelerate your death. Obtain information as to others' feelings. Their perspective may enable you to see the need to continue to live or other ways to hasten your demise. Receive assurance of their love and support in your final decision.

We next turn to consider your death and dying from the perspective of your loved ones.

Notes

1. I have drawn on Stephen Jamison, *Final Acts of Love: Families, Friends, and Assisted Dying* (New York: G.P. Putnam's Sons, 1995), 12-78; Stephen Jamison, *Assisted Suicide: A Decision-Making Guide For Health Professionals* (San Francisco: Jossey-Bass, 1997); Margaret Pabst Battin, "Assisting in Suicide: Seventeen Questions Physicians and Mental-Health Professional Should Ask," chap. 13 in *The Least Worst Death: Essays in Bioethics on the End of Life* (New York: Oxford University Press, 1994), 271-276; Pamela J. Miller, Susan C. Hedland, and Karen A. Murphy, "Social Work Assessment at End of Life: Practical Guidelines for Suicide and the Terminally Ill," *Social Work in Health Care* 26:4 (1998): 23-26; Nathan I. Cherny, Nessa Coyle, and Kathleen M. Foley, "Suffering in the Advanced Cancer Patient: A Definition and Taxonomy," *Journal of Palliative Care* 10:2 (Summer 1994): 57-70.

2. Ronald H. Isaacs in *Miracles: A Jewish Perspective* (Northvale, NJ: Jason Aronson, 1997) presents a useful survey of the role, meaning, and understanding of miracles in the Jewish tradition.

3. Nicholas A. Christakis and Elizabeth B. Lamont, "Extent and Determinants of Error in Doctors' Prognoses in Terminally Ill Patients: Prospective Cohort Study," *British Medical Journal* 320:7233 (February 19, 2000): 469-473. In this study of 343 doctors and 468 patients admitted to hospices over 130 days in 1996, 63% of the physicians overestimated the time of survival, by a factor of 5.3.

4. Sherwin B. Nuland, M.D., *How We Die: Reflections on Life's Final Chapter* (New York: Knopf, 1994). See also Joanne Lynne, M.D. and Joan Harrold, M.D., *Handbook for Mortals: Guidance for People Facing Serious Illness* (New York: Oxford University Press, 1999), 93-118.

5. Jane E. Brody, "Personal Health: When a Dying Patient Seeks Suicide Aid It May Be a Signal To Fight Depression," *New York Times*, 18 June 1997, sec. C10 cites two studies, one of 378 AIDS patients concluding that the strongest predictor of a personal interest in suicide was the presence of depression and another finding that more than one half of suicidal cancer patients who expressed a consistent, unequivocal desire for death were clinically depressed. See also Harvey Max Chochinov et al, "Desire for Death in the Terminally Ill," *American Journal of Psychiatry* 152:8 (August 1995): 1185-1191.

6. I have drawn on James L. Werth, Jr. and Debra C. Cobia, "Empirically Based Criteria for Rational Suicide: A Survey of Psychotherapists," *Suicide and Life-Threatening Behavior* 25:2 (Summer 1995): 231-240; James L. Werth, "Using Rational Suicide as an Intervention to Prevent Irrational Suicide," *Crisis* 19:4 (October, November, December 1998): 185-192; Margaret P. Battin, "Can Suicide Be Rational? Yes, Sometimes," in *Contemporary Perspectives on Rational Suicide*, ed. James L. Werth, Jr. (Philadelphia: Brunner/Mazel, 1999), 13-21.

7. Amy D. Sullivan, Katrina Hedberg, and David W. Fleming, "Legalized Physician-Assisted Suicide in Oregon - The Second Year," *New England Journal of Medicine* 342:8 (February 2000): 598-604; David Brown, "A Picture of Assisted Suicide," *Washington Post*, 24 February 2000, sec. A3; Arthur E. Chin et al, "Legalized Physician-Assisted Suicide in Oregon-The First Year's Experience," *New England Journal of Medicine* 340:7 (February 1999): 577-583; Sam Howe Verhovek, "Oregon Reporting 15 Deaths In Year Under New Suicide Law," *New York Times*, 18 February 1999, sec. Al.

8. Paul J. van der Maas et al, "Euthanasia and Other Medical Decisions Concerning the End of Life," *The Lancet* 338:8768 (September 1991): 672.

9. Harvey Max Chochinov et al, "Will To Live in the Terminally Ill," *The Lancet* 354:9181 (September 1999): 816-819; Erica Goode, "Terminal Cancer Patients' Will to Live Is Found to Fluctuate," *New York Times*, 4 September 1999, sec. A8. A study of physicians eligible to prescribe lethal medications under the Oregon Death with Dignity Act showed that 46% of the patients for whom substantive palliative interventions, such as control of pain or other physical symptoms, referral to a hospice program, or a trial of antidepressant medication, were made changed their minds about physician-assisted suicide. Linda Ganzini et al, "Physicians' Experience with the Oregon Death with Dignity Act," New England Journal of Medicine 342:8 (February 2000): 557-563.

Chapter 9

A Loved One's Perspective on a Patient's Plight

A life threatening illness presents significant challenges for a patient's beloved. They, along with the patient, suffer; they experience anguish, repeatedly. They encounter doubt and confusion caring for a dear one during the dying process and especially near death, caught between hoping for his or her death and wishing that he or she was well and fully back with them.

This chapter begins by examining the physical and emotional strains caregivers face for which they are generally unprepared. It will help you determine whether you are able or want to provide (and continue to provide) home care for someone who is chronically or terminally ill.

Beyond being there at the end, the chapter offers specific suggestions for meeting a dying person's physical, emotional, and spiritual needs. The chapter also examines how love ones can help someone deal with various death moment visions, thereby deepening a soon-to-depart individual's spiritual path.

The Impact of the Initial Diagnosis of a Terminal Illness or a Chronic, Debilitating Condition and Thereafter

Once you get over your initial shock -- this could not happen, it's not true -- an emotional exhaustion, a numbness, some sort of resignation, often sets in on learning of the diagnosis of a loved one's mortal illness or incurable, chronic condition. For most of us, slow acceptance, and in the case of a progressively debilitating condition, adaption, follows our initial denial.[1] Gradually, family members restructure their roles so they can continue to function. They come to accept help from others and publicly acknowledge something's very wrong, physically or mentally, with a loved one.

Learning to live with another's chronic condition characterizes adaption. Family and friends integrate changes caused by the situation into a new lifestyle often shifting their values and priorities.

As the weeks and months pass, fear about the future comes to the fore, characterized by uncertainty about the dying process and one's ability to cope with the multitude of problems lying ahead, in the midst of ever advancing physical or mental symptoms. The future seems to only hold grief and loss. Each day dawns with dread. Will there be another symptom, a new problem, further deterioration?

Living in a permanent state of anxiety results in continuous stress. The mounting perception of hopelessness often yields anger and despair. Despite the acceptance of care burdens and life restrictions, family members and friends often can't do anything to take away a loved one's pain and suffering. They can't change the course of a disease or condition and make things better. The helplessness continues for the rest of a sufferer's life. There is no way out.

Many of us ask ourselves did we in some way cause our beloved's condition? Why does one suffer and not another? Why do the healthy ones escape?

Loved ones feel guilty about their inability to provide perfect physical care as well as a meaningful degree of emotional and spiritual support. When they give more than they should, their guilt often turns toward feelings of resentment.

Economic concerns may exacerbate their fears. They wonder whether they can take unpaid family leave time. Also, will they be able to work part-time and still make the mortgage payments and keep their health insurance?

Although a sufferer may receive care at a hospital, a nursing home, or an inpatient hospice, earlier on in the course of a terminal illness or chronic condition, loved ones focus on care at home. The limited hospital stays caused by the managed healthcare revolution as well as the expense of nursing home stays or assisted living arrangements have placed much greater responsibilities on family members to provide home care, particularly for elderly relatives suffering from a chronic illness, marked by disability and dependency. In fact, family members and friends provide about 80 percent of all long-term care in the United States.[2] Loved ones must contemplate the benefits of and burdens imposed on them of extended home caregiving.

You may face this new role, right now. Before taking it on, ask yourself: What do you expect to accomplish? Are you acting out of a sense of duty, are you seeking fulfillment, or for some other reason?

The Benefits of Providing Informal, Home Caregiving

In a society often marked by an absence of love, compassion and forgiveness, virtues so important to Spiritual Judaism, there is always something tender and moving about the continuity of family life and its bonds. A dutiful child cares for an elderly parent; in later years, for his or her spouse. Care embodies an expression of reverence for another.

Reflect on the benefits both your beloved and you derive from your involvement in another's care. By choosing to be a caregiver, you can help your dear one die at home, free from unwanted medical interventions, relieved of pain as far as possible, warmed by the bright sunshine of your attention.

Caring for another may enrich you in many ways, making you more compassionate, kinder, softer, and more helpful. You may come to feel more deeply and increase your empathy for others. You may come to discover new things about yourself -- your capacity to learn and to listen. You may show strengths you did not know you had that might otherwise have remained dormant. You may learn that you have what it takes. If you take on the burden of caregiving, you will perform a rewarding function, knowing that you have been there for a loved one and "done well." You also come to know a sufferer -- whether a parent, a sibling, or a close friend -- as a person.

Caregivers also learn to rearrange their priorities. You focus on what is important, letting the trivialities and pettiness of daily life drop away. You come to realize your finiteness, the impermanence and fragility of the world. As perhaps never before, you become aware that we all have only a limited time in our present earthly existence. Learning to use your time fully and wisely, you may focus on and achieve a better sense of direction and purpose in your life.

The Dilemmas Caregivers Face

In the twenty-first century, as more and more responsibility for care is placed on patients' families and friends, caregivers, especially women, face complex lives with many competing demands.[3] Beyond their traditional roles of wife, mother, and daughter, women encounter other demands and roles to play. Fewer and fewer occupy the stereotypical roles of full-time wife, mother, and daughter. They have jobs and careers. Older women may have more than one person to care for; a younger caregiver may tend to two or three frail elders.

If you handle the complex caregiving role for someone, especially a loved one suffering from an incurable, debilitating chronic illness, often for a much longer duration than in previous generations, incredible demands may be placed on you. You encounter the economic and cultural changes profoundly impacting traditional family structures, characterized by fewer members and reduced emotional resources. It is difficult to balance your multiple roles including the burdens of caregiving. If you have not previously been involved in it, you will discover the management of care at home often involves assistance with complex medical regimes and diets, concurrent healthcare problems, time-consuming treatments, basic care needs, such as help in bathing, eating, getting dressed or undressed, and the emotional and spiritual reactions of sufferers.

You want to help your loved one have as good a quality of life and level of self-esteem as possible, but at what personal sacrifice to yourself? The occurrence of unexpected crises and acute medical episodes may lead to further stresses and to the possible deterioration of your own physical and emotional health. You may face mounting physical and emotional strains as the caregiving role consumes more and more of your existence to the detriment of other aspects of your life.

Regardless of how you feel about committing weeks, months or even years of home care, it may be a burden you cannot avoid. What is the cost to you -- physically, emotionally, and financially? Will you be able to balance caring for a dear one and at the same time caring for yourself and handling your other responsibilities? Your daily tasks continue -- your job as well as food preparation, cleaning, the laundry, and paying bills.

Except for older caregivers who may have fewer competing time demands because of retirement, time is at a premium. Caregivers must make major life adjustments as new responsibilities accumulate and new roles are assumed. Home care takes time from other tasks. Family life can become chaotic. Caregivers' lives are restricted. They often sacrifice their personal desires and opportunities to socialize with others. Life plans -- the chance to travel or pursue their own interests -- are put on hold. There may be new financial demands and concerns including the diminution of income resulting from absenteeism, a change in work arrangements, or even job loss. They must also deal with the prospect of sidetracking their job or career prospects.

The loneliness and social isolation of caregivers increases as their relationships with others are adversely impacted. Involvement in community, religious, and spiritual activities are restricted.

Sufferers are sometimes consumed by their own health needs that they have little regard left for their caregivers, who must learn to live with another's moods and mood changes, his or her emotional highs and lows. To limit their own emotional losses, caregivers may begin to withdraw more and more.

Caregivers who provide all the home care for a loved one must struggle to keep all aspects of their lives in balance. Overburdened and overwhelmed, care exacts a price, physically and emotionally.

Physical changes abound. These include appetite shifts, overeating or a loss of appetite, leading to significant weight gain or loss, as well as sleep disturbances, marked by difficulty in falling or staying asleep. Caregiving may require heavy physical work, such as lifting or transferring a weak or immobile patient. Consider whether you have the strength to take on the tasks of constant lifting, feeding, bathing, and toileting.

Emotional difficulties may also mount. You may want to scream: "It's harder than paid work. It's certainly more confining. It's all the time and I don't have energy for anything else. My life is shot." You feel trapped, smothered by the responsibility.

Caregivers face stress, resentment, exhaustion, depression, and especially burnout. They may become short-tempered, cry often, or manifest an expressionless face, a flat voice tone. They may overuse sleeping pills, alcohol, or caffeine. They may experience fatigue, characterized by a loss of energy, a continual sense of tiredness, and reduced levels of motivation or concentration. Anxiety is ever present in providing comfort care and in administering medication. They are concerned with their ability to handle emergencies, such as pain or bleeding. Remorse may arise, as well as unresolved guilt distress from future concerns, feelings of hopelessness, helplessness, meaninglessness and futility.

Strategies for Meeting Your Needs as a Caregiver

If you take on the responsibility of providing all the home care for your beloved, you must learn to deal with your own physical and emotional needs. You must set limits. You also need to know when you cannot provide round-the-clock home care.

To deal with your stress, consider what works for you. Do you find stress reduction through: prayer, meditation, breathing techniques, visualization, exercise, walking, listening to music, pursuing a hobby, spending time with friends or engaging in family activities, work? Getting enough rest, following a proper diet and exercising regularly will enable you to cope better. At least once a week, at a set day and time, give yourself a respite.

You need to take time away from your caregiving without feeling guilty. Through your loving detachment, you protect yourself from being consumed by your enormous responsibility.

Arrange for relief help which includes someone else reading to the patient, feeding and bathing him or her, and assisting with personal hygiene. Hospice volunteers typically provide respite caregiving caregivers some free time away from their immediate responsibilities.

Take a break for yourself to restore your perspective and maintain your own physical and emotional health. Take time out to pamper yourself -- see what works for you -- a long walk, a luxurious bath. If possible, get help. Hire a sitter or an aid for occasional days or on a regular basis. Ask for assistance. Involve other family members and friends in the caregiving. Get away on a planned vacation for a weekend or a week. Remember you have a life of your own.

Don't neglect yourself -- spiritually, emotionally, or physically -- so that you become seriously ill or the quality of care you provide degenerates. If you burnout, you are not useful to anyone. Do not endanger your loved one by neglecting yourself.

Consider participating in a support group. As friends and relatives drift away, especially if your dear one's condition is prolonged, do not let yourself become isolated. Join a support group, in person or on-line, composed of those in the same situation who understand the toll caregiving takes on daily lives and relationships.

Support groups help relieve your isolation. Talk with others who understand what you face. Laugh at humorous incidents. By taking an active stance toward problem solving, you often achieve a growing awareness of options and the generation of creative solutions. Giving help to support group members can be as useful as receiving it.

Even if a specific problem cannot be solved, group discussion about a situation may help you feel better. You can express your negative emotions, your guilt, your anger, your resentment, without being judged.

However, participation in a face-to-face support, represents another demand on your time. Rather than turning to an ongoing group, you may want to rely on an informal network of individuals who really are able to listen to what you are going through. Or, look to message boards and chat rooms on the Internet for information, solace and support.

In addition to the stress, resentment, and exhaustion, burnout typically arises from the constant closeness and the need to get along with your beloved on a day-to-day basis. You and your loved one must communicate openly and honestly about your emotions and fears. There may be resistance to doing this. Exploring how a sufferer feels, the losses he or she experiences, may result in both of you taking joint responsibility for your mutual support, thereby enabling you and your dear one to build on your combined strengths.

If possible, try not to take over everything in another's life, thereby harming the patient who becomes even more dependent as well as exhausting yourself. Give help only when asked. Strive to foster as much independence as possible on the part of your loved one. Restore some areas of control, small tasks over which your beloved can maintain complete control. Find ways a sufferer can exert some degree of control over as many choices as possible. Focus on his or her small, readily observable triumphs, helping his or her feelings of powerlessness recede. Ask yourself: do your efforts at too much caregiving and control stem from your own guilt or from your need to feel useful?

Try to spend time with your loved one on meaningful projects; find ways a sufferer can participate and feel useful. Sort through old papers, tape reminiscences, mount photos in a family album. Making progress on a project counters a sufferer's helplessness and his or her accompanying discouragement as life slips away. Encourage the resumption of a previously satisfying activity or the trying of something new. Any of these enable your dear one to focus on something beyond his or her pain, other physical symptoms, and various forms of suffering.

Develop alternative activities in which you and your dear one can both participate. For instance, if he or she can't walk, perhaps you can read aloud to each other. If possible, establish one or more regularly occurring pleasures your loved one can look forward to. Institute a once a week outing, such as a car ride, to provide a sense of anticipation and mental stimulation, promoting greater alertness, sparking memories and new subjects to talk about. In short, these projects, activities, and outings may stimulate a reawakening of your beloved's former self, if he or she is mentally or emotionally able.

You must also learn to set limits if a sufferer becomes abusive, emotionally or physically, to prevent you from becoming even more resentful. Someone who is ill may take out their anger, if not their rage, at their infirmities on the closest target, you -- their home caregiver. Abuse can take an almost limitless number of forms, including waking you up thoughtlessly at any time of the day or night, demanding help beyond your capacity, finding fault with errors made in good faith, screaming at you, blaming you or others for problems caused by the sufferer, complaining about unavoidable or uncontrollable situations.

Clearly define and set your limits. Holding firm represents an act of caring. Do not feel guilty that you are not doing all you should. You can only do so much.

Ultimately, you face a difficult question: are you able to continue to provide adequate, informal home care? How long can you let the caregiving experience go on? When does caregiving reach the point of diminishing emotional and spiritual returns? When is "enough, enough?"

Weeks and months of constant sleep deprivation and disturbances caused by a sufferer needing pain medication or a change of bedding as well help in getting to the bathroom, can wreck havoc on your coping skills. You may turn to increased use of alcohol, medication, or caffeine. Your mounting depression, if untreated, can result in compromised care, mental or physical illness, or even premature death. You may need to place a loved one in another setting.

Sufferers typically want home care from family members or friends over placement in another venue. However, if the care burdens and demands become too great, or the patient's condition deteriorates markedly, consider asking others for help, getting paid-at-home caregivers, or placing your loved one in a nursing home or an inpatient hospice. Ask yourself: Am I and the other family members able to work together in providing care? Can family members reach a consensus on a course of care? Or do intra-family conflicts result in an inability of family members to agree on a course of care? The best care may be in an out-of-home setting. You may want to place the sufferer in a nursing home or an assisted living facility for a time-limited trial period. Find out how to qualify your loved one for long-term care provided by Medicaid in your state.

When your loved one becomes terminally ill and then slips into the dying process, be certain that his or her physical, emotional, and spiritual needs are met.

Suggestions for Meeting a Patient's Physical Needs

Someone who is gravely ill should be made as comfortable as possible thereby lessening any unnecessary pain and suffering. Whether an individual dies at home, an in-patient hospice, a nursing home, or a hospital, strive to see that the dying person's physical care needs are met. This may require continuous presence of family members and friends throughout the day.

As life ebbs for the terminally ill, focus particular attention on the use on pain medication. Make certain that your beloved does not experience, if at all possible, severe, uncontrolled, intolerable pain and suffering. Concerns about drug usage, including unreasonable fears about addiction to pain control meditation, may cause physicians to underutilize painkillers. For the fatally ill, these fears are unnecessary and simply inappropriate. Do not be insensitive to your loved one's needs to control pain. Take steps to ensure that pain control is adequate. Sometimes this entails moving your loved one from a hospital to a hospice. Medication not obtainable under hospital policy, geared to long-term survival, is obtainable in a hospice, devoted to keeping comfortable those with short life expectancies.

It is paramount that a dying person's pain be adequately controlled. In nearly all situations, this is now medically feasible. Thus, pain medication should be given as your dear one, if lucid, desires. Remember to consider the side effects. The use of painkillers may render a patient unconscious. As developed in Chapter 5, be concerned about a physician sedating your loved one to unconsciousness, particularly from the perspective of Spiritual Judaism, thereby cutting off his or her ability to experience the presence of death moment visions. Also, ask healthcare professionals to attempt to teach a terminally ill patient to deal with pain and suffering through relaxation techniques or breathing exercises.

In addition to focusing on controlling and managing your loved one's pain, make certain that he or she is comfortable. A limitless number of physical concerns may arise, including personal hygiene, nourishment, breathing and bowel movement difficulties, bed sores and itching, cramps in feet and legs, positional discomfort, mouth and skin care, nausea and vomiting, as well as sleep disorders. Ask healthcare professionals to deal with all of these physical needs. The requisite medical technology and knowledge currently exist to control just about every form of physical distress among the dying.

In addition to addressing your beloved's physical discomfort, his or her emotional and spiritual quandaries must be dealt with. Be sensitive to the need to provide continued emotional and spiritual support.[4]

Suggestions for Meeting a Patient's Emotional and Spiritual Needs

The ongoing agony experienced by someone suffering from the debilitating consequences of an incurable, chronic disease or someone who is terminally ill, often hooked up to tubes and monitors in a sterile hospital room, offers the potential for a beautiful sharing experience. New horizons of emotional and spiritual possibilities for awareness and transcendence exist beyond the outwardly bleak concerns.

Those diagnosed with a severe chronic condition or a life threatening illness often are jolted into a new mindfulness about their lives. As discussed in Chapter 3 and 7, what a teacher their sickness is.

Living with an incurable, debilitating condition or a mortal illness and ultimately, the process of dying, life's final chapter, no matter how messy, offers sufferers opportunities to grow within themselves and with others. Death and the dying process can be transforming and liberating -- emotionally and spiritually.

How can you create this emotionally-satisfying, spiritually-oriented environment, marked by time for reflection, reconciliation, and ultimately, closure? Basically, listen to a sufferer's spiritual questions and encourage their open expression. At the bedside, be present for and learn to listen to -- really listen to -- your loved one, to what is said and what is unstated, but implied. "Be there" as a sympathetic ear and "go with the flow." Allow a dying individual to set the pace and to bring up whatever he or she wants to talk about or needs to say -- thoughts, fears, hopes, regrets, feelings about death and dying, good and bad memories. It is important to make a sufferer feel safe, no matter what he or she reveals. If a response is desired, try to give the reassurance and approval that are needed.

Telling funny stories and jokes can be helpful. Laughter causes relaxation and certain other physiological changes; it can be comforting provided the vibration does not actually cause any pain in the belly.

Encourage your loved one to offer the affirmative or petitionary prayers, the prayers of surrender, or cry out to God, as detailed in Chapter 7. Pray with your beloved and outside his or her presence. Guide a sufferer through meditations and visualizations. Ask for prayers from your congregation and other groups who maintain a prayer list.

Offer Prayers Outside a Sufferer's Presence

You can offer prayers outside the presence of the sufferer. Jews have traditionally offered the *Mi-Shebeirakh* prayer, "May God Who blessed our ancestors, bless and heal --, a sick person," on behalf of others outside their presence.

The *Mi-Shebeirakh*, a holistic prayer for a full healing (*refuah shlayma* in Hebrew) -- a spiritual healing, a healing of body, mind, and soul, the attaining of wholeness -- asks God's blessing and compassion and for a sufferer's restoration and strength as follows:

> May the One Who blessed our ancestors Abraham, Isaac, Jacob, Sarah, Rebecca, Rachel, and Leah, bless and heal ---, who is ill.
> May the Holy One of Blessing shower abundant miracles on him/her, fulfilling his/her dreams of healing, strengthening him/her with the power of life.
> Merciful One: restore him/her, heal him/her, enliven him/her, send him/her a complete healing from the heavenly realms, a healing of body and a healing of soul, together with all who are ill, soon, speedily, without delay; and let us say: Amen!

The *Mi-Shebeirakh* is recited in the synagogue after the reading of the

Torah. If a sufferer cannot be present at the worship service, a close relative or friend is called up to the Torah for an honor (*aliya* in Hebrew). The prayer is offered after the completion of the *aliya* to the Torah reading, filling in the name of the person who is ill. The prayer can also be said before and after surgery, during treatments, or on admission or discharge from a hospital.

In addition to the *Mi-Shebeirakh* prayer, as part of the *Shemoneh Esreh* -- the most important portion of the traditional Jewish worship services next to the *Shema* -- Jews recite the *Refaeinu* prayer, a petitionary prayer calling for healing of those who are sick and relieving all who experience pain.

> Heal us, God, and we will be healed; save us and we will be saved, because You are our praise. Bring a full healing for all our pains and sufferings, because You are God, the most powerful, faithful, and compassionate Healer. God, please heal --- [designate your beloved]. Blessed are You, God, Who heals the sick.[5]

Use Guided Meditations

A guided meditation represents a way of helping a loved one. In this instance, the spiritual journey is led by you, as a guide offering a focused message, taking your beloved, who is guided, to a place where he or she has the opportunity to meet with God. A guided meditation thus provides an opening beyond one's ordinary state of consciousness. As an inward spiritual seeking, it serves an instrument of attuning to the Divine Presence at the core of human nature. We affirm the essential goodness of the human personality and believe the meditation can evoke that Presence. A guided meditation affords a sufferer the opportunity to experience a deeper and more profound state of being.

In a guided meditation, for instance the Guided Angel Meditation set forth below, the guide serves as the facilitator. For a successful guided meditation, the guide-facilitator not only needs to direct the process but also to enter into the spirit of the meditation.

Although most Jews in modern times are uncomfortable with the idea of angels, biblical and rabbinic literature contain numerous references to various angels, but not the Hollywood variety with halos and wings.[6] In the Torah, the term "angel" generally connotes a messenger. Angels are spiritual forces given human form. An angel stopped Abraham from sacrificing Isaac. (Genesis 22:11-18). Angels appeared on Jacob's ladder. (Genesis 28:12) These are some of the Hebrew Bible's nonhuman messengers.

Biblical literature also refers to other, rather strange kinds of angels. The prophet Isaiah described the seraphim, the fiery angels with their six wings. (Isaiah 6:2). The prophet Ezekiel experienced a vision of the Divine chariot-throne moved by four strange, four-faced winged creatures. (Ezekiel 1:4-21).

In short, angels fill the Jewish tradition. Although portrayed as having a wide range of powers, they usually, but not always, represent spiritual forces for goodness. Angels are sent to help us.

You can guide your loved one through the Guided Angel Meditation, twice daily, if possible, for ten to fifteen minutes each time. Remember: be patient.

Guided Angel Meditation

Introductory Instructions. As a guide, try to create a warm, welcoming atmosphere, an environment of serenity and spaciousness for the journey within. Lower the lights, if possible. Candles can set a mood that enhances meditation.

Ask your beloved to: close your eyes, sit or lie quietly, calm and relax your body by breathing in and out normally, feeling where the breath flows into and out of the body. Adjust the breaths so that the in and out breaths are the same length thereby bringing about both a relaxation of the body and an alertness of the mind. (Obviously, you need to vary these instructions depending on your dear one's physical condition. Be aware that, for some people, paying attention to the breath produces tension and causes the breath to become irregular and shallow.)

Invoke the angel Michael -- the angel of love and kindness -- on your right side. Ask Michael to be with you, because sometimes your own love fails, when you're unkind or judgmental. Tell Michael to please help you to be truly loving and lovable. Ask Michael that you wish to receive an experience of being cared for with tenderness and generosity, which will warm you more than you could have ever imagined.

Then, invoke the angel Gabriel -- the angel representing the strength and courage of God, Who helps us overcome fear -- on your left side. Ask Gabriel to help you overcome your fears related to death and dying. Tell Gabriel that you wish to draw strength and courage from God to overcome the challenges that you face.

Invite Raphael, the angel of healing -- the angel, who represents the healing power of God -- who is behind you, to come into your body and mind. Name your particular ills, discomforts and emotional needs. If you believe in miraculous cures and are praying to experience one, tell Raphael so, and express you motivation and your intention. If you are finishing your commission for this life, tell Raphael you want to see him clearly and you want to experience a wholeness of body-mind-spirit.

Imagine the angel Uriel, the light of God, in front of you. Ask Uriel, who provides insight and understanding that come from outside our own minds, to help you know and understanding what's happening.

Feel the presence of these four angels. Call on each of them. They're there for you.

Finally, imagine the Divine Radiance above your body flowing through your body. That radiance is the Shekhinah, the feminine aspect of God. Allow the radiance to surround and permeate you with love, to encompass you with a protective inner peace, and to infuse into you the undeniable sense of the Presence of God.

Help is all around you.

The angels will remain with you as you slowly open your eyes and perceive the physical world of God's creation. Observe the beauty of it and feel the happiness of having loved ones around you.

Concluding Instructions. Offer these instructions. Now invite your beloved to come back to the here and now. Say: Take time to ease yourself back. Slowly bring your awareness back into your being. Feel yourself back in the room and open your eyes.

Use Guided Visualizations

Visualization can be a powerful goal-setting technique for anyone, even someone who is encountering a life threatening illness. Making a mental picture of what one wants is often the first step to attaining it.

Visualization works best when one imagines a specific, favorable experience. The visualization process forces one to identify what he or she wants to achieve. The clearer the goal, the more reachable it often becomes.

As with a guided meditation, in a guided visualization, the guide serves as the facilitator. The guide-facilitator needs to direct the process and enter into the spirit of the visualization.

If you, as a guide, can be with your loved one, use the following guided visualization for ten to fifteen minutes, once or twice a day, for three weeks. Again, the guide and the sufferer should be patient.

Guided Visualization for Recovery

Introductory Instructions. Both you and your beloved should relax your bodies, eliminating all tensions from mind and body, and close your eyes. You, as the guide, should remain active and awake.

Visualize your loved one as the recipient of God's curative powers.

For a physical ailment, visualize a stream of curative powers coming from the Eternal and flowing into your dear one's body, penetrating and saturating the ailing body part, purifying and carrying away the pain and suffering. Visualize your beloved one becoming completely well and in perfect health and well-being.

For a mental illness, visualize your dear one as filled with joy, calmness, and equanimity, as radiant, happy, full of optimism, with his or her mental agony eliminated, the storm in his or her mind cleared away, with tranquility and peace of mind restored.

Concluding Instructions. Invite your beloved to come back to the here and now. Tell him or her: take time to ease yourself back; slowly bring awareness back into your being.

You can also use the following visualization for your beloved outside your presence, once or twice a day, for ten to fifteen minutes, for at least three weeks, if possible. Be patient.

Distant Visualizations for Healing and Recovery

Introductory Instructions. Place yourself in a prayerful state of mind, eliminating extraneous thoughts. Relax your body and mind, and close your eyes.

Visualize your loved one as present, seated opposite in a relaxed position, eyes closed, body at ease. Visualize him or her surrounded by a bright, healing light. Imagine that he or she is healed, restored to wholeness.

If the affliction is physical, visualize the restoration as coming from God in the form of a stream of light, penetrating into the affected part of the body and purifying the body from all pain and suffering.

If the affliction is mental, visualize rays of joy and tranquility radiating from God, saturating your dear one's mind and restoring his or her inner peace and wholeness.

Concluding Instructions. Come back to the here and now. Slowly bring awareness back to your body and mind. Feel yourself back in the room and open your eyes.

On completing this visualization, you may want to recite the *Refaeinu* prayer, set forth earlier in this chapter, indicating the name of your dear one.

Encourage Forgiveness

During the process of dying, as part of the acceptance of death, often individuals need to clean up and heal old, previously unfinished emotional and relationship "baggage." Open up to your loved one, perhaps broaching topics you long wished to discuss. Be particularly sensitive to a dying person's efforts to communicate previously unexpressed feelings and emotions, such as guilt, jealousy, greed, anger, desire, or anxiety, or a need to come to terms with others.

The dying process can be a profound time for forgiveness and possibly reconciliation as well as emotional and spiritual transformation. Encourage your dear one, if he or she is at all receptive, to make up with family members and friends, by addressing failed relationships, old grievances, and hurts inflicted on or by others. This suggestion is not easily made, requiring great delicacy. By being more open-hearted, he or she may be ready to ask for forgiveness from others and to send forgiveness to others as well as to himself or herself. As discussed in Chapter 7, a dying person often realizes the importance of rectifying incomplete relationships so he or she departs earthly life in peace.

Although forgiveness represents an important aspect of Spiritual Judaism, as we all recognize, forgiveness is often quite difficult. Each of us continues to fear being hurt or rejected again. We may be unable to let go of our past perceptions. What has been done to us in the past may approach being unforgivable.

Encouraging an admission of past mistakes and asking for forgiveness is often quite powerful. It opens the possibility for healing old wounds and tapping, from the viewpoint of Spiritual Judaism, the power of love and compassion. By facilitating the reconciliation between estranged children, parents, siblings, and others, the quest for forgiveness often enables a terminally ill person to reach closure with and open unconditionally into love for his or her closest relatives as well as friends.

Acting as a guide, you can use the Guided Forgiveness and Lovingkindness Meditation - Visualization to facilitate the process of forgiveness and possibly reconciliation before your beloved dies, bringing lasting healing to previously troubled relationships. As a guide, you can use this either as a meditation or as a visualization. Take a terminally ill person through this meditation or visualization for ten to fifteen minutes, once or twice daily, if possible. Again, be patient.

Guided Forgiveness and Lovingkindness Meditation - Visualization

Introductory Instructions. As a guide, try to create a warm, welcoming atmosphere, an environment of serenity and spaciousness for the journey within. Lower the lights, if possible. Candles can set a mood that enhances meditation or visualization.

Ask your loved one to: close your eyes, sit quietly, calm and relax your body by sitting, reclining or lying down, breathing in and out normally, feeling where the breath flows into and out of the body. Adjust the breaths so that the in and out breaths are the same length, thereby bringing about both a relaxation of the body and an alertness of the mind. (Obviously, you need to vary these instructions depending on your beloved's physical condition).

Ask your loved one to feel surrounded by warmth and love -- allow any anger to dissolve into the warmth and love. With each breath, breathe in warmth, feel the warmth nourishing you.

Breathe in love and feel the openness that love creates in you. Allow the warmth and love to give rise to forgiveness. The power of forgiveness is so great.

Ask your dear one to contemplate forgiveness -- its meaning and what it might mean to bring forgiveness into one's life.

Then guide the sufferer to visualize another person whom you resent. With a new state of openness, invite that person into your heart. Notice whatever blocks their approach to your heart -- the problem, the hurt, the fear, the anger, or whatever. Enter into and continue a dialogue with that person, until there's nothing more to say. Now, try to let that person through to your heart. Let go of the pride that holds on to resentment. Allow the pain of old hurts to dissolve. In your heart, say: "I forgive you for whatever you did in the past, whether intentionally or unintentionally, through your deeds, words, or thoughts, that caused me pain or hurt." Repeat the words: "I forgive you." Allowing the forgiveness to grow, let go of your resentments and open unconditionally into love and compassion.

Then, repeat this entire sequence for others whom you resent.

Next, visualize someone who resents you -- someone whom you have caused pain. Someone who has put you out of their heart. Within a new state of openness, invite that person into your heart. Notice what blocks their approach to your heart -- your fear, your guilt, or whatever. Try to let that person through to your heart. From the bottom of your heart, ask for their forgiveness. Say: "I ask for your forgiveness for what I did in the past, whether intentionally or unintentionally, through my deeds, words, or thoughts, that caused you pain or hurt." Repeat the words: "Please forgive me." Again, let yourself be touched by the possibility of forgiveness. Ask him or her to let you back into their heart.

Then, repeat this for others whom you may have hurt.

Close each occasion of a forgiveness meditation-visualization with this guidance. Let your heart fill with forgiveness and lovingkindness for yourself. Repeat: May I be happy and at peace. May I be free from anger, pain, fear, guilt, and doubt. May I be filled with love. May I know that I am secure in God's love. I am a good person. The power to give and receive forgiveness is growing in me. God's Light is increasing in me. Wait in silence for some while before the concluding instructions.

Concluding Instructions. Offer these instructions. Now invite your loved one to come back to the here and now. Tell him or her: Take time to ease yourself back. Slowly bring you awareness back into your being. Feel yourself back in the room and open your eyes.

Death Bed Rituals in the Jewish Tradition

In the Jewish tradition, a terminally ill individual may pray, meditate, and visualize. You may offer prayers on his or her behalf as well as use guided meditations and visualizations. Let's consider each of these and their role in facilitating your loved one's tranquility and the transition of his or her soul into the postdeath realms.

The Death Bed Confessional Prayer

No one special form of Jewish deathbed confessional existed in ancient times. The traditional Jewish deathbed confessional (*Viddui*) has been in use for about eight hundred and fifty years since the time of the medieval philosopher Nachmanides, who lived from 1194 to 1270 C.E. Once widely known and used, thc *Viddui* fell into disuse throughout most of the twentieth century. Only now is it being reclaimed; many dying persons seek reconciliation with God.

The Deathbed Confessional Prayer is outwardly directed. Based on a sentence in the Book of Proverbs (28:13), "People who confess and forsake their sins, will obtain mercy from the Eternal," this prayer enables a dying individual to speak directly to and make peace with God. Through the deathbed prayer, a dying individual confesses to the Eternal his or her sins, acknowledges his or her guilt, and expresses feelings of regret for failing to live up to his or her potential or fulfill his or her obligations. In accounting to the Holy One for a life that is about the end, he or she asks for and indicates a willingness to receive God's forgiveness.

The Deathbed Confessional Prayer, which follows, can be read by or to your loved one. If you read it to him or her, say it slowly with warm emphasis and conviction. It is brief and moving. Assure your beloved that many have recited it and survived.

> *Deathbed Confessional (Viddui)*. I acknowledge unto You, O Eternal my God and God of my ancestors, that both my cure and my death are in Your hands. May it be Your Will to send me a perfect healing. Yet if my death be fully determined by You, I will in love accept it at Your hand. May my death be an atonement for all the sins, iniquities and transgressions of which I have been guilty against You. Grant me the abounding happiness that is treasured up for the righteous. Make know to me the path of life. In Your presence is the fulness of joy; at Your right hand bliss for evermore.
>
> You, Who are the protector of the bereaved and the helpless, watch over my loved ones with whose souls, my own is linked. Into Your hand I commit my spirit; redeem it, O Eternal God of truth.[7]

The deathbed confessional serves several purposes. First, it represents an individual's turning from evil. As a petitionary prayer, the confessional asks for something we want. A gravely ill person, striving to "make right" with the Eternal, offers repentance and seeks forgiveness from God.

Second, the deathbed confessional also serves as an affirmative prayer to God: Your will be done, O Eternal.

Third, as we have discussed, your dear one, if possible, should try to settle all major emotional issues and achieve closure before his or her demise. By focusing on significant interpersonal relationships and how he or she feels about each, the recitation of the confessional may trigger one final attempt by a gravely ill person to make amends and achieve a reconciliation with family members and friends.

Fourth, the confessional prayer may also enable a dying individual to explore his or her inner life -- feelings about God and the fate of his or her soul -- as well as the meaning of his or her life. In asking for forgiveness of oneself - perhaps for past actions inconsistent with one's personal values, he or she may also realize the presence of God's unconditional love for all of us.

The Deathbed Confessional (*Viddui*) can be used not only to ask for forgiveness from God but also to seek forgiveness from and of other humans. Listening to a deathbed confession, particularly as an expression of interpersonal forgiveness, takes considerable sensitivity. Remember that your dear one may not want to reveal well-kept secrets, the scars of failed relationships, or hurts inflicted on others, that generate feelings of guilt and emotional distress. Provide a safe space for the expression of the regrets, fears, or sadness resulting from past actions, words, or thoughts.

Use Guided Meditations

Dying individuals often find two meditations, the Deathbed Confessional *(Viddui)* and the Guided Angel Meditation, to be of considerable help. You can assist a gravely ill individual, who is lucid, to use the *Viddui* prayer as a guided meditation to aid in the departure of the soul from his or her physical body and the accompanying transfer of consciousness. According to Jewish sages, the *Viddui* helps clear a path for the soul to exit one's body. The deathbed confessional may also be used as a guided meditation for an unconscious person. Whether as a prayer or a meditation, the confession of sins is said to facilitate the transition of a dying person's soul from the World of the Living to the World of Souls. It helps usher one's soul to the next realm.

Dying individuals receive comfort also from the Guided Angel Meditation. Surrounded by angels, they feel in the arms of safety as their life ebbs. Try to take your dear one through the Guided Angel Meditation often.

Use Guided Visualizations

By altering one's ordinary perspective of reality, a guided visualization helps a dying person travel on an inner journey to the postdeath realms and freely form his or her own internal images of the afterlife. It also assists him or her explore these other realms thereby lessening fears of the unknown.

If requested by your loved one, enter into a dialogue and explore his or her beliefs about the afterlife. Offer your beloved the opportunity, if desired, to become knowledgeable about the Jewish concept of the afterlife. In addition to using the next visualization, a gravely ill person could read (or be read) the portions of Chapter 3 dealing with the World of the Souls not only as a map of the afterlife but also to help send the soul on its journey and find its way in other realms.

The Spiritual Journey Visualization provides visual (nonverbal) spiritual support for a dying person, by enabling him or her to see a place not visible to anyone else, to explore beliefs about the afterlife, to recognize the existence of a transcendent realm, and to surrender to the unknown. A glimpse of the afterlife provides peace and comfort.

Guide a mortally ill individual through this visualization for ten to fifteen minutes, twice daily, if possible. Be patient.

Spiritual Journey Visualization

Introductory Instructions. As a guide, try to create a warm, welcoming atmosphere, an environment of serenity and spaciousness for the journey within. Lower the lights, if possible. Candles can set a mood that enhances the visualization.

Suggest to your dear one: close your eyes, sit quietly, calm and relax your body by sitting, reclining or lying down, breathing in and out normally, feeling where the breath flows into and out of the body. Adjust the breaths so that the in and out breaths are the same length thereby bring about both a relaxation of the body and an alertness of the mind. (Obviously, you need to vary these instructions depending on your loved one's physical condition.)

Ask your loved one to feel from the inside your own death, what you think will happen at the death moment. Specifically, invite the exploration of the transcendent realms. Experience yourself as being a true image of God, full of life, love, and joy. Feel the lightness, the freedom, the release and happiness, the certainty of life forever in the Divine. Experience the transfer of your consciousness and the ongoing journey of your soul.

Especially, feel how God surrounds and immerses you in radiant love and compassion, unconditionally. You are perfectly safe. Stay where you are for as long as you like. Wait in silence before proceeding.

Concluding Instructions. Offer these instructions. Now invite your dear one to come back to the here and now. Take time to ease yourself back. Slowly bring you awareness back into you being. Feel yourself back in the room and open your eyes.

Afterwards, welcome, but do not press, your beloved to verbalize, if possible, this visualization. The Spiritual Journey Visualization and the ensuing verbalization will enable you to better provide support for departure of the dying person's soul as it begins its afterlife journey. Accept and validate what is told to you; ask for more details. However, if the visualization has been successful it may not be easy to verbalize it. Verbalization runs the risk of objectifying and rendering less real, less personal, this important experience.

Dealing with Death Moment Visions

When deceased family members and friends visit a dying person, strive to validate his or her visions and experiences and try to honor his or her inner, subjective realities. Calmly explain that one or more visions are part of the dying process, as discussed in Chapter 4, thereby alleviating deathbed fears and making it easier for the gravely ill individual to die peacefully. He or she is not alone; he or she is getting ready for his or her afterlife journey. Continually respect the wishes and needs of someone who is terminally ill.

Specifically, assist your dear one facing death to deal with: the life review; the encounter with previously departed relatives and friends as well as angels; and the Clear Light. As awareness increases, a transformation occurs -- a dying person generally becomes more comfortable and peaceful.

Hallucinations can sometimes be dealt with by first entering into the scene your beloved is experiencing and then gradually changing it to something normal, pleasant, and real. Be careful not to discredit a death moment vision as a hallucination. The latter is unpleasant for a sufferer; it is puzzling, frustrating, and anxiety-provoking. The former is uplifting, reassuring, enlightening, and joy-provoking.

Facilitating a Life Review

If possible, try to facilitate a life review, as a way of helping a dying individual sort through what has gone before, particularly his or her unresolved life experiences, engage in the emotional and spiritual preparation for death, and clear the path for the hereafter. A life review also helps renew a sense of vitality, provides a clearer sense of a personal philosophy of life, and enables a gravely ill person to share his or her personal history and legacy with family members and close friends. It also assists a sufferer with his or her existential struggles.

Encourage a life review, either in the form of a monologue or a dialogue between you and your dear one, if he or she is at all receptive. As detailed in Chapter 7, a life review helps a dying person find and pull together the threads of identity running through a life, explore who he or she is, directly and honestly, and give the meaning and purpose of his or her existence. It aids your loved one come to terms with his or her life, experience a sense of serenity in having done what he or she could with what he or she was given, and perhaps gives rise to a sense of gratitude for his or her life. By typically focusing on relationships and the small gestures that make us human, it offers the chance to come to terms with one's inevitable frustrations and disappointments. It may help a dying person establish a degree of realistic hope, replacing his or her despair.

A life review may not only contribute to an acceptance of one's imperfections but may also serve as a key to emotional and spiritual growth, including the resolution of past conflicts, the forgiveness of self and others, the possible reconciliation with loved ones, and the atonement for past wrong doing. Facing the inevitability of death may encourage thinking about the past, working it through, leading to a new openness of communication, an illumination of the past with a new found love and forgiveness, resulting in offering an apology or expressing gratitude. However, if there has been a past trauma or abuse, it is probably best not to force such memories.

A comprehensive life review encompasses:

- Happy moments and sad occasions;
- Expressions of gratitude and appreciation of goodness and beauty in life, including the experience of love;
- Accomplishments and virtues, times of growth, and instances of overcoming a limitation or a challenge;
- Regrets, disappointments, grievances, old hurts, unrealized hopes and

dreams, undeveloped talents, tasks not completed, missed opportunities, failed relationships, and hurts inflicted on or by others;

Important people, whether from a positive or a negative standpoint, in one's life;

Final expressions of emotions and feelings as well as previously unrevealed family secrets.

A sense of how God has been present in and guiding life all along, and through all its experiences has brought one to the state in which the next stage of existence can be approached with inner peace and confidence.

Gently, and as sensitively as possibly, ask your loved one open-ended questions, such as: Is there anything you hold against others (or you think they hold against you)? What is stuck in your craw? Can you (and do you want to) bring these matters to a resolution? Although some risk exists that the life review may aggravate a dying individual causing additional and unnecessary suffering, a pattern of worthwhileness and meaningfulness often emerges from these open-ended questions and the accompanying answers. Reflecting back to your dear one his or her words may allow a pattern of meaning to emerge. Think about how the world been a better place because you have been here. A dying person often sees how much he or she accomplished and did for others -- through marriage, raising children, participation in various organizations, a multitude of little things that cheered others. Think how you have helped, supported, affirmed, and encouraged those whose path crossed yours.

You may find the following guided meditation and journaling exercise useful in facilitating a life review. Entering into the spirit of the meditation, guide a dying individual through this meditation for ten to fifteen minutes, once or twice daily, if possible. Be patient.

Guided Life Review Meditation

Introductory Instructions. As a guide, try to create a warm, welcoming atmosphere, an environment of serenity and spaciousness for the journey within. Lower the lights if possible. Candles can set a mood that enhances meditation.

Ask your loved one to close your eyes, sit quietly, calm and relax your body by sitting, reclining or lying down, breathing in and out normally feeling where the breath flows into and out of the body. Adjust the breaths so that the in and out breaths are the same length thereby bring about both a relaxation of the body and an alertness of the mind. (Obviously, you need to vary these instructions depending your beloved's physical condition).

Invite the contemplation of what you are grateful for, including, happy times, good friends, special moments, love, compassion, and forgiveness.

Give thanks to deceased family members and friends, mentors and teachers, asking them to help you cross over.

Then, invite each special living person separately to enter into your open heartedness and engage in a dialogue with you. Invite the saying of separate good-byes and thanks to each special person.

Next, invite the contemplation of moments and memories associated with frustration, anger, guilt, remorse, or anxiety. These form the unfinished relational business needing closure.

Concluding Instructions. Offer these instruction. Now invite your beloved to come back to the here and now. Tell him or her to take time to ease yourself back. Slowly bring your awareness back into your being. Feel yourself back in the room and open your eyes.

A dying individual may find it helpful to make notes on their earthly journey, distinct memories and the accompanying states of mind, whether in a journal, on separate pieces of paper, in some sort of visual form, or on an audio or videotape. This can be a particularly liberating exercise. In whatever permanent mode, a life history as a record -- the transmission of knowledge and wisdom -- can be passed down to the next generation; young children or grandchildren can read it when they are older as a treasured heirloom. Leaving a written message or some type of tape expressing love and encouragement often helps survivors surmount their grief.

Journaling Exercise

Acting as guide, ask your loved one to record on paper, in prose, poetry, or letters (or notes) to family or friends, visually in the form of drawings, or on an audio or videotape, memories as well as past and present states of mind, emotions, and feelings. Ask for the noting of regrets, persons harmed, suffering created, unfulfilled hopes and dreams, and unkept promises. Also ask for accomplishments, happy times, and high moments.

If your beloved wishes assistance, let him or her verbalize the life review and you write it down. The life review can also take the form of an audio or videotape.

As gently as possible, suggest that your dear one make amends to the appropriate people, either personally, face-to-face, over the telephone, or in writing, as best as he or she can. A message of love and hope can be written or dictated.

If desired, save the journal, the pieces of paper, or the audio or videotape as a family history memorializing recollections and closely guarded family secrets. Or, you may destroy the journal or the scraps of paper by tearing or burning. Likewise, the audio or videotape may be destroyed.

In connection with the life review, you may want to guide the soon-to-depart through the Guided Forgiveness and Lovingkindness Meditation-Visualization, set out earlier in this chapter, as a technique to ask for and extend forgiveness. Working out troubled family relationships helps a dying person achieve not only a measure of inner peace but also offers the possibility of reconciliation with others.

Do not pressure someone who is gravely ill to engage in an oral or written life review. Don't push, but don't wait until the last few days. Listen unconditionally and in a nonjudgmental manner. Ask questions. You can only provide a safe space, which may be difficult in a busy and often intrusive hospital environment, in which a terminally ill individual can discuss, orally, in writing, or on audio or videotape, the events and relationships of a lifetime, one-by-one, express what is in his or her heart and ask for forgiveness for past hurts and harms to and from others. Let the one who is dying control the dialogue.

Your dear one may be unable to capture these experiences in words. If so, suggest that he or she use, if physically or mentally able, the Life Roadmap Exercise contained in Chapter 7.

The earthly life review will not only assist a dying person to question and broadly reflect on the meaning not only of his or her life overall but also will help achieve perspective on his or her present pain and suffering. This technique may hopefully help one achieve an inner peace of mind with all that has been lived through during a lifetime.

Also, ask your loved one to create an ethical will by writing a letter (or talking into a tape or video recorder) and describing his or her personal history, values, beliefs, hopes, and fears. There is no special format; let it come from the heart. Preparing an ethical will offers significant opportunities for self-affirmation and closure. It provides a means to express what is most important and "bequeath" these values to survivors. An ethical will gives your dying beloved something to do each day, as well as providing a spiritual legacy for his or her descendants in a format that will be treasured long after death. It gives others a vivid sense of the meaningfulness of one's life, glowing evidence of the wonder of God's manifestation in a human being.

Visualizing Deceased Family Members, Friends, and Angels

Visualizing contact, now and in the future, with deceased family members and friends as well as angels open new vistas for exploring the meaning of eternal life and the soul's postmortem journey. Those who are gravely ill typically interact with invisible, significant others in their lives who are already deceased.

The dying process and the moment of death are not lonely. We have companions and guides as we embark on our afterlife journey from this world to the next.

If a gravely ill person is receptive, guide him or her through the following visualization, for ten or fifteen minutes, daily. Be patient.

Guided Visualization of Deceased Family Members and Friends

Introductory Instructions. As a guide, try to create a warm, welcoming atmosphere, an environment of serenity and spaciousness for the journey within. Lower the lights, if possible. Candles can set a mood that enhances meditation.

Ask the dying individual to close your eyes, sit quietly, calm and relax your body by sitting, reclining or lying down, breathing in and out normally, feeling where the breath flows into and out of the body. Adjust the breaths so that the in and out breaths are the same length thereby bring about both a relaxation of the body and an alertness of the mind. (Obviously, you need to vary these instructions depending on your beloved's physical condition).

Ask your loved one to imagine your guardian angel or another angel, perhaps one of the four angels from the Guided Angel Meditation, earlier in this chapter.

Inviting communication with the guardian angel (or another angel), ask: When did the angel come into your life? What is it doing for you now? And what will it do for you in the future?

Focusing on complete relaxation, invite the guardian angel (or other angel) to describe various stages of the soul's afterlife journey, the death moment and the immediate postdeath transition, particularly deceased family members and friends who will serve as guides in the postmortem realms.

Concluding Instructions. Offer these instructions. Now invite your dear one to come back to the here and now. Tell him or her to take time to ease yourself back. Slowly bring you awareness back into your being. Feel yourself back in the room and open your eyes.

Surrendering To and Entering the Clear Light

Gently urge the dying person to surrender and enter the intense Clear Light, invisible to everyone else, appearing just before or at the death moment or immediately thereafter. Following the example of the Baal Shem Tov, set forth in Chapter 4, encourage your loved one to let go of earthly attachments and desires and slowly and consciously exit the earthly realms. Facilitate the process of dying when death is imminent as characterized by the gradual shutting down of various life functions.

Obviously, the timing of this exercise represents a difficult judgment call, as a terminally ill person may still have weeks or days left prior to his or her demise. However, a glimpse of the Clear Light seems to bring peace and comfort to many who are dying.

Disidentifying with the Body

In addition to encouraging a life review, the visualization of previously deceased relatives and friends as well as angels, and the surrender to and the entering into the Clear Light, facilitate a dying person's disidentification with his or her physical body and attachments to the earthly plane. By striving to break the linkage with his or her body, one ceases to identify with the material dimension of his or her being as well as the earthly realm and begins to focus awareness on his or her timeless, immortal soul and its postdeath journey in the World of the Souls. Recognizing that our earthly body is not all of what we are as humans, and indeed not the essence of who we are as persons, the reduced attachment to the physical, materialistic aspects of life assists the soul to leave the body and opens each of us to the next state of our being.

You may want to offer or help a sufferer with the following prayer:[8]

Letting Go Prayer

Dear God,
As my earthly
time nears an end,
Let me learn to let go
of all my bonds with this world,
of my attraction to physical
indulgences and material objects,
of my envy of others,
of my regrets of all
that might have been.

The following guided meditation (or visualization) helps encourage the process of letting go by setting in motion the process of inner liberation and facilitating identification with the spiritual dimensions of one's inner life. Remember: letting go takes time. Each of us needs time to overcome our attachments to the material world, to our physical body, our thoughts, our emotions, and to the roles that have defined us.

Guide your beloved through this meditation (or visualization) for ten to fifteen minutes once or twice daily, if possible. This is the exercise to practice for months before dying. If it is not practiced well beforehand, it is far more difficult to do near the time of death.

Guided Bodily Disidentification Meditation (or Visualization)

Introductory Instructions. As a guide, try to create a warm, welcoming atmosphere, an environment of serenity and spaciousness for the journey within. Lower the lights, if possible. Candles can set the mood that enhances meditation or visualization.

Ask your loved one to close your eyes, sit quietly, calm and relax your body by sitting, reclining or lying down, breathing in and out normally, feeling where the breath flows into and out of the body. Adjust the breaths so that the in and out breaths are the same length thereby bring about both a relaxation of the body and an alertness of the mind. (Obviously, you need to vary these instructions depending on your dear one's physical condition).

Invite the feeling of your body. Feel the weight of your head. Feel the weight of your arms and hands. Feel the weight of your torso. Feel the weight of your legs and your feet. Feel the pull of gravity on your body.

Open your heart to subtler and lighter sensations; experience your immortal soul.

With each in breath, see how it is received by the soul. The soul uses the breath to sustain the physical body. But the soul does not need the breath to sustain it.

Then imagine that each breath is your last breath. The connection between your soul and your body is severed.

Let your last breath go, forever.

Let go gently and die. Let go of your attachments, your desires, your fears, your thoughts. Let yourself die and go gently into the Clear Light. See the Clear Light all around you.

Be your soul floating free from your body. You may want to look down and see the body you have left.

With an open heart, let go of your identification with your body and all things that hold you back. Let your soul float free. Let your body die. Let your soul be free from this earthly incarnation.

Forget the body and realize yourself glowing with holiness and happiness in the Clear Light. Wait in silence for some while.

Concluding Instructions. Offer these instructions. Now invite your loved one to come back to the here and now. Tell him or her: Take time to ease yourself back. Slowly bring your awareness back into your being. Feel yourself back in the room and open your eyes.

The life review, the visualization of deceased relatives and friends as well as angels, the disidentification with the physical body and the entering into the Clear Light, help dissolve a dying person's fear of death, provided he or she is receptive. They open the possibility of and prepare the way for a more tranquil withdrawal from earthly life and entry into the new phase of existence, the World of Souls.

Some Questions If You Are Asked By a Loved One Who Wants to Accelerate the Transition of Life

A sufferer may ask you about accelerating the transition of life, by his or her own hand, or securing the assistance of a physician or someone else, perhaps you. Before you say or do anything, ask yourself:

1. Have you provided whatever emotional and spiritual support as well as practical help you can offer so that you are certain nothing more can be done? Obtain all possible information about your loved one's physical condition, including his or her diagnosis, treatment options, prognosis, and alternative techniques to alleviate pain and suffering. Accompany your beloved on his or her next medical appointment. You may want to speak privately with his or her physician. Ask the patient to give the physician permission.

2. What is the sufferer's emotional state? Does your loved one suffer from depression creating a tunnel vision in which he or she sees only bleak alternatives? Talk to others, including the patient's physicians, and

obtain their opinions. You may need to recommend or demand that your dear one seek counseling and take antidepressant medication. Or, you may feel that spiritual issues should not be covered over with chemically induced euphoria.

3. Have you helped your loved one achieve a true healing -- a wholeness of body-mind-spirit?

4. Have you manipulated or coerced your beloved in anyway?

A request for an accelerated death often triggers a challenge to your values and beliefs. Consider the following:[9]

1. Are you uncomfortable with your loved one's impending death? Are you in denial, angry, fearful, guilty, nervous, sad, or depressed?

2. What are your beliefs about the sanctity of biological life?

3. Does each of us have the right to decide matters of life-and-death for ourself, to end his or her biological life, or request help in making his or her transition? If so, under what conditions?

4. How do you view suicide or aid-in-dying? Wrong under all conditions? Why? Or, sound? If so, under what circumstances?

5. Do you feel it is right for you to help end another's life on his or her request? If so, under what conditions?

6. Do you believe in the immortal soul, the afterlife, and/or reincarnation? What do you believe about the impact of suicide or aid-in-dying on the soul and the afterlife?

7. What are your reasons for saying to a loved one go ahead or agreeing to assist in his or her demise: love and compassion; unwillingness to see further needless pain and suffering; physical exhaustion as a caregiver; feelings of helplessness; an inability to do more; or what else? Or, out of guilt, are you insisting that a loved one, perhaps a parent, spend his or her last days in an intensive care unit at a cost of tens and tens of thousands of dollars? Are you afraid that if you agree to facilitate the transition, others will say you did it to save the money?

8. Do you feel comfortable in helping your dear one die? Do you view the request as an honor, or as a burden? Do you look at it favorably or negatively? Do you think your assistance will bring you future regrets, or will you view it positively, as an act of love and compassion?

9. Why is your beloved consulting you? Were other, closer family members or friends previously consulted? What aspects of the situation did they consider that you may be overlooking? Is there someone else more appropriate to help in the process? What about his or her own

physician? Are you afraid that if you agree, you risk criminal prosecution?

10. What are your loved one's motives for wanting to end his or her life? Whose idea is it? Is there any possibility of emotional or economic coercion by you or others? Is there a desire to relieve you or others of a financial or an emotional burden?

11. Analyze the financial implications. Do you or others stand to gain financially, in any way, through an early death? Conversely, will a prolonged dying process create any type of financial hardship for you, your loved one, or others?

12. Have you (and other family members and friends) had the opportunity to achieve emotional and spiritual closure with your beloved? Do any emotional loose ends or unresolved interpersonal issues still exist?

13. Consider others' needs and interests. For example, if you have siblings and a parent asks you alone for advice, your input goes beyond your relationship with your parent. Let the feelings of your siblings enter into the decision-making equation. Give your siblings ample warning, so they can resolve any of their own unfinished emotional business and achieve closure with a parent who has asked for your help. What if a parent asked you because you alone could be trusted to do what the parent wants?

14. What would be expected of you with respect to aid-in-dying? What does assistance with another's death consist of? How involved do you want to be? Will you be there only to offer emotional support, or will you be more involved, possibly to administer the pills, to put a bag over the patient's head for purposes of asphyxiation, or to give a lethal injection? If so, what is your fallback strategy if the method selected is unsuccessful? Have you considered other techniques? If so, what do they require of you? Are you emotionally prepared for what may occur? Do you even know what sorts of things may happen?

15. Have you openly shared your concerns with your dear one? Do you accept his or her decision and regard as appropriate the reasons, the timing, and the method?

16. Is your loved one's end of life decision enduring? Is it explicit and persistent? Has it been fully discussed with you on several occasions? Has it been written down in the patient's hand and dated?

To help a beloved in making an end of life decision, keep open your lines of communication with him or her. Engage in an honest dialogue.

Be There at the End

The Jewish tradition teaches that each of us should die in dignity, surrounded by his or her loved ones. A dying person should not, if at all possible, make the passage out of this earthly life unaided, however his or her physical end occurs.

Do not abandon your dear one. Do not leave a dying person, whether in a hospital, a nursing home, an inpatient hospice, or at home, alone and scared. A gravely ill individual needs to be surrounded by family and friends so that he or she does not feel abandoned or isolated. Rather, provide the bright sun of loving attention. Do not underestimate the importance of human warmth for these near death. Being with someone when he or she is dying represents an act of lovingkindness, so important from the perspective of Spiritual Judaism. Through your words, deeds, and thoughts, express that you will continue to be with him or her. Even if you do not have a chance to say all the things to each other you might have hoped, try to walk the last mile together, thereby bringing about closure and a lasting healing to your relationship. Surround your soon-to-depart beloved with tranquility and help usher his or her soul to the next dimension.

Opening your heart and offering your full support, strive to send your unconditional love, compassion, and acceptance. Often sitting quietly and holding a hand (or stroking the face) is sufficient. Touching conveys an important message, "I'm with you." Make your dear one feel loved, accepted, and understood. Offer your heartfelt support and reassurance. Say "It's OK. You can let go. I'll be all right."

Following the model of the Baal Shem Tov's departure from earthly life, as discussed in Chapter 4, transmit a sense of equanimity and a peaceful acceptance of death. Try to communicate an awareness that, according to the Jewish tradition, death, particularly the moment of death, will be, for most of us, a peaceful, painless experience.

Do not send "negative" thoughts or feelings, such as fear, sadness, or attachment. Through your attitude and verbalizations as well as your accompanying actions and emotional expressions, strive to convey your open-hearted love and confidence.

Even if your beloved is in a coma or a vegetative state, try to communicate with him or her through various means, including touch, eye contact, music, or loving and compassionate thoughts. It is still not too late for you to use your mind and heart in positive ways. Express your regrets, saying, "I'm sorry." Tell a parent or sibling, "I love you." Express love and compassion through your heart.

Give your dear one permission to die, thus providing great relief. Reassure him or her that the survivors will be all right. He or she need not worry about you or others. If there is someone in the family who needs care, or someone for whom the dying had a responsibility, assure the patient that that person (or animal) will be well look after. Do not neglect pet relationships, often very important to both parties. Remember that the animal will grieve, perhaps seriously. The pet needs to know that its beloved had died, not abandoned it. The dying person may want the pet to be with him or her.

Offer a dying person -- most know they're dying -- the calm certainty of knowing that, according to Jewish tradition, he or she is, and will continue to be, safely held in the Eternal's loving arms. In time, his or her soul will experience healing, rebirth, and ultimately be united with God. Soft music and calm voices help a sufferer relax.

Say your tearful, last "good-byes," until there's nothing left unsaid or undone. Everyone present experiences great grief at the impending physical separation. Tears flow freely with remembrance and memories.

If, while capable of medical care decision-making, a loved one avoids discussing his or her preferences regarding emergency medical care or the use of life sustaining technology, try to open a discussion by asking, "Do you fear death or the process of dying?" This question generally lets individuals express their fears and concerns. Explain that signing a written advance care directive, including a healthcare proxy, which we turn to in the next chapter, makes it easier for a sufferer's loved ones and helps avoid unnecessary, "last ditch" measures.

Notes

1. David M. Luterman, *In the Shadows: Living and Coping with a Loved One's Chronic Illness* (Bedford, Mass.: Jade Press 1995), 1-20.

2. Ken Dychtwald, *Age Power: How the 21st Century Will Be Ruled by the New Old* (New York: Tarcher/Putnam, 1999), 144.

3. Wendy Lustbader and Nancy R. Hooyman, *Taking Care of Aging Family Members: A Practical Guide* (New York: The Free Press, 1994), 19-41.

4. Adapted from Lewis D. Solomon, *The Jewish Book of Living and Dying* (Northvale, NJ: Jason Aronson, 1999), 66-75, 81-91, 110-119.

5. Adapted from Dr. Joseph H. Hertz, *The Authorised Daily Prayer Book*, rev. ed. (New York: Bloch, 1985), 141.

6. In *Ascending Jacob's Ladder: Jewish Views of Angels, Demons, and Evil Spirits* (Northvale, NJ: Jason Aronson, 1998) Ronald H. Isaacs offers an overview of the Jewish world of angels.

7. Hertz, *Authorised Daily Prayer Book*, 1065. Essays and other prayers for the death moment are collected in *Jewish Insights on Death and Mourning*, ed. Jack Riemer (New York: Schocken, 1995), 48-80.

8. *The Gentle Weapon: Prayers for Everyday and Not-So-Everyday Moments: Timeless Wisdom from the Teachings of the Hasidic Master Rebbe Nachman of Breslov*, adapted by Moshe Mykoff and S.C. Mizrahi with the Breslov Research Institute (Woodstock, VT: Jewish Lights Publishing, 1999), 108.

9. I have drawn on Stephen Jamison, *Final Acts of Love: Families, Friends, and Assisted Dying* (New York: G.P. Putnam's Sons, 1995), 190-222.

Chapter 10

Planning Ahead: Advance Care Directives and Organ Donations

I am a strong advocate of thinking and making decisions about end of life care while you are relatively healthy, before death is imminent, not when terminal illness forces admission to a hospital. Considering your options, talking them out, and planning ahead provides a source of reassurance and peace of mind by reducing your anxiety, and helps you better prepare for your demise. In addition to fostering autonomy by encouraging more thoughtful choices, giving you more control over how you live even if you are very ill and letting you avoid what you regard as an undignified, lingering dying process, advance planning may enable you to live more comfortably at the end of your days. It enables you to let your loved ones know what you want and what is important to you, thereby sparing them the burden of selecting alternatives without this knowledge. Do not force your loved ones (or a judge, if there is a dispute between or among your family members) to guess at your wishes and make difficult, often wrenching, medical care decisions for you.

If you are unable to express your wishes, tough choices often must be made. What kind of medical care do you want (or not want)? More specifically, what procedures or treatments do you want (or not want) if your physicians say you are terminally ill or your condition is hopeless? Do you want every possible intervention tried even if none is likely to work? Whom you want to make important healthcare decisions for you if you are unconscious or otherwise lack medical decision-making capacity?

After providing a brief overview of the American legal background, this chapter presents the views of the Jewish tradition on advance care directives. My analysis includes a discussion of both a healthcare proxy letting you designate a substitute medical care decision-maker and a living will enabling you to state what medical procedures or treatments you do and do not want under certain conditions. Practical planning suggestions are also provided. We will also discuss organ donations.

Most of us find it difficult to think about the end of our life and the process of dying. We do not want to confront our own mortality. We do not want to face the prospect of serious future illness or the loss of our decision-making capacity. We do not like to make decisions ahead of time about these matters or even contemplate them. Young, vigorous, healthy individuals believe they have plenty of time to ponder what they want done in the event of a medical catastrophe. To jar you out of your complacency, let's see what happens if you do not plan ahead. Reading about what Nancy Cruzan's family went through may impress on you the importance of executing a written advance care directive.

Disaster Strikes and Horror Results From Failing to Plan Ahead

Nancy Cruzan lost control of her car on a country road, when she was 25. She was thrown about thirty-five feet from her overturned auto, landing face down in a water-filled ditch. Her heart stopped. When help arrived, her brain had been without oxygen for several minutes. At least twelve to fourteen and possibly twenty minutes later, paramedics were able to restart her heart, but they could not undo the damage to her brain. As a result, she was in a persistent vegetative state. Her eyes opened and wandered, but could not focus. Her brain stem kept her body breathing without a respirator. Lacking a swallowing reflex, she was given food and water by a feeding tube surgically placed in her stomach. Gradually over the next eight years, her body became rigid; her hands and fingers curled up. She alternated between incontinence and the opposite.

After several years of hoping for and expecting Nancy's demise, her parents went to court to remove the feeding tube. The Missouri Supreme Court refused. Because Nancy was incompetent to refuse life sustaining treatment and reasoning that the state has a strong interest in preserving life, the court would give permission to withdraw the life sustaining treatment only if "clear and convincing" evidence existed that this was what Nancy would have wanted. No such evidence was presented to the court.

Nancy's parents appealed to the United States Supreme Court, asserting that their daughter had a constitutional right to be allowed to die. In 1990, the Court held that each state could provide its own standards as to when a patient is not competent to express his or her own wishes.[1] A state, like Missouri, if it wishes, could refuse to allow a medical intervention to be removed unless "clear and convincing evidence" exist that the patient would have wanted life sustaining treatment to be withdrawn. When the evidence of a patient's desires is unclear or unconvincing, a state may assert, according to the High Court, its interest in the protection and preservation of human life by requiring the continuation of artificial hydration and nutrition.

Ultimately, the tragic situation had a merciful ending. Shortly after the United States Supreme Court reached its decision, Nancy's friends recalled that she had told them things indicating that she wished to die, if she were in such a situation. The State of Missouri did not oppose her parents' renewed application to terminate artificial feeding and hydration. At a subsequent state court hearing, the judge concluded that "clear and convincing" evidence existed of Nancy's desire not to have her life sustained in this situation and allowed the feeding tube to be withdrawn. Nancy died twelve days after the tube was removed; however, her body had existed in a persistent vegetative state for more than eight years.

The moral of this tale: express your wishes about your end of life care now, before a cognitive impairment occurs. Document your wishes in writing.

American Legal Background: Advance Care Directives

State legislation regarding healthcare decision-making has sought to encourage the statement of preferences regarding the withholding or withdrawal of treatment if one becomes terminally ill or lacks decision-making capacity. Motivated by the *Quinlan* case, in 1976 California became the first state to legalize an advance care directive, a signed, written document, in which individuals could indicate how they want to be treated if they become ill and are unable to express their own wishes.

Spurred on by the *Cruzan* decision, the United States Congress enacted the Patient Self-Determination Act of 1990.[2] All healthcare facilities, including hospitals, nursing homes, and inpatient hospices, receiving federal government funding must now give patients written information regarding their right to make medical decisions, including the execution of an advance care directive. Specifically, these facilities must: inform each patient at the time of admission about their state's advance directive legislation; ask whether a patient has completed a directive; and document in patients' records whether or not each patient has executed a directive. In addition to maintaining written policies and procedures to implement patients' rights to accept or refuse life sustaining treatments and execute directives, these facilities must provide patients with written information regarding their policies and procedures as well as the right of admittees to accept or refuse medical interventions. It is an institutional responsibility, rather than one imposed on individual physicians practicing at that facility.

Today, every state has its own advance care directive legislation; however, large discrepancies exist from one state to another. Although every jurisdiction has legalized some form of directive, a crazy quilt of state statutes and judicial interpretations exists. Although a brief overview follows, you must consult your own attorney.

There are two basic types of advance care directives: first, a healthcare proxy (or medical power of attorney) and second, a living will. A healthcare proxy, authorized by statute in every jurisdiction in the United States (except Alaska), enables you to give another person the legal power to make medical care decisions for you when you no longer can. You must figure out, ahead of time, who will be your voice -- a family member, a close friend, a rabbi or an attorney -- to make treatment decisions if you are no longer able to decide for yourself, even if you are not terminally ill. You must also choose a deputy, a second person, who will serve if the first is unable.

A few state statutes limit the ability of surrogates to refuse certain types of life sustaining treatments. These restrictive statutes expressly prohibit the withholding or withdrawal of life prolonging interventions under certain conditions. Some twenty other states, although expressly or implicitly permitting the withholding or withdrawal of life sustaining procedures, prohibit surrogates from authorizing the withholding or withdrawal of artificial food and water under certain conditions.

In addition to executing a signed, written document, a healthcare proxy, make certain that your surrogates, who will make medical care decisions on your behalf, understand your treatment choices and your values. Later in this chapter, we will see how you can inform your designees regarding these matters.

Even if you have not executed a valid healthcare proxy, you may have some protection, because some thirty-five states have enacted family succession laws[3] empowering family members, in a designated order of succession, to make decisions regarding specific treatments for patients with certain medical conditions. Some statutes either require a lack decision-making capacity (or communication skills) or a terminal illness; others require both. Some statutes apply in quite narrow circumstances, for example, to decisions regarding cardiopulmonary resuscitation; or they may apply only to those who are hospitalized or who reside in skilled nursing centers or intermediate care facilities. A patient's spouse usually heads the list of family members empowered to make decisions, followed by adult offspring, parents, and adult siblings. Obviously, if you think you might not agree with your next of kin's decisions or believe that he or she is not suited to the task, then make sure of your protection by executing a healthcare proxy, recognized by statute in forty-nine states.

The other legal instrument you should prepare is a living will. It gives your written instructions for medical treatments if you are terminally ill or unable to express your wishes because you are in an irreversible coma, a persistent vegetative state, or otherwise unable to communicate your wishes. This type of document lets you specify what kinds of medical interventions you do want and those you do not want.

All jurisdictions in the United States, except Massachusetts and New York, have some type of living will legislation. These statutes are not uniform. Almost all provide a pre-approved model, a very generally worded form, rather poorly guiding protected decisions; only a few do not provide such a model.

Typically, the statutes provide that a living will takes effect only if a patient is terminally ill, or in an irreversible coma or a persistent vegetative state. The definition of terminally ill varies widely, ranging from "imminent" death to death within a specified number of months. Weeks or months may pass before a doctor will declare a prognosis "terminal." The requirement of an imminent death is problematic, for an individual, if vegetative or in a coma, can live for an indeterminate period of time with medical treatment. A coma often is not labeled irreversible until every available intervention has been exhausted. Physician certification is usually required with respect to your inability to make your own medical care decisions.

Some state laws restrict the right to refuse medical treatments, particularly artificial nutrition and hydration. These usually require that a living will must specifically refuse artificial nutrition and hydration or that your proxy document specifically empower your healthcare agent to refuse tube feeding; otherwise it must always be provided.

Remember that your state's living will statute does not provide the exclusive means of exercising your rights. For example, some may want to refuse treatments even if they are not terminally ill or in a persistent vegetative state, for instance, if they suffer from severe Alzheimer's disease. The legislation generally acknowledges that different versions of advance care directives, other than a pre-approved form, enable patients to exercise their rights to refuse various specific types of interventions. Thus, your directive can be more detailed and extensive than the model form your state provides that nevertheless can serve as a useful starting point for preparing your document.

A carefully drawn directive not conforming to your state's statute (or a statutory form) is legally valid. Why? State courts must recognize nonconforming directives based on judge-made (common) law supporting the twin rights of informed consent and refusal of treatment and after the *Cruzan* decision, a right under the United States Constitution, namely, a liberty interest in freedom from bodily intrusion. Jurisdictions may, however, establish their own standards to test the validity of nonconforming directives. Only a few states embrace the "clear and convincing" standard. Courts in the others use the more permissive substituted judgment or best interests standard. Most state courts permissively view directives as taking many forms and containing many different choices.[4]

State law determines the execution procedures and witness requirements which vary widely. Advance care directives must be written, signed, and generally witnessed. States typically require a person executing a directive to be at least 18 years old and of sound mind. Some states require the document to be notarized.

If you move to another state, make certain your new jurisdiction recognizes your existing directive as binding. State laws vary. Some states recognize a validly executed directive in another state. Others do not. You must make a new one.

Many statutes offer a single statutory form combining both a proxy directive and instructive directions. The proxy directive provides a decision-maker, who can make decisions when needed, someone who can see the situation and discuss it with your physician. The instructive directions inform and guide the surrogate.

Despite the legal recognition of some type of advance care directive in all states, a widespread reluctance to use it still exists. Only about 20-25% of adult Americans have executed some type of directive.[5] However, a much higher proportion of terminally-ill patients, between 40 and 50%, have advance care directives.

Take advantage of modern statutes validating advance care directives. Contemplating this type of document provides the basis for an exploratory conversation, a dialogue, between you, your loved ones, and your physician, about a future time when end of life decision-making will be critical. Implement your instructions, desires, values, and preferences in a signed and witnessed written instrument. Remember: you may revoke your directive at any time, even if at revocation your medical decision-making capabilities are diminished, provided you still are competent.

American Legal Background: Postmortem Organ Donations

Organ transplantation has saved the lives of thousands of critically ill people. Because of the number of illnesses and diseases that currently cannot be adequately treated by any procedure other than organ transplantation, the demand for transplantable organs remains high. As each day passes, the medical known-how improves and the quantity and variety of transplanted human organs increase. However, the number of organs available for donation lags behind both medical advances and the demand. Due to the shortage of willing donors, thousands of American adults and children die each year.

All states have adopted some form of Uniform Anatomical Gift Act,[6] in some instances with a degree of variation, enabling a person, at least eighteen years old, to make a postmortem anatomical gift of his or her body, in whole or part. To donate organs on your death, you must sign a written document, which some jurisdictions require to be witnessed, containing broad language authorizing the use of organ, tissues, and body parts for transplantation as well as for therapy, medical research or education. (An alternative procedure exists if you are unable to sign the document). Most states have established a means for licensed drivers to signify their wish to become organ donors on their demise. Organ donor registration cards typically appear on the reverse side of a driver's license. All hospitals must inquire whether a patient is an organ donor and place a copy of the documentation in one's medical records.

Family members may also make a postmortem gift of a departed's organs, unless a previously indicated refusal exists. Most states have enacted one of two types of laws designed to bring home to families the need and opportunity for donation. Under a required request statute, hospital administrators (or their designees) must make an explicit request to family members when a patient has died (or is near death) to donate all or part of a deceased body unless consent has been explicitly refused. A routine inquiry statute requires a hospital to advise a patient's family that they have the opportunity to make a gift of organs and allows them a choice between opting for or refusing a donation. A small number of states allow a healthcare proxy to make organ donations following one's demise.

The Jewish Tradition and Living Wills

The Conservative Movement and Reform authorities agree that Jewish law permits living wills and encourage their use. Although two leading Orthodox organizations, The Rabbinical Council of America (an organization for ordained Orthodox rabbis) and Agudath Israel of America (an organization for Orthodox Jews) have developed their own living will forms and recommend their limited use, traditionalists continue to oppose the execution of a refusal of treatment type of living will.

Drawing on a theme previously developed in Chapter 6, Rabbi J. David Bleich writes that humans do not have the right to decide issues regarding the quality of life. He argues that God provides medical innovations for patients' benefit.[7] Medical procedures and treatments are designed to save human lives. A physician must utilize all available means to prolong lives. Only experimental or hazardous treatments are not mandatory because they may shorten one's existence. According to Bleich, under no circumstances may a physician listen to a patient's request to withhold or withdraw treatment, even if he or she pleads for death. Thus, under Jewish law, a sufferer cannot previously state a wish to refuse or stop medical interventions, unless, as discussed in Chapter 5, one has become a *goses*. Accordingly, Bleich recommends against the execution of a living will providing for the refusal of medical interventions, one asking physicians to refrain from acting by withholding or withdrawing procedures or treatments. He would, however, approve of a directive requesting physicians to do everything medically possible.

Like Bleich, fellow traditionalist and medical doctor, Fred Rosner, although taking a somewhat more moderate stance, advises against the execution of a refusal type of living will because one does not have a "right to die." According to Jewish law, Rosner reasons, a patient may not choose when or how to die. Consonant with the sanctity of biological life principle, he notes that life-and-death decisions are within God's domain and out of human hands. Only the Eternal gives and takes biological life.

Rosner also points out that significant problems often arise with respect to advance care directives. Patients may change their minds while the document is in effect, yet fail to revoke it. Individuals are often misled into thinking that having a living will provides a dignified, painless, natural death. Rosner notes that the execution of this type of document does not guarantee a "good death." A refusal type of living will also may preclude from taking advantage of innovative procedures along with advanced pain therapy. In sum, Rosner pointedly writes, "The living will only protects refusal of treatment but does not guarantee a peaceful easy death."[8]

Rosner asserts, however, that Jewish law does not require the prolonging of suffering. Thus, a patient may, in certain circumstances, refuse medical treatment. Seemingly, this opens the way for the execution of a living will dealing with the withholding or withdrawal of interventions, at least under limited conditions. However, Rosner concludes, "From the moral viewpoint, the living will denies the preciousness and infinite value of human life. Here is where the 'slippery slope' begins."[9]

Although approving the use of living wills, a difference of opinion exists between Conservative Rabbis Elliot N. Dorff and Avram Israel Reisner with respect to authorizing the withholding or withdrawing of certain medical interventions. Rabbi Dorff writes that living wills are "acceptable halakhically in those areas where we determine that a person may choose among forms of therapy,"[10] as discussed in Chapter 5. In support of his conclusion, Dorff relies on Rabbi Seymour Siegel, who nearly a quarter of a century ago stated, "What the Living Will makes possible is the giving of the privilege to the patient himself to stop those things 'that delay the soul's leaving the body.'"[11] Thus, when death is imminent and medical procedures cannot provide a cure, Dorff concludes, it is best to follow a patient's expressed wish to discontinue treatment and allow him or her to die naturally.

Rabbi Reisner also encourages the use of living wills, reasoning that they allow individuals to assert their autonomy and affirm life, yet recognize death in its time.[12] During the process of writing a living will, one must weigh one's end of life choices and make personal healthcare decisions. For Reisner, it is halakhically important that an individual make these decisions based on the belief about what God has in store for him or her. One chooses or rejects various medical procedures with the knowledge of ultimately facing God's judgment. No one else can really stand in the shoes of one who makes such a decision.

According to Dorff, as discussed in Chapter 5, one may accept or refuse treatments, including artificial nutrition and hydration, medication, and technological devices, when suffering from a terminal illness. At this point, continued medical interventions become hindrances to dying. A patient may thus forego procedures or treatments merely extending life without hope for cure. It is best, Dorff concludes, to follow a sufferer's express wish to withhold or discontinue interventions and allow the patient to die naturally.

In contrast to Dorff, Reisner does not believe that Jewish law provides as great a latitude to the wishes of someone who is terminally ill. As noted in Chapter 5, according to Reisner, one may not refuse medication or artificial nutrition and hydration, particularly through IV tubes, when they serve as effective measures to sustain life. However, he concludes that in a living will one may halahkically refuse mechanical interventions artificially prolonging the process of dying.

Both Dorff and Reisner distinguish between hindrances to the process of dying and intentionally ending one's life. A patient may not use an advance care directive to end life intentionally.

In an effort to harmonize the divergent opinions of Rabbis Dorff and Reisner, the Conservative Movement's Committee on Jewish Law and Standards concluded that one may decide which rabbinic opinion better fits the patient's understanding of Jewish law and ethics.[13] Although Dorff and Reisner disagree on certain points, they agree on the halakhic validity of living wills. Thus, the Committee has upheld the use of living wills, within specified limitations under Jewish law.

Conservative rabbis recognize and approve of the execution of a healthcare proxy. According to Reisner, a surrogate "functions as an extension of the patient." Although proxies have been legally assigned by sufferers, halakhically they are limited in their decision-making. A surrogate, Reisner notes, "must proceed with extreme caution and humility," however difficult this is in real life, not presuming to know the patient's position, especially concerning that one's personal dialogue with the Creator.[14]

However, Dorff and Reisner differ as to the resolution of a conflict between how a proxy judges a patient's wishes and the way in which the surrogate interprets an advance care directive. Dorff concludes that the proxy should have the final say in interpreting a sufferer's wishes. If a conflict persists, Reisner maintains that the written directive should be decisive.[15]

According to Reform authorities, a living will implements a patient's wishes for a "peaceful release" when one becomes a *goses*, that is, when no hope for his or her recovery exists.[16] If respiration and circulation are maintained only through artificial means, a living will may provide for the removal of mechanical devices. At this point, "natural independent life" no longer exists. Thus, in accordance with a living will, physicians may withdraw treatments and life-support systems, provided the patient is "dead" under the whole brain definition of death discussed in Chapter 4, but not before, if, for instance, he or she is in a persistent vegetative state. These Reform rabbis do not view living wills as encouraging physician-assisted suicide or voluntary active euthanasia, acts they view, as considered in Chapter 6, as prohibited under Jewish law based on the sanctity of biological life principle.

Spiritual Judaism encourages the use of advance care directives. In brief, as developed in Chapter 5 and 6, one may not only authorize the withholding or removal of any form of medical intervention, including artificial nutrition and hydration, but also accelerate the transition of life. Thus, one may use an advance care directive to implement his or her wishes, bounded by the virtues of love, compassion and forgiveness, the search for meaning and purpose in one's life, and a belief in the soul's immortality.

The Jewish Tradition and Postmortem Organ Donations

According to the Jewish tradition, the treatment of a human body after death depends on three principles: giving every sign of respect and dignity to a cadaver; not benefitting from a corpse; and providing an immediate burial. As the author of the Book of Deuteronomy (21:23) states: "One's body shall not remain all night upon a tree, but you shall surely bury the dead the same day." The Babylonian Talmud (Sanhedrin 47a) construes this phrase as prohibiting any action disgracing a deceased, for example, any physical disfigurement. Thus, Jewish sages found an obligation to provide dignity to a corpse and a corresponding aversion to any interference with the dead, even after the soul has left the physical body. A prohibition exists against mutilating a dead body (Babylonian Talmud Hullin 11b). The Babylonian Talmud (Avodah Zarah 29b) prohibits deriving any benefit from the dead. Also, the Babylonian Talmud (Sanhedrin 46b-47a) indicates that the burial of the dead may not be delayed, as befitting a sacred object, unless waiting would bring honor to the deceased. These general rules concerning the disposition of one's final remains may, however, be set aside in order to save a life, which overrides all other considerations.[17] As we will see, traditional and more liberal commentators differ markedly on the application of these general principles to postmortem organ donations.

Many traditional authorities permit an exception to these general principles only if an intention exists to bring a direct benefit to a known and present recipient who faces a real threat to his or her life. Thus, according to Rabbi Bleich, organs may be removed for transplantation after death only in order "to cure or alleviate a life threatening condition from which the recipient suffers."[18] Because organ donor cards provide authorization for the postmortem use and study of organs even if another's life is not threatened and make no provision for the ultimate return of organs for burial, Bleich concludes, "Jews cannot sign such a blanket authorization without violating religious principles,"[19] at least as he sees them. Based on the need for a known recipient awaiting a transplant, Bleich also disapproves of donations to organ banks where organs are stored for an indeterminate amount of time until a recipient is identified.

Traditional rabbis disagree as what constitutes a "threat to life" in order to suspend the general rules pertaining to the disposition of one's final remains. For some, blindness, necessitating the transplantation of the clear, thin membrane covering the lens of an eye, allowing light to enter the lens, may not meet the life threatening test. Most, however, permit corneal transplantation, conditioned on the donor giving his or her permission prior to death, because blindness increases one's odds of experiencing a serious, if not a fatal, accident. Even if a potential recipient has one working eye, and thus a threat to life may not exist, the corneal implantation may be allowed by some authorities who consider that the transplanted cornea is still a living organ; thus the prohibitions against ritual defilement, deriving benefit from the dead, and delaying burial are inapplicable. Because of the large number of visually impaired and the assumption that a recipient is readily at hand, most traditionalists even allow postmortem donations to eye banks.[20]

Far less doubt about the "threat of life" criterion exists among traditionalists with respect to postmortem kidney transplants, undertaken when both of a recipient's kidneys are so diseased that they are unable to perform their usual waste removal functions. Even if a potential recipient has access to kidney dialysis, a danger to life still exists. Thus, traditionalists set aside the general rules concerning the dead thereby permitting a postmortem kidney transplant to an identified recipient in order to save that person's life.[21] The same principle also applies for heart transplants, subject to the ongoing dispute among traditionalists, as in Chapter 4, regarding designating a donor as dead. In practice, donor hearts are taken from brain dead patients. Thus, heart transplants under Jewish law from a donor's standpoint are predicated on the acceptance of brain death as the standard for the determination of death.

Traditionalists also disagree about the meaning of a "present recipient." With today's advancement in communications and transportation, a potential recipient is "present" even if hundreds or thousands of miles away from a donor.[22] Thus, for example, the entire United States is generally viewed as "right there" with respect to a donor. However, if the organ is to be stored in an organ bank (except for corneal transplants) for most traditionalists the general prohibition against dishonoring the body cannot be overcome.

Conservative Rabbi Elliot N. Dorff maintains that the strong principle of saving another's life through organ donation suspends the general rules concerning a dead body. Transplantation neither desecrates the body nor does it lessen the respect for the dead. Delaying burial for this purpose, for Dorff, enhances the respect for a decedent. Donating one's organs, in addition to saving lives and honoring the deceased, prevents the desecration of God's name. Dorff's concern centers on the negative perception by gentiles of Jews who do not engage in the cadaver organ donation.[23]

The Conservative Movement's Committee on Jewish Laws and Standards has ruled that organ donations after death represent not only an act of kindness but also constitute a "commanded obligation" designed to save human lives. Failing to participate in organ donations after death amounts to violating the commandment: "Do not stand idly by your neighbor's blood" (Leviticus 19:16). Reasoning that we must use all available resources so that another's life will not be lost, Conservative Jews must indicate their commitment to saving others' lives by consenting to postmortem organ donations on their driver's license, on a signed organ donor card, or granting consent when required by physicians or hospitals. This obligation also applies to healthcare proxies and next of kin who are legally empowered to make such a decision on behalf of a dying person.[24] Withholding consent, according to the Conservative Movement, violates Jewish religious law. Disregarding the traditionalists' general requirement of a specific recipient who suffers from a life threatening condition, The Rabbinical Assembly has also validated postmortem donations to organ banks.

Similar to Conservative authorities, Reform rabbis in a series of responsa conclude that any of a dead body's rights are set aside out of desire to help fellow human beings and an overwhelming concern to save lives.[25] Organ donations bring honor to the deceased. Thus, organ banks are permissible conditioned on storing and handling the organs with care and respect as well as disposing of the unused organs with reverence.

Furthermore, the prohibition against benefitting from the dead is avoided because the transplanted organ is not ingested as food. When the organ is inserted into the body not as food, Jewish laws are more permissive, according to one Reform responsum.[26] When transplanted, an organ is integrated into the recipient's body. Because the transplanted organ does not die, it does not require burial according to the general rules pertaining to the decedent's body.

Spiritual Judaism encourages postmortem organ and whole body donations to a specific recipient, to organ banks, or for medical research and education. Donations serve, in accordance with the virtues outlined in Chapter 2, as significant acts of love and compassion. In the event any of us does not execute an organ donor card or grant consent when admitted to a medical facility, family members should provide for the gift of organs after our demise.

Some Planning Suggestions for Preparing an Advance Care Directive

As you look to preparing an advance care directive, let's consider four points: first, the need for a directive; second, selecting a proxy; third, providing your surrogate with specific instructions; fourth, giving your designee a statement of your values and beliefs.

The Need for an Advance Care Directive

Advance care directives offer many benefits. Through a signed, written document you can make your medical wishes known in advance, thus the term "advance care directive." Planning ahead helps you formulate preferences for future medical care. In undertaking the planning process, you are more likely to raise end of life questions and begin a dialogue with your primary care physician before a serious illness or accident. Engaging in the planning process promotes a shared understanding of your relevant values and preferences by you as a prospective patient (when you are in an upright rather than in a horizontal position) with your family members, loved ones, and physicians. It reduces the burden on and the potential for conflict between (or among) your relatives at a future time when you lack decision-making capacity. It also avoids over or under treatment when you no longer are able to indicate what care you consider worthwhile.

Most of us want to retain control over end of life decision-making while we are able to do so. By "control" most of us do not have in mind micromanaging treatment choices, although some may have particular things they want done or avoided. It is not like ordering take-out food. A sense of control connotes your views being respected and followed. We also want our designated proxy to retain control over our medical care when we are unable to do so.

Selecting a Healthcare Proxy

In contrast to a living will, a healthcare proxy provides greater flexibility. Living wills may take an either-or approach to medical treatment, overlooking the reality that a severely ill patient might possibly benefit from a temporary intervention, such as a ventilator, which then can be withdrawn. Often, a reliable benefit/burden determination cannot be made in advance. Thus, placing a decision in a proxy's hands allows a trial intervention to be stopped after a specified time has elapsed or when reasonable medical judgment shows the intervention not to be beneficial, for instance, when it only prolongs the dying process.

A proxy can also respond to changing medical conditions or unforeseen developments, interpret your desires and instructions, even if not clearly expressed, and, in theory, help ensure that your wishes are carried out. Your surrogate can consider all the specific details of your situation before making any decision.

With an agent in whom you have confidence, medical care determinations can be made based on the circumstances at the time of crisis, rather than being bound by decisions made in the past. Seeing your condition and discussing the various alternatives with physicians, your proxy can more easily make these choices, rather than your having to imagine and anticipate so much.

Despite these benefits, the designation of a surrogate faces several nagging and troublesome questions. Does your proxy fully understand your healthcare preferences? If so, will he or she carry them out? Or, will that individual simply defer to a physician or the perceived "head of the family"?

You need to designate the right person as your proxy, an agent who is mentally and emotionally capable of making difficult choices, someone who will carry out your wishes. You need someone you trust to make potentially difficult decisions for you. If there is no one close to you whom you can trust to act as your surrogate, do not execute a healthcare proxy.

Your designated surrogate may misconstrue his or her responsibility. Your agent should represent your preferences, not his or her own. A proxy may make decisions with a minimal understanding of your values and wishes. At worst, a surrogate may exercise his or her own judgment without any regard to what a patient wants, ignore explicit wishes, or confuse one's own personal desires with a sufferer's. In short, your proxy may not share or accurately reflect your values, goals of care, or specific treatment preferences.

In the absence of quite specific guidance, studies indicate that many surrogates often are unable to choose consistently the treatment option conforming to a patient's preferences.[27] There seems to be a bias toward aggressive medical intervention and a reluctance to refuse care, whether from guilt, an inability to "let go," or fear of being blamed for the patient's death. Even with detailed instructions, proxies may experience difficulties in letting go.

In *Patrimony: A True Story*,[28] a magnificent memoir of his father, the novelist Philip Roth recounts how he decided that "everything" need not be done to postpone the inevitable. Herman Roth, the author's eighty-six-year-old father, had a nonmalignant tumor pressing against the brain stem that could have been excised by surgery. Although the operation had a 75% survival rate (and would have been paid for by Medicare), it required either one eight to ten hour operation or two seven to eight hour operations several months apart; the recovery period would take a period of some months. The elder Roth would need to learn how to walk again. The surgeons were ready to do the operation. They confidently asserted that Herman would be worse off without it -- an argument that is sometimes heard, even when the merit of a procedure is debatable. The senior Roth, with his family's agreement, did not want it. Son Philip had his father sign a living will, refusing "mechanical respiration when I am no longer able to sustain my own breath." Yet the end proved to be an ordeal. According to Roth:

> Early on the morning of his death, when I arrived at the hospital emergency room... I was confronted by an attending physician prepared to take "extraordinary measures" and to put him on a breathing machine. Without it there was no hope, though, needless to say -- the doctor added -- the machine wasn't going to reverse the tumor.... And I, who had explained to my father the provisions of the living will and got him to sign it, didn't know what to do.... How could I take it on myself to decide that my father should be finished with life, life which is ours to know just once? Far from invoking the living will, I was nearly on the verge of ignoring it and saying, "Anything! Anything!"[29]

Provide your proxy with the needed guidance, through specific instructions regarding your decision-making preferences and a written statement of your values and beliefs. When the time comes, however, you must trust your surrogate to follow your wishes and let go, no matter how difficult this may be. As Philip Roth tells us:

> I asked the doctor to leave me alone with my father, or as alone as he and I could be in the middle of the emergency room bustle.... I thought about the misery that was sure to come, provided he could even be kept alive on a respirator. I saw it all, all, and yet I had to sit there for a very long time before I leaned as close to him as I could get and, with my lips to his sunken, ruined face, found it in me finally to whisper, "Dad, I'm going to have to let you go." He'd been unconscious for several hours and couldn't hear me, but shocked, amazed, and weeping I repeated it to him again and then again,

until I believed it myself.[30]

Indicating Your Specific Instructions: Intervention Options or Treatment Goals

You can use one or both of two modes of guidance -- intervention options or treatment goals -- to provide written instructions to your proxy and your physicians. Although you cannot anticipate all the eventualities or contingencies that may arise at the end of your life or plan for them specifically, try to make certain that your directive is as clear and as comprehensive as possible. Often living wills are imprecise and difficult to apply. Beware of general expressions, such as "I desire not to have my dying prolonged without dignity," or "I do not want to undergo needless suffering." Many terms, such as "heroic," "extraordinary," or "aggressive" treatment, are hard to interpret. Lacking a commonly understood content, they mean different things to different people. They lead to misunderstandings and misinterpretations.

Even using these vague terms, however, performs a useful function. They dispel the notion that you seek maximum medical maintenance. They reflect your concern about indignity in the dying process. They alert physicians to the underlying message: "Please don't do useless things to me that won't do any good."

Intervention Options

Looking beyond these general statements, it is hard to compose a document covering your approach to interventions in future situations, especially in the ever-changing world of medical care and technology, resulting in the dramatic transformation of therapeutic options. It is difficult to give directions about a complex and subtle process. Assessing the benefits and burdens of any specific procedure or treatment is rather daunting and bewildering. Nonphysicians do not know much about life-support systems and other medical care options. However, some indication is better than none. Talk it over with your primary care physician. Get his or her input.

Ask about what sorts of things they are apt to do to you in a hospital and how are they experienced by patients. Question nurses. Talk with other families. Once you find out about the relevant interventions, you will need an attorney to draw up the document. Review your directive with your current physician periodically and amend it as needed.

In thinking about and then embodying your preferences in your advance care directive, two types of life sustaining interventions are noteworthy. First, as we have seen in Chapter 5, the withholding or withdrawal of artificial nutrition and fluid remains controversial, particularly from a Jewish legal standpoint. As a practical matter, physicians may be reluctant to withhold or withdraw tube feeding from an unconscious or vegetative patient unless he or she has left specific instructions to do so. In your document, specify what you want done with respect to the artificial nutrition and fluids. Rather than an either-or approach, consider whether you want a feeding and a hydration tube introduced for a trial period so as to determine its effectiveness, using reasonable medical judgment.

Second, interventions to fight disease encompass both invasive and noninvasive measures. In addition to major surgery, invasive treatments include: a respirator, a mechanical means to breathe for you if your lung function is inadequate; kidney dialysis, a machine to clean your blood when your kidneys no longer function properly; monitoring by means of catheters to watch your heart and kidney functions; and intravenous (IV) lines to administer drugs as well as water, electrolytes, sugar and proteins. Noninvasive treatments include oral antibiotics to treat infections as well as chemotherapy and radiation to fight cancer.

Express your wishes regarding invasive and noninvasive interventions with respect to a variety of medical conditions in case you become terminally ill or are mentally unable to do so.[31] Do you want these various procedures or treatments in any case, or only for a specified trial period to determine their benefits and burdens, using reasonable medical judgment?

There may be some procedures you do not want, such as a ventilator or artificial feeding, under any circumstances. What is it about these therapeutic options that makes them so undesirable that you want to forgo them? Or, are there specific conditions under which they are to be forgone? Who will determine these conditions?

Are there any procedures or treatments you would want regardless of the situation? Why? Specify these interventions.

You can be as detailed and explicit as you like. The more exactly you spell out your wishes, the clearer your intentions will be to your healthcare providers. If you want to leave room for your proxy's own best judgment, then say that too, indicating the circumstances under which it will apply.

It is not easy to make a well-informed judgment regarding the multitude of options, in advance, on the basis of your limited knowledge, even with the assistance of your primary care physician. It is difficult to delineate ahead of time what degree of pain and suffering you are willing to experience and at what threshold you want to avoid continuing your ongoing agony. Thus, it is probably easier to focus on treatment goals, rather than on specific interventions and the conditions under which they would (or would not) be administered.

Treatment Goals

At least five medical treatment plans, each with various goals, exist. First, use all possible efforts including invasive and noninvasive measures, to preserve earthly life for as long as possible. Second, attempt a cure, but subsequently reevaluate the plan of treatment. This option is not, however, available with respect to cardiopulmonary resuscitation, surgery, or diagnostic tests. Third, comfort care as well as artificial nutrition and hydration, but not other types of medical treatment including interventions for curable infections and organ dysfunctioning. Fourth, only comfort care. Fifth, some form of physician aid-in-dying.

You may want to consider each of these five options in the context of the following seven situations:[32] First, you are terminally ill, unconscious, death is expected soon, even with the most extensive medical treatment.

Second, you are in an irreversible coma or a persistent vegetative state, there is no reasonable hope of regaining awareness and higher mental functions, but life-support mechanisms could keep your body alive for years.

Third, you are in a coma and have a small possibility of recovering fully, a greater possibility of living with permanent brain damage, and a much larger possibility of dying.

Fourth, you are in a state marked by the advance loss of mental capability, for instance, as a result of Alzheimer's disease or a stroke, that cannot be reversed. You cannot recognize or communicate with those close to you. You can do almost nothing for yourself. With medical treatment, your body could survive for some time period.

Fifth, you are in a state of permanent, but not total confusion, for instance, as a result of Alzheimer's disease or a stroke. You are legally "incompetent." You cannot recognize people or interact with them in any meaningful way. Although others take care of you, you're "pleasantly" senile. You are not in distress and are able to experience some of life's daily satisfactions, such as listening to music. You are diagnosed with a terminal illness.

Sixth, you are frail, chronically ill, and uncomfortable, able to engage in only a limited range of activities. You become temporarily unconscious, as a result of a sudden, acute illness that is likely to be fatal unless vigorously treated. Intensive care in a hospital offers only a small chance of recovery to your former condition, with the greater likelihood that you will end up worse off than before or will die.

Seventh, you unexpectedly suffer a serious injury or illness. With intensive care, you have less than a 5% chance of a good recovery. Even if you survive, you will most likely (95%) have permanent, serious brain damage.

Because estimates indicate that Alzheimer's disease strikes about 11% of those over sixty-five, and approximately 48% of those over eighty-five,[33] I strongly suggest that your advance care directive deal with your treatment goals in the context of moderately advanced Alzheimer's disease (and dementia) as well as chronic, progressive, debilitating physical conditions that are not immediately fatal. Remember that with Alzheimer's sufferers gradually lose their memory and other mental and bodily functions sinking into dementia and ultimately, death. Along their downhill slide, they lose the capacity for interaction with family and friends; they cannot think, play a game, read, or converse with anyone; they live in a world without purpose, one often filled with horrendously threatening paranoid delusions. They pass their last few years in a vegetative-like state, bedridden, restricted in mobility, incontinent. None of their personality traits is evident. Do you want to continue to live as an empty human shell who can't move?

Recent scientific evidence indicates that tube feeding does not make people more comfortable. Most advanced demented patients who are tube fed do not live longer than those who are not; they still have lung problems resulting from choking on their saliva and stomach secretions.[34]

With the increasing chance your life will end in confused dementia and dependence, do you want to cut short your distress if you suffer from: mild, moderate, or severe Alzheimer's? Remember: although Alzheimer's is an incurable illness, its time line is slow and unpredictable. It is difficult to spell this out in advance. Also, what if you experience vascular dementia, a series of tiny strokes gradually destroying your brain?

Draft your treatment goals in consultation not only with your attorney but also with your primary care physician. Remember: you want your proxy to be able to use your directive and have it applied in a hospital context without the need to go to court.

Additional Thoughts on Your Specific Instructions

Whether your directive provides a set of intervention options or sets forth more general treatment goals, you must face the possibility that when your instrument becomes operative, if you were able to think about it again, you might have changed your mind. A crisis can alter everything when you know your diagnosis, options, and prognosis. The insults of age, such as incontinence at forty, may be acceptable when you are seventy, eighty, or ninety. A low quality of life may otherwise become acceptable; a poor quality of life might not seem so bad if that is all you have left. You may be willing to put up with a lot more pain and suffering to live a little longer. You may change your mind about what type of life is worth living.

Terminal patients sometimes cling to any glimmer of hope. It is difficult for many in such a condition to believe that nothing more can be done to keep them alive, even a little bit longer. In one study, seriously ill sufferers evidenced a willingness to grasp at any hope to prolong life. Fifty-eight percent of the two hundred and forty-four surveyed with end stage heart, lung, or liver disease, metastatic cancer or lymphoma, indicated that they would want life sustaining treatments continued even if it prolonged their life for just one week.[35]

In thinking about your advance care directive, carefully reflect on whether you really want the wishes you express today to be applicable when your health is really different. Do you think age or sickness would change your mind about what constitutes a tolerable quality of life for you? Are you prepared to "let go?" What may seem futile to you now as a healthy person, may seem like one last chance for a little more "life" latter on.

Do Not Resuscitate Orders

In considering a variety of intervention options or treatment goals, you need to deal with Do Not Resuscitate (DNR) orders. Such an order forbids Cardiopulmonary Resuscitation (CPR) used to restart a heart that has stopped beating. Many people are trained to do this. They may use basic techniques, such as chest compression to squeeze the heart or mouth-to-mouth breathing to push air into the lungs, or advanced measures, such as medication or defibrillation, using powerful electrical shocks to start the heart beating again.

Do you find any of these procedures disturbing? Why? Do you want someone to disrupt your "date with death"? Do you fear the pain resulting from any technique, particularly, chest compression, as paramedics crack your ribs in order to jump-start your heart? Do you worry about severe brain damage if you survive or a long stay in an intensive care unit after resuscitation, perhaps with mechanical ventilation or other invasive procedures? If so, make certain that your physician and your loved ones know that you do not want resuscitation attempted. Remember: in the absence of a DNR order, healthcare professionals, in particular, a new group of providers, emergency medical technicians, will attempt resuscitation on anyone whose heart or breathing stops.

If you do not want to be resuscitated, have your physician sign an out-of-hospital DNR order and put it on your refrigerator or next to your bed. Many states have legislation authorizing the use of nonhospital DNR orders. This is a large sign, not easily overlooked. Most of these jurisdictions issue an approved identifier, such as a bracelet, indicating your wishes. Find out about your state's policies. Warning: an emergency medical technician responding to a 911 call will not follow your advance care directive, regardless of what it says about CPR. You need a nonhospital DNR order and you must post it where emergency personnel will be sure to see it.

If hospitalized or admitted to a nursing home, ask for a DNR order, indicating that you do not want CPR to be provided in the event you suffer cardiac arrest or your pulmonary functions cease. Ask your physician to place this order ahead of your admission. When you arrive, you (or your proxy) should make certain that the DNR order is in place. When you get to your room, you (or your surrogate) should again ascertain that your DNR order is in place. Make sure that the facility follows its normal procedures, typically identifying DNR patients with a bracelet. Remember: a DNR order is not the same thing as an advanced care directive. If you are hospitalized or in a nursing home and you want to limit (or eliminate) CPR, your physician must write a DNR order.

A degree of caution is in order concerning DNR orders. In Chapter 5, I have already mentioned the findings of a massive study of more than nine thousand terminally ill patients in five U.S. hospitals. This study generated widespread concern about deficiencies in end of life decision-making and care in hospital settings.[36] The presence of advance care directives, for example, had no impact on DNR orders and end of life care. The study found that nearly half of the patients who orally indicated that CPR be withheld did not have a DNR order written during their hospital stay. Only 47% of those who did not want CPR had physicians who were aware of their preference. Depending on their medical specialty, doctors took an average of twenty-two to seventy-three days to write DNR orders after patients had requested them. Among those who died with a DNR order, 46% were written within two days of death, indicating they probably had received much futile treatment.

Remember: your proxy as well as your primary care physician must serve as your advocates with respect to your preferences regarding DNR orders. If at all possible, make your wishes clear and be certain they are implemented.

Describing Your Values and Beliefs

Discuss what you want by way of medical treatments with your physician, close family members, other dear ones and the person (or persons) you designate as your proxy. Although difficult to initiate, these conversations are extremely important. Discuss and clarify your values and beliefs. Communicate what is most important to you. These deep convictions can help guide others, especially your primary care physician, in treating you and determining a course of care. Ask your physician, close family members, and proxy if they will support you in the way you desire.

Consider using a written values questionnaire focusing on the premises and processes you would use (and you would want your agent to use) when deciding on medical interventions at the end of your life. Talk things over with your proxy, family members, and physician. Discuss your values and beliefs touching on illness, the dying process, and death.

Write out your answers to the values questionnaire and give them to your family members, especially your surrogate who will speak for you regarding your wishes when you cannot.

In formulating your statement of values and beliefs, consider the following:[37]

First, what do you value most about your life? What goals do you have for the future? Do you value the length or the quality of your life, if so, in what sense?

Second, how do you feel about death and dying? Do you fear death and the process of dying? What was your reaction to the death of a loved one?

Third, should biological life, in particular, your life, be preserved as long as possible? Do you want life-support to be vigorously maintained until you are really in extremis, until death is unpreventably imminent, without regard to your condition, your chances for recovery, or the cost of any procedures and treatments?

Fourth, what will be most important to you when you are dying -- the absence of pain, physical comfort, the presence of family members? Or, do you want a good quality of life, in all its various dimensions, even if this means you may not live as long as you possibly could?

Fifth, what conditions are worse than death? Do you fear indignity more than death?

Sixth, what life prolonging procedures or treatments should no longer be used under what physical or mental conditions, such as severe, unrelenting pain, physical immobility, physical helplessness (complete or particular aspects, such as incontinence or incapacity to feed yourself), mental incapacity (unawareness of surroundings, an inability to appreciate important relationships, or to think well enough to make everyday decisions or understand a newspaper), or various forms of physical, emotional, and spiritual suffering, including dependency, frustration, anxiety, embarrassment, or hopelessness? Would you temporarily accept a medical procedure or treatment if you faced any of these physical or mental conditions? How much pain and risk would you accept if your chances for recovery were good (at least fifty-fifty) or poor (less than one in ten)?

Seventh, do you want financial considerations to enter into decisions about your medical care? Would you want less money spent on you so more funds will be available for your spouse, children, other relatives, significant others, or close friends?

Eight, do you want the emotional burden your condition can impose on your loved ones, resulting from a prolonged deathwatch or the care of an extremely deteriorated person, to be considered? Do you have a distaste for the eroded image left in your loved ones' memories?

Ninth, what other beliefs or values do you want to be taken into account by those making medical decisions for you?

Some Concluding Thoughts

Designate one proxy (and a backup) to avoid confusion if more than one family member or loved one wants to make healthcare choices for you. Naming one agent (and a substitute) avoids that hazard.

Prepare written, informative instructions, goals, and values for your agent. Do not rely on prior oral conversations because memories fade and can be disputed. Written directions serve as a check on your proxy's personal predilections and ensure that he or she knows something about your wishes.

Combine in one document the proxy designation with some form of treatment preferences. In addition to naming a surrogate (or surrogates), provide specific instructions as to your basic perspectives if you become terminally ill or you lack the mental capacity for medical decision-making. Your written answers to a values questionnaire gives your surrogates relevant information regarding your values and beliefs. Your specific instructions and values statement helps physicians make immediate decisions if your agent is unavailable for any reason. Be certain your physician knows how to reach your deputies. Be sure that both proxies keep you informed on their whereabouts.

Select a primary care physician who will respect your judgment about the kind of life you want (or do not want). You want someone who will honor your wishes as expressed in your directive, who will respect your preferences about how you want to be treated. Also, ask your doctor if he or she can continue to be your advocate even if one or more specialists will treat you. Most important, you want a physician who sees you as a human being, with a mind and a soul, not just someone who suffers from a rampaging disease, such as cancer, to be treated surgically or pharmacologically. If your doctor is unable to comply with your wishes and your values, find another primary care physician.

Give copies of your executed advance care directive to your proxy, your physician, and your family members. You (or your surrogate) should make certain this document is part of your medical records and that it is properly recorded on your medical chart. On admission to a hospital or during hospitalization, your surrogate should inform the hospital staff of your views, as contained in your instrument. All physicians caring for you should know that there is a directive and understand your specific wishes. You (or your proxy) should make certain that the notation alerting the hospital staff you have prepared a directive does not get lost when you are transferred from one unit to another. Your surrogate should have extra copies to give out.

What if a medical emergency occurs while you are out-of-town? An advance care directive may be of limited value in such a situation. Also, even if an acute medical problem occurs locally, the attending physician, for instance, in an emergency room, may be unaware of your wishes. If you are admitted to a hospital, your directive likely will not be on record.

To deal with this contingency, carry a card in your wallet indicating that you have executed an advance care directive and its location. You may want to take a photocopy of your directive with you at all times. Or, carry a "living will" card containing a toll-free number for a central registry supplying callers with full text of your instrument in an emergency.

Review your directive every few years; more often, if your health is declining. A time of transition, such as the death of a loved one or a serious health scare you encounter, should trigger a reevaluation. Is your proxy designation up to date? What do you want for yourself in the future, in terms of options or treatment goals? Is your statement of values and beliefs current?

Remember: you can alter your directive. It is not some sort of irrevocable, unchangeable document. As long as you are alert, even if your mental capacity is diminished, you can change your directive at any time. You can revoke an old instrument and execute a new one. If you do, be sure to tell everyone who has copies of your old directive that you have canceled it and have written a new one. And, of course, supply the pertinent parties with legally valid copies of the new instrument.

Do not wait until you are elderly or facing a serious illness to think about what medical interventions you want (or do not want) in critical or terminal situations. Contemplating these issues while you are healthy gives you and your loved ones the opportunity to prepare for a serious medical emergency. Use a values questionnaire, set forth earlier in this chapter, to stimulate discussion with your dear ones and help clarify your preferences. Use a directive to leave instructions for your care if you are unable to speak for yourself. Everyone, young or old, sick or healthy, should execute a written advance care directive, combining a living will and a healthcare proxy. This document enables you to face the dying process and death, providing guidance for your surrogate to make medical care decisions for you if you lack decision-making capacity or face a terminal illness.

Do not force family members and loved ones to make difficult medical decisions for you when you lack decision-making capability or become terminally ill without prior guidance from you. Start by obtaining your "official" or the generally accepted form from your state. Also, obtain various forms from nonprofit advocacy groups. Aging with Dignity (www.agingwithdignity.org) lets you download a free, reader-friendly plain-English version, *Five Wishes*, that is valid in 33 states and the District of Columbia. (You can write to Aging with Dignity, P.O. Box 1661, Tallahassee, FL 32302-1661, (telephone (850)681-2010, or fax (850)681-2481). Another organization, Choice in Dying (telephone (800) 989-9455 or www.choices.org), provides advance care directives geared to specific states.

Various branches of Judaism offer advance care directive forms. There are two types of Orthodox forms, one promulgated by the Rabbinical Council of America, 305 Seventh Avenue, New York, NY 10001 (telephone (212)807-7888, fax (212)727-8452) expounds a specific position, advising its followers to execute a living will in accordance with the Council's mandates. This form permits a patient in an irreversible coma or a persistent vegetative or an irreversibly brain-damaged patient, who is unable to recognized people or communicate in any fashion but who is not terminally ill, to refuse life sustaining treatment. Another, issued by Agudath Israel of America, 84 William Street, New York, NY 10038 (telephone (212)797-9000, fax (212)269-2843), for use in New York State, provides general guidelines, reserving the ultimate decision-making to an individual's preselected rabbi.

There is also a Conservative form, Jewish Medical Directives for Health Care, approved by The Committee on Jewish Law and Standards of The Rabbinical Assembly, distributed by the United Synagogue Book of Service, 155 Fifth Avenue, New York, NY 10010 (telephone (212)533-7800 ext. 2000, (800)594-5617, fax (212)253-5422 or e-mail booksvc@uscj.org). A Reform version is set out in "Responsa 156. Living Will (1989)," contained in Walter Jacob, *Questions and Reform Jewish Answers: New American Responsa* (New York: Central Conference of American Rabbis, 1992), 254-255, and is available from Central Conference of American Rabbis' website (www.ccarnet.org) or by e-mail (info@ccarnet.org).

Organ donor cards are provided by The Rabbinical Assembly (Conservative Movement), 3080 Broadway, New York NY 10027 (telephone (212)678-8060, fax (212)749-9166, e-mail (rabassembly@jtsa.edu) and the Union of American Hebrew Congregations (Reform Movement), Department of Jewish Family Concerns, 633 Third Avenue, New York, NY 10017 (telephone (212)650-4294, fax (212)650-4239, e-mail (deptjewfamcon@uahc.org). The living will forms prepared by two Orthodox organizations, the Rabbinical Council of America and Agudath Israel of America, respectively, provide for organ donations, conditioned on rabbinical concurrence.

Notes

1. *Cruzan v. Director, Missouri Department of Health*, 497 U.S. 261 (1990).

2. 42 U.S.C. §§ 1395i-3, 1395l, 1395cc, 1395bbb.

3. Alan Meisel, *The Right To Die*, vol. 2, 2nd ed. (New York: Wiley Law, 1995) 268-269, § 14.10.

4. Ibid., 25-30, § 10.12.

5. Ezekiel J. Emanuel and Linda L. Emanuel, "The Promise of a Good Death," *The Lancet* 351:9114 (May 1998): SII 21-SII 29; Nancy M.P. King, *Making Sense of Advance Directives*, rev. ed. (Washington, D.C.: Georgetown University Press, 1996), 186.

6. 8A Uniform Laws Annotated 19 (Uniform Anatomical Gift Act 1987) and 63 (Uniform Anatomical Gift Act 1968).

7. J. David Bleich, *Bioethical Dilemmas: A Jewish Perspective* (Hoboken, NJ: KTAV, 1998) 74-75; J. David Bleich, *Judaism and Healing: Halakhic Perspectives* (New York: KTAV, 1981), 137-139.

8. Fred Rosner, "Jewish Perspectives on the Issues of Death and Dying," *The Journal of Halacha and Contemporary Society*, no. 11 (Fall 1985): 67-68.

9. Fred Rosner, "Ethical Dilemmas in Medical Practice," in *Jewish Values in Health and Medicine*, ed. Rabbi Levi Meier (Lanham, MD: University Press of America, 1991), 134-135.

10. Elliot N. Dorff, "A Jewish Approach to End-Stage Medical Care," *Conservative Judaism* 43:3(Spring 1991): 39; Elliot N. Dorff, *Matters of Life and Death: A Jewish Approach to Modern Medical Ethics* (Philadelphia: Jewish Publication Society, 1998), 169.

11. Dorff, "A Jewish Approach," 39. Dorff cites Seymour Siegel, "Jewish Law Permits Natural Death," *Sh'ma* 7:132 (April 1977): 96-97.

12. Avram Israel Reisner, "A Halakhic Ethic of Care for the Terminally Ill," *Conservative Judaism* 43:3 (Spring 1991): 66-68.

13. The Committee on Jewish Law and Standards, The Rabbinical Assembly, *Jewish Medical Directives for Health Care*, ed. Rabbi Aaron L. Mackler, 1994.

14. Reisner, "A Halakhic Ethic," p. 67.

15. "Jewish Medical Directives for Health Care."

16. Central Conference of American Rabbis (CCAR), "Responsum 156. Living Will (1989)," in Walter Jacob, *Questions and Reform Jewish Answers: New American Reform Responsa* (New York: CCAR, 1992), 258-259.

17. Basil F. Herring, *Jewish Ethics and Halakhah For Our Time: Sources and Commentary*, vol. 2 (Hoboken, N.J.: KTAV, 1989), 105-115, 125; Rabbi Reuven Frank, "Halachic Aspects of Organ Transplants," *The Journal of Halacha* and *Contemporary Society*, no. 5 (Spring 1983): 45-64.

18. Bleich, *Judaism and Healing*, 165, 129-133, 162-168.

19. Ibid., 165.

20. Fred Rosner, M.D., *Modern Medicine and Jewish Ethics*, 2nd ed. (Hoboken, N.J.: KTAV, 1991), 283-286; Fred Rosner, "Organ Transplantation in Jewish Law," in *Jewish Bioethics*, ed. J. David Bleich and Fred Rosner (New York: Hebrew Publishing, 1979) 361-364; Herring, *Jewish Ethics and Halakhah*, 109; Dr. Immanuel Jakobovits, *Jewish Medical Ethics: A Comparative and Historical Study of the Jewish Religious Attitude to Medicine and Its Practice* (New York: Block, 1975), 285-286.

21. Rosner, *Modern Medicine and Jewish Ethics*, 286; Rosner, "Organ Transplantation," 364-365.

22. Herring, *Jewish Ethics and Halakhah*, 108, 125.

23. Dorff, *Matters of Life and Death*, 226-230.

24. Rabbi Joseph H. Prouser, "*Chesed* or *Chiyuv*?: The Obligation to Preserve Life and the Question of Post-Mortem Organ Donation," Committee on Jewish Law and Standards, The Rabbinical Assembly, December 1995; Resolution Adopted, "Organ and Tissue Donation" in *Proceedings ofThe Rabbinic Assembly*, vol. 52, ed. Rabbi Jules Harlow (New York: The Rabbinic Assembly, 1991), 279.

25. CCAR, "Responsum 78. Banks for Human Organs (1986)," in Walter Jacob, *Contemporary American Reform Responsa* (New York 1987), 131-132; CCAR, "Responsum 84. Transplanting the Eyes of Deceased Persons (1953)," in *American Reform Responsa: Collected Responsa of the Central Conference of American Rabbis 1889-1983*, ed. Walter Jacob (New York: CCAR, 1983), 287-288; CCAR, "Responsum 85. The Use of the Cornea of the Dead (1956)," ibid., 288-291.

26. CCAR, "Responsum 86, Surgical Transplants (1986)," ibid, 294-296.

27. Jeremiah Suhl et al, "Myth of Substituted Judgment: Surrogate Decision Making Regarding Life Support is Unreliable," *Archives of Internal Medicine* 154:1 (January 1994): 90-96.

28. Philip Roth, *Patrimony: A True Story* (New York: Simon and Schuster, 1991).

29. Ibid., 232.

30. Ibid., 232-233.

31. Linda L. Emanuel and Ezekiel J. Emanuel, "The Medical Directive: A New Comprehensive Advance Care Planning Document," *Journal of the American Medical Association* 261:22 (June 1989): 3288-3293; Linda Emanuel, "The Health Care Directive: Learning How to Draft Advance Care Documents," *Journal of the American Geriatrics Society* 39:12 (December 1991): 1221-1228. According to one study, the use of pre-drafted advance treatment directive containing a range of illness scenarios and including stated choices, coupled with inferring unstated choices from stated choices, "allay some concern that prior preferences cannot take all relevant decisions into account." Linda L. Emanuel et al, "Advance Directives: Can Patients' Stated Treatment Choices Be Used to Infer Unstated Choices?" *Medical Care* 32:2 (February 1994): 103.

32. Adapted from Vermont Ethics Network, "Medical Situations & Their Treatment," worksheet 2 in *Taking Steps to Plan for Critical Health Care Decisions* (Waterbury, VT: Vermont Ethics Network, 1992).

33. Denis A. Evans et al, "Estimated Prevalence of Alzheimer's Disease in the United States," *The Milbank Quarterly* 68:2 (1990): 273-274.

34. Muriel R. Gillick, "Rethinking the Role of Tube Feeding in Patients with Advanced Dementia," *The New England Journal of Medicine* 342:3 (January 2000): 206-210. See also Thomas E. Finucane, Colleen Christmas, and Kathy Travis, "Tube Feeding in Patients with Advanced Dementia: A Review of the Evidence," *Journal of the American Medical Association* 282:14 (October 1999): 1365-1370.

35. Marion Danis et al, "A Prospective Study of the Impact of Patient Preferences for Life-Sustaining Treatment and Hospital Cost," *Critical Care Medicine* 24:11 (November 1996): 1811-1817.

36. The SUPPORT Principal Investigators, "A Controlled Trial to Improve Care for Seriously Ill Hospitalized Patients: The Study to Understand Prognoses and Preferences for Outcomes and Risks of Treatment," *Journal of the American Medical Association* 274:20 (November 1995): 1591-1598. The SUPPORT study investigated critically ill, hospitalized patients, about 25% of whom died during their hospital stay.

37. Adapted from Vermont Ethics Network, "Values Questionnaire," worksheet 1 in *Taking Steps*; David J. Doukas and Laurence B. McCullough, "The Values History: The Evaluation of the Patient's Values and Advance Directives," *The Journal of Family Practice* 32:2 (1991): 145-153; Pam Lambert, Joan McIver Gibson, and Paul Nathanson, "The Values History: An Innovation in Surrogate

Medical Decision-Making," *Law, Medicine & Health Care* 18:3 (Fall 1990): 202-212.

Chapter 11

Conclusion: Our Search for a "Good" Death

We live in a society marked by a denial of death. We seek to avoid any thought of our own mortality. Television and the movies do not portray a typical demise from a progressive, chronic disease at an old age, after a substantial period of frailty and disability. We spend billions each year to conquer, or at least, postpone death.

We celebrate the young. Print and visual media portray a world of the active and youthful who never get sick and do not die. We all desire longevity.

We are also reluctant to talk about death. We usually speak in hushed euphemisms of someone having "passed away" or "not making it," rather than saying he or she died. We do not want to talk about it. Our unspoken fear, on the part of patients, families, and physicians, leads to often fighting death to the end.

In this book, you have come face to face with death and the dying process. There is one more question I want to pose: What do you consider a "good" death, or more accurately, a "good" dying process?

When we come to grips with death -- your death -- you want a "good" death, with the manner and timing as if you were free to choose. Most of us would, from my experience, want a gentle and dignified death. We want to die in relative physical comfort, with little or no pain and discomfort, and in a clear state of mind.

We imagine dying in our sleep -- going to bed and not waking up. Or, collapsing from a massive heart attack while we are out walking the dog. As so envisioned, we are able to retain our sense of dignity and control until the end. We want to avoid making our exit during our final days or weeks tethered to machines in a hospital intensive care unit. We do not want a lonely, protracted high tech demise.

In the twenty-first century, these idealized notions of death will constitute the exception, not the general rule. Because of medical innovations, most of us face a long period of physical or mental decline. Yet, as we contemplate the ebbing of life, we resist the idea of a lingering dying process, one that is emotionally and spiritually degrading. We rebel against the thought of the ever greater loss of independence in our everyday life. We abhor increased reliance on others to provide care, especially in the personal, intimate tasks of daily living. Many of us regard adult dependency as undignified. It is seen as leading to a loss of self-esteem by those requiring care, no matter how willingly and lovingly administered.

Only you and your loved ones can reach a decision about how you chose to face these lifestyle changes from a prolonged decline and the accompanying emotional and spiritual difficulties. Some may see these transformations and quandaries as opportunities for emotional and spiritual growth, learning patience and living with dependency, and enabling others to express their love and compassion. For others, the possibility and fear of severe suffering -- physical, emotional, or spiritual -- often creates dread, dominating the experience of dying and limiting the opportunities for personal development. They may find their impairments so great that life is no longer worth living. They are concerned about losing control in the face of serious illness or an incurable, debilitating condition.

Dying well is not easy. It has a number of dimensions -- physical, emotional, and spiritual. Most of us want to die in relative physical comfort -- out of physical pain and suffering as much as possible and mentally alert as long as possible. Most of us would want to use life prolonging medical interventions as long as they produce a reasonable quality of life (at least in terms of our own values and goals) and a reasonable level of function. Then, I suppose, many of us would want to turn to high quality hospice-style terminal care at home. But the process of dying is much more complex than its mere physical aspects. It also has its emotional and spiritual dimensions.

We want to bring our personal and business relationships, activities, and strivings to a close. We want to die supported by and connected to the important persons in our life, to strengthen family bonds and come closer to these essential people. We need to settle unfinished emotional and relational business with these significant people. It is a time for the resolution of a number of personal matters. It is not easy, when you are dealing with pain and other physical symptoms.

To achieve emotional closure, we need time to share openly our thoughts and feelings and enter into a dialogue with our loved ones. We want to be able to open our hearts, to reminisce, to talk about and relive past, happy moments. Families and friends want to express their love and sadness at the impending loss and say their final goodbyes so that they too feel a sense of completeness in their relationship. All of us want to die within a circle of human companionship and caring.

We also want to have time to attempt to deal with and resolve our spiritual quandaries, to put our life into perspective and gain some understanding of its meaning and purpose. Many of us want to ask: What is the sum of my life? Where is it going in the time left, beyond the flow of the weekly calendar?

Within your physical and mental limits, it is a time to complete projects and perhaps learn new things or engage in uncharted activities. You might, for instance, want to indulge in creative endeavors, such as painting or sculpture, even if you have never considered yourself an artist. It is never too late to find meaning in your life, to do one noble act, to make provisions for a postmortem organ donation, to express unconditional love, to forgive someone, to ask for forgiveness, and possibly achieve a reconciliation with estranged family members and friends. Accepting the finiteness of earthly life, you may gain a sense of self beyond the loss of your physical body, recognize a transcendent realm, and surrender to the unknown.

In short, a "good" dying process enables us to achieve a sense of emotional and spiritual completion and fulfillment and allows us to "let go." Dying a "good" death takes courage, emotional and spiritual insight, interpersonal communication as well as sufficient time and energy.

After a sufferer's long deterioration, if the dying process is "successful," survivors generally feel relieved on his or her demise, able to move through and grieve their loss serenely. Ultimately, they too are able to let go and get on with their lives.

Despite our idealized notions of a "good" death, survivors generally are shocked if a healthy loved one dies suddenly without warning. Time spent dying can assist family and friends to learn the lessons of love, compassion, and forgiveness. With an unexpected demise, they do not have a chance to be prepared, to say their goodbyes, to ask for forgiveness, and achieve closure; acceptance and closure come far more slowly, long after a beloved one is gone.

The process of dying, with all its attendant pain and suffering, provides opportunities for spiritual growth and development, provided our physical agonies are dealt with. Triggering a spiritual awakening, the dying process can be transforming and liberating. It can be a time for seeking meaning and a sense of completion in life.

A "good" dying process, whether medically prolonged, merely natural, or accelerated, offers the opportunity for saying our goodbyes and "I love you," and addressing our deepest emotional and spiritual needs. It is a time to strengthen bonds with loved ones, to learn to forgive, and to close the door to regrets and resentments.

In the twenty-first century, when facing physical or mental disintegration or terminal illness, many of us may desire the comfort of choice at the end of life. Fearing a technological death, where medical powers are not in our mastery, many may want some measure of control over the circumstances of their dying process. They may wish to die in their own time and on their own terms, avoiding a lengthy physical or mental decline leaving them isolated and degraded.

I hope you see my desire to open the window to choice at the end of life -- a very private, quite complex endeavor -- as enhancing our autonomy bounded by the virtues of love, compassion, and forgiveness. A "good" death, whether a prolonged "natural" demise, a medically managed or an assisted exit, represents a time for achieving meaning in life and closure. Let us hope that there is nothing (or nearly nothing) left unresolved. A "good" death enables everyone -- the sufferer and his or her loved ones -- to be emotionally and spiritually prepared for what happens, to be able to accept that this is the conclusion of one's present, earthly journey but not the dissolution of one's soul, which is immortal.

Dying represents a stage of living, enabling us to conclude our existence in this world well. One of the great challenges of the twenty-first century centers on how we can civilize death and dying so as not to make them a source of dread. Perhaps, in some small way, this book will help you see death and dying not as a source of terror, but rather as a deep mystery.

Closure in earthly life does not mean a door slamming shut, locking out our hopes, forever sealing our unfulfilled desires, blotting out our personal consciousness. Rather, if we find meaning and purpose in life, use this new found wisdom to reframe our current situation, no matter how outwardly bleak, and are able to express our unconditional love and forgiveness of others, so important from the viewpoint of Spiritual Judaism, even if we exhibit these virtues only at the very end, death may be welcomed as an appropriate and timely finale to a life fully lived or one seemingly cut far too short, yet one that has made its contribution to the great, ongoing creative work.

Through a "good" death, we may come to appreciate the impermanent nature of all earthly things. Everything in this world changes and is in flux; everything coming into being passes away. In so doing, it contributes to the melody, as each note gives place to the next. The transcendent meaning of our existence -- our immortal soul -- creates a context in which death is not an enemy; rather, it represents a sacred moment.

Selected Bibliography

Battin, Margaret Pabst. *The Least Worst Death: Essays in Bioethics on the End of Life*. New York: Oxford University Press, 1994.

Benson, Herbert, M.D. with Marg Stark. *Timeless Healing: The Power and Biology of Belief.* New York: Scribner, 1996.

Byock, Ira, M.D. *Dying Well: The Prospect for Growth at the End of Life*. New York: Riverhead, 1997.

Cousins, Norman. *Anatomy of an Illness as Perceived by the Patient: Reflections on Healing and Regeneration*. New York: Norton, 1979.

Dorff, Elliot N. *Matters of Life and Death: A Jewish Approach to Modern Medical Ethics.* Philadelphia: Jewish Publication Society, 1998.

Ellenson, David H. "How to Draw Guidance from a Heritage: Jewish Approaches to Mortal Choices," in *Contemporary Jewish Ethics and Morality: A Reader*. Edited by Elliot N. Dorff and Louis E. Newman. New York: Oxford University Press, 1995.

Frankl, Viktor E. *Man's Search for Meaning*. New York: Washington Square Press, 1984.

Jacob, Walter and Moshe Zemer, eds. *Death and Euthanasia in Jewish Law*. Pittsburgh: Rodef Shalom Press, 1995.

Jamison, Stephen. *Final Acts of Love: Families, Friends, and Assisted Dying*. New York: G.P. Putnam's Sons, 1995.

Knobel, Peter. "Suicide, Assisted Suicide, Active Euthanasia, A *Halakhic* Inquiry" in *Death and Euthanasia in Jewish Law and Responsa*. Edited by Walter Jacobs and Moshe Zemer. Pittsburgh: Rodef Shalom Press, 1995.

Lynn, Joanne and Joan Harrold. *Handbook for Mortals: Guidance for People Facing Serious Illness*. New York: Oxford University Press, 1999.

Meier, Levi, ed. *Jewish Values in Health and Medicine*. Lanham, Md.: University Press of America, 1991.

Quill, Timothy E., M.D. *Death and Dignity: Making Choices and Taking Charge*. New York: Norton, 1993.

Quill, Timothy E., Bernard Lo and Dan W. Brock. "Palliative Options of Last Resort: A Comparison of Voluntarily Stopping Eating and Drinking, Terminal

Sedation, Physician-Assisted Suicide, and Voluntary Active Euthanasia." *Journal of the American Medical Association* 278:23 (December 1997): 2099-2104.

Raphael, Simcha Paull. *Jewish Views of the Afterlife*. Northvale, N.J.: Jason Aronson, 1994.

Reynolds Price. *Letter to a Man in the Fire: Does God Exist and Does He Care?* New York: Scribner, 1999.

Sherwin, Byron. "A View of Euthanasia." In *Contemporary Jewish Ethics and Morality: A Reader*. Edited by Elliot N. Dorff and Louis E. Newman. New York: Oxford University Press, 1995.

Solomon, Lewis D. *Jewish Spirituality: Revitalizing Judaism for the Twenty-First Century*. Northvale, N.J.: Jason Aronson, 2000.

_____. *The Jewish Book of Living and Dying*. Northvale, N.J.: Jason Aronson, 1999.

Index